Family-Centred Perinatal Care

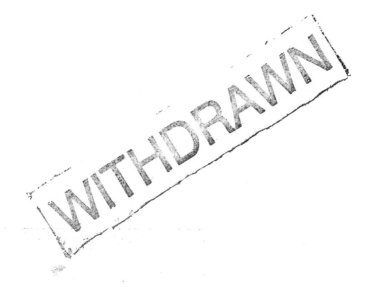

Family-Centred Perinatal Care

Improving Pregnancy, Birth and Postpartum Care

Beverley Chalmers, DSc(Med), PhD
Kingston, Ontario, Canada

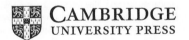

CAMBRIDGE
UNIVERSITY PRESS

University Printing House, Cambridge CB2 8BS, United Kingdom

One Liberty Plaza, 20th Floor, New York, ny 10006, USA

477 Williamstown Road, Port Melbourne, vic 3207, Australia

4843/24, 2nd Floor, Ansari Road, Daryaganj, Delhi – 110002, India

79 Anson Road, #06–04/06, Singapore 079906

Cambridge University Press is part of the University of Cambridge.

It furthers the University's mission by disseminating knowledge in the pursuit of education, learning and research at the highest international levels of excellence.

www.cambridge.org
Information on this title: www.cambridge.org/9781316627952
DOI: 10.1017/9781316809662

© Beverley Chalmers 2017

First published 2017

Printed in the United Kingdom by Clays, St Ives plc

A catalogue record for this publication is available from the British Library

Library of Congress Cataloging-in-Publication Data
Names: Chalmers, Beverley, author.
Title: Family-centred perinatal care : improving pregnancy, birth, and postpartum care / Beverley Chalmers.
Description: Cambridge, United Kingdom ; New York : Cambridge University Press, 2017. | Includes bibliographical references and index.
Identifiers: LCCN 2016047636 | ISBN 9781316627952 (pbk. : alk. paper)
Subjects: | MESH: Perinatal Care | Pregnancy | Patient-Centered Care | Professional-Family Relations | Attitude of Health Personnel
Classification: LCC RG627 | NLM WQ 210 | DDC 618.3/206–dc23
LC record available at https://lccn.loc.gov/2016047636

ISBN 978-1-316-62795-2 Paperback

• •

For Bernie
With love, respect, admiration and a lifetime of thanks.

Contents

Foreword

Despite my appreciation of former research and writing by the author, I did not really look forward to reading *Family-Centred Perinatal Care*. The term 'family-centred childbirth' has become somewhat hackneyed, ubiquitous in the daily press, the theme of innumerable magazine articles and books, no longer even mildly controversial. I thought there was no more to say about it. How wrong I was!

The problem is that old people like me, who had once pioneered in a cause and were proud of the progress it has made, are not always aware of the extent to which the imaginative insights and dedication of a new generation could take it. Reading this book has shown me how much more has been accomplished and how much more remains to be done. Writing this Foreword gives me the opportunity not only to show my appreciation for what Beverley Chalmers and her co-workers have achieved in furthering family-centred care but also to review the worldview in which the concept arose.

Two major movements in maternity care occurred during the first half of the twentieth century. The emphasis initially was, quite properly, on safety. It was the rare woman who did not personally know someone who had lost a relative in childbirth. Maternal mortality was counted in per cents rather than in per 100,000 as today. My father's mother died in childbirth, as did so many other women. Each woman giving birth must have worried about her own safety, each partner about the risk to a loved one. Soon, however, advances in medical care rapidly reduced the danger of death during childbirth, and attention shifted, beginning to focus on reducing the pain of labour and delivery. The infamous practice of twilight sleep was imported from Germany about 1915. It was initially opposed by the medical community because of the associated hazards but was soon adopted, acclaimed and came to be used almost universally. It was at its peak in the late 1940s when I began my medical career.

It is hard to believe now, but the picture is still vivid in my memory. A woman was admitted to hospital when her labour began; she was separated from her partner and loved ones, stripped of her clothing and dressed in what is euphemistically called a 'gown' (wide open in the back). She was taken to a labour ward in a wheel chair, where she heard other women screaming in pain, and put to bed, where she would remain until taken by stretcher to the delivery room. She was given an enema (needed or not), and her pubic hair was shaved. She was given her medication according to the routine orders of her doctor, irrespective of her needs or desires: a barbiturate (or paraldehyde or chloral hydrate) to make her sleepy, an opiate (Demerol, or morphine, or heroin [it was legal at that time]) to obtund her pain, and an amnesiac (scopolamine) so that she would not remember the pain. When her cervix was fully dilated (determined by repeated rectal examinations), she was transferred by stretcher to a steel delivery table in a room furnished like a surgical operating room. Her wrists were strapped in leather handcuffs to the sides of the table, her legs were trussed up in the air in stirrups and she was put to sleep with open-drop ether or chloroform so that her baby could be delivered by forceps. She was then transferred to a postpartum ward and kept there for 10 days. Her baby was taken from her, kept in a separate nursery and brought to her for carefully scheduled formula feedings (breastfeeding was discouraged because the amounts taken could not be readily measured). At the end of her hospital stay, she was discharged from the hospital and left to her own resources, expected to be a mother and to know how to look after her baby.

Although there were a few fledgling attempts to change some of these practices during the 1940s and 1950s, they remained essentially omnipresent throughout what we proudly called the developed world. Pregnancy, childbirth and postpartum care remained firmly and unequivocally hospital- and professional-centred.

Although the term was not yet popularized, family-centred care started, timidly and tentatively, in the 1960s. Childbirth classes began to include partners as well as pregnant women, and a few hospitals began to allow husbands and significant others to be with their wives or partners during labour, and eventually during delivery. There were no adverse effects on outcomes. Controlled trials of many degrading conventional practices, such as pubic shaving and routine enemas, showed that they conferred no benefits. They were gradually discarded. Physiological or less intrusive chemical methods of pain relief were developed which allowed women to be awake and aware during childbirth. Family-centred care was at first grudgingly accepted and then popularized, acclaimed and claimed. It was, however, still narrowly conceived and spottily implemented.

This was the situation when Beverley Chalmers began her research, first in South Africa, then in Canada and now throughout the world with the World Health Organization (WHO). She has developed and implemented demonstration programs in truly family-centred care for pregnancy, birth and postpartum programs that serve as examples, and exemplars, of what can be achieved in 'the real world'. She and her colleagues have significantly and importantly added to the modest improvements in care that we early advocates struggled to initiate. This research and these projects are the subject of this book.

It is still a work in progress. There is a long way to go, but research and practice such as Beverley Chalmers has carried out and described here so eloquently may bring us closer to where we hope to be. She has shown how women, their babies and their families can become the central actors in the drama of birth, while professionals play their important but secondary roles as facilitators.

Murray Enkin, CM, MD, FRCSC
Victoria, British Columbia, Canada

Preface

As a child, I learned that it is important, and morally appropriate, to give credit to those from whom one has learned and not to 'kick over the ladder after you have ascended it'. This Preface describes how this book came to be written and acknowledges the many colleagues, family members and friends whose thoughts have contributed greatly to this work.

This book is an amalgamation and culmination of more than 40 years of work dedicated to mothers, their newborns and their families, as well as their care providers. It draws from many of my 280-plus publications, including a number of books, book chapters and peer-reviewed journal articles, on pregnancy, birth and postpartum care. It also draws heavily on my life experiences devoted to strengthening maternal and newborn care in the context of the family. The academic content of this book reflects a model that we should strive towards for evidence-based, psycho-socially sensitive care during pregnancy, birth and the post-partum period. The boxed texts included throughout reveal personal events, observations and experiences that have contributed to my thinking on these issues throughout my lifetime.

I have benefitted enormously from others' knowledge. In my early research years, academic giants such as John Kennell, Marshall Klaus, Doris Haire, Niles Newton and Anne Oakley inspired me. Murray Enkin and Iain Chalmers revolutionized perinatal care by setting evidence-based standards, challenging me to seek ways to integrate a family-centred approach with excellence in clinical care. James McIntyre and Keith Bolton in South Africa shared clinical, research and teaching opportunities with me that have remained valuable for more than 30 years. My international consulting skills were initially honed by Marsden Wagner (then Regional Advisor for Maternal and Child Health at the World Health Organization's Regional Office for Europe), who threw me in at the deep end of the former Soviet Union – at my request – leaving me to sink or swim. This was a valuable and appropriate way to test my mettle in the pioneering world of inter-cultural collaboration, cooperation and confrontation. I learned an enormous amount from Marsden in terms of both what works best and what does not. I learned further lessons in family-centred care from courageous caregivers working in sometimes repressive systems such as Agnes Gereb in Hungary, Octavian Bivol in Moldova, and Adik Levin in Estonia, all three struggling to reform Soviet-era legacies. Agnes Gereb, an obstetrician in Hungary, whom I met in the 1990s, was imprisoned for assisting mothers to give birth at home when they refused care from their country's technologically focussed caregivers. In the same decade, Octavian Bivol (a senior advisor with the United Nations Children's Fund [UNICEF]) was singularly impressive in his ability to inspire a national perinatal care reform program that whole-heartedly, rapidly and comprehensively incorporated family-centred care approaches that changed childbirth care for millions of mothers in his country. One chapter of this book (Chapter 15) outlines the amazing scope of the changes he and Professor Petru Stratulat of the Ministry of Health of Moldova encouraged and facilitated. Adik Levin in Estonia pioneered the Humane Neonatal Care Initiative (HNCI) in the 1970s under the Soviet healthcare system that virtually excluded mothers (let alone families) from neonatal inten-sive care unit (NICU) settings. He gained special permission to incorporate mothers into the NICU environment not just as visitors but as an integral part of the care-giving team. I met Adik in 1992, and we have collaborated ever since. Most recently, I assisted him to co-ordinate a global petition from hundreds of neonatal caregivers that was submitted to the United Nations (UN) Committee on the Rights of the Child, imploring them to include the rights of the preterm and sick baby (and their family) into the UN child rights declarations. We published a book together in 2001, entitled *Humane Perinatal Care*, that is now out of print. This book exposed a more sensitive and normative approach to neonatal care as well as to prenatal, birth and postpartum care of mothers and their families, giving equal emphasis to both topics. The present book has developed from this earlier text, with one chapter (Chapter 5) now being devoted to family-centred neonatal care and the remaining text dealing with the multiple other aspects of family-centred care that arise during pregnancy, birth and postpartum. I will remain ever grateful to and inspired by these great pioneering minds for their example, ideas, approaches – and friendship. Others, too numerous to mention here, have contributed to my academic and personal development over the past decades and hence to the development of this book: I am sincerely grateful to them all.

I would also like to thank those who have assisted with the review and publication of this book. Professor Mahmoud Fathalla (former president of the International Federation of Obstetricians and Gynaecologists (FIGO) and director of the UNDP/UNFPA/WHO/World Bank Special Programme of Research, Development and Research Training in Human Reproduction – among other titles) provided immensely valuable constructive feedback during the final stages of writing this book; Dalia Jeckaite (midwife and international perinatal health consultant) gave thoughtful consideration to the penultimate version of the book; Diony Young (former editor of the journal *Birth: Issues in Perinatal Care*) gave me careful editorial advice; Anne Biringer (family medicine, Mt. Sinai Hospital, Toronto, Canada) made me rethink many of my earlier writings; Dana Chalmers (Vancouver, Canada), whose critical readings challenged almost every sentence I wrote and whose careful typesetting made a world of difference; and Murray Enkin (one of the founding fathers of evidence-based perinatal care and a justly deserved recipient of the Order of Canada) graciously wrote an apt Foreword to the text, wisely setting the scene for its contents.

I remain, also, forever indebted to my husband and our three daughters, who have supported my decades-long journey into family-centred perinatal care. My husband, Bernie, deserves particular thanks. We have shared our lives for more than 45 years, although it hardly seems like 45 months. He has shared my numerous highs and lows, my inability to say no to challenges and the consequent scrapes that I get into; provided wise counsel throughout; and supported and encouraged me to travel to unknown, frequently inaccessible and some-times hostile war-torn destinations, often alone. My gratitude to him, admiration, and love are immeasurable.

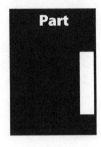

Part I

Overview

Chapter

1

Executive Summary

Family-centred care during pregnancy, birth and the postpartum period can be defined as care offered to the woman and her supportive family members that is evidence-based, psycho-socially sensitive, multi-culturally adapted, inter- and multi-disciplinary and utilizing only essential and appropriate technology. At first glance, it may appear that all our healthcare services fulfil this promise. After all, we are all nice to patients and their partners, we all have professional guidelines based on evidence and we all (or nearly all) use translators to assist us in providing care in diverse languages with which we are unfamiliar. On closer examination, however, as this book shows, we have a long way to go before we are truly family-centred. We have yet to implement our evidence-based guidelines (where these exist); we have yet to truly integrate women and their families, and particularly partners, into care; and we have yet to understand that the woman giving birth is not only a uterus, vagina and perineum carrying a fetus but a person with hopes, wishes, expectations, feelings and a family. Like those imprisoned in the ignorance of Plato's allegorical cave (*The Republic, c.* 360 BCE), exposing ourselves to the light of new and different ideas about perinatal care will be painful, at times threatening and certainly challenging. Just as care in the mid-1900s, described by Murray Enkin in his Foreword to this book, was regarded as state-of-the-art practice, so too is care today regarded as 'as good as it gets'. This book challenges this conviction.

Many of the issues raised in this book are controversial. Solutions to the challenges raised may be difficult to implement, especially for those who are resistant to change. Caution, care and sensitivity to the needs of both caregivers and families are needed when implementing changes, but failure to do so is no longer an option if we truly value family-centred care.

A family-centred approach to perinatal care incorporates a number of principles. These apply to the care of women having either vaginal or caesarean births and to those experiencing optimal as well as adverse maternal or neonatal outcomes. The principles of family-centred care are divided into 10 that focus on the needs of families and 10 that emphasize the caregivers' role – the '10:10 Principles'. Each of the chapters in this book addresses one or more of these principles. Key points are highlighted in summary textboxes at the end of each chapter. A selection of these points is included with each principle listed next.

The 10:10 Principles of Family-Centred Perinatal Care

Family-Centred Principles

1. *Care addresses the needs of women, their newborn/s and their chosen family supports during pregnancy, birth and postpartum.*

- Our emphasis on technological development in recent decades has benefitted many, but is accompanied by a loss of concern and respect for women's psychological, social and intellectual needs. We need to give birthing, and babies, back to families.
- The 10:10 Principles of family-centred perinatal care apply to the care of women having either vaginal or caesarean births and to those experiencing optimal as well as adverse maternal or neonatal outcomes.
- Family-centred care incorporates care for all those the woman regards as significant others.
- This book addresses family-centred psycho-socio-cultural and clinical issues occurring primarily during pregnancy, birth and the first few months after birth. All healthcare, however, for example, cardiovascular, respiratory, neurological, endocrine, and not only reproductive healthcare, should be family-centred.

2. *Care is sensitive to the individual psychological and social needs of women and their families – as perceived by them – including their needs for knowledge, emotional support and spiritual considerations.*

- The clinical birth environment is stressful for many women and their families. Maintaining a quiet, gentle, supportive, encouraging environment for both vaginal and caesarean births is a requirement.
- Encouraging skin-to-skin care from the moment of delivery, not separating mother and baby, and breastfeeding when the baby shows signs of readiness for a feed can make the experience of vaginal and caesarean birth that much more psychologically satisfying for mother, partner and baby.
- The more positive women's ratings are of their interactions with their caregivers, the higher will be their ratings of satisfaction with their labour and birth experience.
- Behind every stillbirth, miscarriage, birth of a baby with an anomaly and even difficult birth, unwanted caesarean section, failure to breastfeed successfully, or similar, severe or less severe, adverse outcome of childbearing lie real people with hopes, feelings, wishes, expectations and dreams.
- Psychological support may be needed at many stages of the perinatal and parenting periods. Perinatal psychologists can play an important role in providing supportive care.

3. *Care is culturally sensitive and informed.*

- The world is increasingly multi-cultural, revealing diversity of ethnic origin, religion, race and language. Cultures differ significantly in their beliefs regarding health and illness, as well as in their attitudes and practices regarding childbearing.
- Childbirth is the greatest leveller we have; we are all equal in this experience.
- We can learn a great deal from alternate cultures' approaches to healthcare.
- Cross-cultural challenges regarding perinatal care occur both when caring for women from different countries who live in our own country and when working in countries other than our own.

4. *Care is individualized to meet each family's needs.*

- There is no universal 'best' approach to perinatal care.
- It is possible to highlight *universal needs of women* in childbirth rather than *universal means of satisfying them* using Maslow's model of a need hierarchy.

5. *Families are cared for with respect and with concern for their dignity.*

- A women giving birth is not just a uterus, vagina and perineum.
- Excluding psycho-social concerns from perinatal care results in less optimal biological care.
- Women and their families wish to be cared for with sensitivity, respect for their dignity, concern for their cultural, religious or ethnic needs, and with gentleness as well as evidence-based, but individualized, care.
- Lack of respect for a woman's dignity, privacy and confidentiality may result in emotional abuse: non-dignified care is commonly reported around the world.

6. *Families are encouraged, prepared and supported to be actively involved in the care of their newborn, whether a healthy term infant or a sick or preterm baby requiring intensive clinical care.*

- Prenatal preparation classes for families provide cognitive, behavioural and emotional support for families. Families need to be prepared to care actively for their newborns from the moment of birth.
- In most countries, no specific training is provided for prenatal educators, and there is little or no standardization of the content of programs.
- The Humane Neonatal Care Initiative (HNCI) includes the mother, her baby and her partner in a rooming-in neonatal intensive care service, with direct parent care of the sick or preterm newborn and close skin-to-skin mother- and/or father-baby contact with breastfeeding (or breastmilk feeding) from birth until discharge. Except for technical medical and nursing care, mothers are taught and expected to provide all the infant's care and to stay in the NICU until discharge.
- Distinctive to Levin's HNCI approach, and differing from Kangaroo Care's primary focus on skin-to-skin care and breastfeeding, is the concept of constant mother/family-centred care rather than nurse/physician-centred care.

7. *Families take an active role in decision-making about their care, based on evidence-based information, provided without either covert or overt coercion, and with full knowledge about the potential adverse effects of any care procedure.*

- Making decisions about their transition to parenthood is central for all childbearing families.
- Facilitating 'informed choice' has long been a basic tenet of family-centred care. Care choices should be offered to the woman/family in an objective manner based on the best available evidence and should be devoid of coercion or 'informed coercion'.
- A woman and her family have a right to refuse consent for care. In family-centred care, the needs and expectations of the mother are a priority with respect to her care. Once the baby is born, the needs of the newborn become a priority with regard to the baby's care.

8. *Families are offered knowledgeable and appropriate care to support breastfeeding and, when needed, alternate feeding methods.*

- Uninterrupted skin-to-skin mother– and/or parent–infant contact, for the first hour or more after birth, is the goal to strive for in both vaginal and caesarean births both to optimize family experiences and to support breastfeeding.

- Mothers and babies and, ideally, partners should room-in together after birth. Essential for effective breastfeeding, rooming-in promotes mother–infant (and father–infant) attachment and develops confidence regarding infant care.
- The Baby Friendly Hospital Initiative (BFHI) and the Code of Marketing of Breastmilk Substitutes are a core component of family-centred care. To be truly 'baby friendly,' however, hospitals need to incorporate breastfeeding support together with 'friendly' or psycho-socially supportive evidence-based obstetric and neonatal care which is respectful of the rights of babies as well as of their parents.
- Most of the Ten Steps of the BFHI apply to NICU care, although some modifications and/or additions are needed.

9. *Feedback from families is encouraged and facilitated and is monitored and rigorously evaluated by caregivers and the healthcare facility.*

- Conducting national surveys of women's experiences of their perinatal care is essential. Evaluating psycho-social and cultural issues in perinatal care is difficult, but that does not justify their omission.
- There is a need for a uniform international perinatal assessment process that includes a careful analysis of the family-centredness of care.
- It is not only the mother's experiences that are of importance in family-centred data monitoring but also those of her chosen family support persons.
- Maternity hospitals should conduct local surveys of women's and their partner's experiences of their perinatal care in order to monitor and evaluate their own particular policies and practices.

10. *Information about mothers, partners and their infants is strictly confidential.*

- All aspects of clinical and psychological care must remain confidential.
- Caring for families whose babies are sick or preterm is psychologically challenging. As with all parents, information about their baby, the aetiology of its clinical needs, its treatment or prognosis and the parents' and caregivers' roles in the care of the infant should be handled with sensitivity to privacy needs and should remain strictly confidential.

Caregiver-Centred Principles

1. *Care is based on the best available evidence-based information.*

- Despite evidence-based guidelines, childbirth practices and policies differ – sometimes widely – both between countries and across regions within countries.
- Evidence-based practice applies to all families regardless of socio-economic status or other discriminatory variables.
- We need to designate personnel who are responsible for disseminating current research findings within healthcare facilities, implementing them and taking action to ensure that these findings are followed.

2. *Pregnancy and birth are regarded as healthy, normal life events with caregivers remaining vigilant for deviations from normal.*

- Definitions of 'normal birth' vary widely across Canada, the United Kingdom (UK) and the World Health Organization (WHO). Most women's births do not meet the criteria specified as 'normal birth'.

- There is wide disparity globally in both the number and types of interventions proposed for routine prenatal care.

3. *Interventions are used only when essential.*

- Many technologies used in perinatal care confer no clinical benefit, and some may be harmful.
- Countries adhering to a high-technology model of care sometimes report poorer maternal child health outcomes than others that rely less on the use of technology.
- Global reports of optimal caesarean section rates have found no reductions in maternal and neonatal mortality and morbidity when frequency of caesarean section was more than 15%. An increased rate of intervention is associated with higher mortality and morbidity in mothers and neonates.

4. *Care is interdisciplinary requiring integration among caregivers.*

- Primary care practitioners such as midwives and family physicians ideally care for normal pregnancies and births: the development of complications requires referral to specialists. Midwifery care is rated more highly by mothers than care by other providers.
- Every maternity care setting should have access to trained perinatal psychologists to provide support and care for women, their families and their healthcare providers.
- Care of families during the perinatal period requires inter-professional contact, communication, coordination and collaboration. This model should be initiated during undergraduate training and continue into later years of specialization.

5. *A holistic approach to care is expected of all care providers regardless of disciplinary background.*

- Holistic, sensitive, caring support, together with respectful treatment that is considerate of biological, emotional and intellectual needs of women and their family members, should be offered by *all* caregivers for *all* pregnant and birthing women regardless of the normality of their birth experiences or the degree of complication they develop.
- Routine, clinically focussed perinatal care is not sufficient: women need social, cultural and psychological support; relevant and timely information; concern for potential pathology; and an individualized approach to care.
- We need to heed the voices of women and their families.

6. *Professional education of caregivers should include the diverse principles of family-centred care as outlined in this book.*

- Inter-professional, psycho-social and cultural issues involved in clinical practice should be integrated into mainstream medical teaching programs.
- Instead of teaching obstetrics separately from neonatology, the care of the mother and baby and the interaction between the two requires a more closely integrated teaching model. Combined care requires combined teaching.
- Little formal training is available for perinatal psychologists. Psychologists with a thorough knowledge of perinatal practices who are a part of the perinatal care team and who focus on the emotional and intellectual challenges faced by couples and caregivers are urgently needed.

7. *Families are entitled to full, open and honest communication about all aspects of their care and are entitled to apology in the event of avoidable negative outcomes.*

- Women – and their partners – may benefit from debriefing regarding their pregnancy and birth experiences.
- Discussion of difficult experiences might do more to prevent litigation than to precipitate it.

8. *Care respects the reproductive and sexual rights of women and their families.*

- The incidence of violence against women and children provides a shocking reminder of the progress that we have yet to make in providing a respectful and healthy social environment. This concern is global.
- Political systems play a significant role in determining whether childbirth is supportive or abusive of mothers and their families.
- Discriminatory care, based on social and personal characteristics of women, occurs.

9. *Care is always non-abusive.*

- All forms of abuse may occur during perinatal care. Abuse is inappropriate, whether it is psychological, social, sexual, physical, emotional, financial or medical.
- Some situations are regarded as abusive by women but are, or were at the time of their experience, considered necessary or beneficial by caregivers. In many developed societies these practices have been discontinued, although not completely and not everywhere.
- Women who experience abusive birth procedures continue to require obstetrical care for future pregnancies as well as gynaecological care between pregnancies and after their childbearing years. Their trust in caregivers may be lost.
- Comments passed, and actions taken, in the operating theatre when a woman is anaesthetized may be inappropriate and disrespectful of patients, harmful to students and derogatory towards colleagues.

10. *Aggregated information about family-centred, psycho-social and clinical practices and outcomes is made publicly available and accessible regardless of socio-economic or educational background.*

- An efficient system of national and regional perinatal data collection that is reliable, timely and standardized is necessary for effective monitoring and evaluation of perinatal care and the development of national guidelines.
- Perinatal data collection has traditionally focussed on clinical events or practices. Psycho-social and cultural issues are not usually included, although they should be.
- Providing transparent, 'psycho-social and clinical perinatal practices and outcomes reports' for families as well as for caregivers is long overdue.

An Introduction to Family-Centred Perinatal Care

Principle:
- Care addresses the needs of women, their newborn(s) and their chosen family supports during pregnancy, birth and postpartum.

Overview

'Family-centred care' has become a familiar phrase in today's maternity services, although its precise definition is challenging.[1] More concerning is that its actual implementation, despite its being a current fashion in care, is still inadequate. This book defines family-centred care, examines its many facets in depth, provides available evidence-based knowledge supporting its benefits, outlines how it can and probably should be implemented and provides examples of how and where this has been done.

Outline

Defining Family-Centred Perinatal Care

A Holistic Approach

Defining Health

The 'Family'

The Timeframe of Family-Centred Maternal and Newborn Care

The 10:10 Principles of Family-Centred Perinatal Care

I have been fortunate to be able to collaborate with colleagues from multiple cultures, countries and religious backgrounds in the course of my career. I have lived and worked in Canada, South Africa and Denmark and travelled and worked extensively in perinatal care in 19 countries of the former Soviet Union and in a number of Central African, South American and a few Asian countries in addition to North American and European centres. I have co-authored books and articles with Jews, Muslims and Christians and with those who are strong adherents to religious belief and those who reject such considerations. My concern with a family-centred, holistic approach to childbearing has emerged from these rich and varied experiences. A broad approach to humanity is needed if cultural respect and collaboration are to be facilitated, just as a broad approach to childbearing is necessary to meet widely differing women's and caregivers' expectations. Highlights from my decades of experience in striving towards the attainment of family-centred care in many parts of the world, both developed and developing, have been included throughout this book in text boxes. These allow for the realization that family-centred care is not simply an academic construct but also a series of real-life actions taken to implement a system of care that values not only clinical excellence but 'whole-family well-being.'

> When first embarking on studies in perinatal health, I read an obstetrics textbook, a midwifery manual and books written for mothers. The impact was mind-blowing and directed my life's work in this field. It was almost impossible to accept that all three were describing the same experience. Exposing all newcomers to this broad field of perinatal healthcare in this manner, whether medical, nursing, midwifery or social scientist, might provide a valuable entry point to the study of family-centred childbirth care.

Defining Family-Centred Perinatal Care

Family-centred care during pregnancy, birth and the postpartum period can be defined as care offered to the woman and her supportive family members that is evidence-based, psycho-socially sensitive, multi-culturally adapted, inter- and multi-disciplinary and utilizing only essential and appropriate technology. Each of these concepts is examined extensively in this book.

Alternate definitions exist. *The Canadian National Family-Centred Maternal and New-born Care Guidelines*[2] defines family-centred care as '[a] complex, multidimensional, dynamic process of providing safe, skilled and individualized care. It responds to the physical, emotional, psycho-social and spiritual needs of the woman, the newborn and the family'. The Transforming Maternity Care Vision Team in the United States emphasizes the mother rather than the family and provides an alternate definition:

> [T]he goals for maternity care are best met by implementing a holistic, relationship-based model of care that is woman-centred, inclusive, and collaborative. Caregivers are included as dictated by the health needs, values, and preferences of each woman, taking into account her social and cultural context as she defines it, and given consideration for evidence of effectiveness, value, and efficiency.[3]

Common to most definitions of family-centred care is the understanding that, for most women, pregnancy and birth are normal, healthy life events, although it is recognized that family-centred care is applicable not only to healthy mothers and babies but also to mothers and newborns requiring specialized care such as surgical delivery[4] or intensive care.[5] Implementing family-centred care occurs at many levels of the care environment ranging from the individual to the departmental and organizational. It is not a specific set of procedures or practices but an approach that guides policy and program development, facility design, decision–making and daily activities throughout the healthcare environment.[6]

This lack of a clear definition has resulted in many, if not most, hospitals and care facilities claiming to be 'family-centred' even though there is no standard set for such accreditation. While some, no doubt, do aspire to being truly family-centred and incorporate all or many of the principles outlined in this book, most, in all probability, are not.

The Canadian national guidelines, entitled, *Family-Centred Maternal and Newborn Care,* are currently being revised for the fifth time in as many decades. The oversight committee for the revision of the guidelines was rather dumbfounded to find that a literature search revealed few, if any, sound and accepted definitions of 'family-centred care', despite all of us 'knowing' what we meant by the term. We are still grappling with the meaning of this term after almost 50 years of its use. Families are likely to have even greater difficulties assessing which care facilities they could use are truly 'family-centred'.

A Holistic Approach

Since childbirth became a medicalized, and usually hospitalized event, a century ago,[7] women, their babies and their partners have been relegated to a somewhat peripheral role within the clinically focussed hierarchy of medical care. Reinstating women, babies and partners from the secondary role to which they are assigned to a central role within perinatal care services is the purpose of this book.

The mother, her partner and her newborn are the sole reason for the establishment of the whole structure of perinatal and reproductive healthcare services, and consequently, such services should be totally directed towards best meeting their cognitive, emotional, social, cultural and spiritual needs, as well as their biological needs, during the transition to parenthood. This primary reason for the existence of obstetrics, midwifery and related services is frequently forgotten, underplayed or neglected. Women, their partners and their babies are the most important people in this experience. Their families, available and appropriate technology or facilities, and the caregivers who are best able to give them supportive care surround them and serve them. These include, for example, midwives, nurses, family physicians, obstetricians, neonatologists/paediatricians, doulas or companions, childbirth educators, social workers, community healthcare services and traditional birth attendants.

Defining Health

As long ago as 1948, the WHO Constitution[8] defined health as '[a] state of complete physical, mental and social well-being and not merely the absence of disease or infirmity'.

Since then, there has been an increasing awareness of psycho-social issues in addition to biological concerns in the care of women during pregnancy, birth and the postpartum period. This development underlies the fundamental tension between a medical and a psycho-social approach to childbearing: the perception of pregnancy and birth as a normal physiological process (a 'well role') or as an illness requiring close medical management (an 'ill role').[9] An increasing recognition of the psychological and social components of a family's transition to parenthood, in addition to their physiological basis, has resulted in a gradual change from physician-centred to baby- and/or mother-centred, then to woman-centred and, more recently, to family-centred care. Despite these developments, there are still many unaddressed issues for women, their families and professionals regarding their care.

The 'Family'

The concept of 'family' is not limited to those with marital or biological ties: families may be nuclear or multi-generational; headed by couples, single parents or various forms of shared parenting groups; may have same-sex or heterosexual parents; may include alternate gendered partners; may include children; or may involve additional support people or friends. Family-centred care incorporates care for all those whom the woman regards as significant others. Offering family-centred care recognizes the strengths and needs of women and their families and the essential roles that family members and friends play in the promotion of health and the management of illness.[10]

The Timeframe of Family-Centred Maternal and Newborn Care

The concept of family-centred care has extended the timeframe usually considered as encompassed by maternal and newborn care. Until recently, this care has focused on the pregnancy, birth and 6-week postpartum period. Today, this timeframe may be extended both before and after these limits to encompass preconception care; care during pregnancy and birth; care for mother, father and baby for at least 6 months postpartum (incorporating the period of exclusive breastfeeding with the additional understanding that the birth is not over until the baby is weaned); and inter-pregnancy care. Some consider that family-centred maternal and newborn care originates during adolescence, continues through pregnancies and inter-pregnancy periods, and concludes only with menopause. A truly family-centred approach will consider this lifetime framework, a focus on all family members and recognition of cognitive, emotional, social, spiritual and biological needs for families in transition to parenthood.

For practical reasons, this book addresses family-centred, psycho-socio-cultural and clinical issues occurring primarily during pregnancy, birth and the first few months after birth. It also does not address the expectation that all healthcare, for example, cardiovascular, respiratory, neurological, endocrine, and others, and not only reproductive healthcare should be family-centred.

I recall speaking to a professor, who was singularly influential in my life, about my academic life goals when I was in my early twenties. The research objectives that I outlined to him then have remained fairly consistent over my lifetime. I am grateful that he did not scoff at my lofty goals (and particularly point 6 below) when I precociously verbalized my hopes. These goals focussed on six basic aims that are all incorporated into the concept of family-centred care during the transition to parenthood and have led to the thoughts discussed in this book:

1. To examine childbirth primarily from a psycho-social perspective but to integrate this viewpoint with the many related disciplines that are involved.
2. To examine in more depth some issues within the field of reproductive health that appear to have particular relevance to current experiences or which appear to have been neglected or misunderstood.
3. To examine not only the perceptions of women and their families as receivers of care but also to understand the views of caregivers.
4. To explore issues involved in education regarding childbirth both for families and for professionals.
5. To explore differences and, more particularly, similarities between cultures regarding their experience of pregnancy, birth and the early postpartum period.
6. To influence globally, through this research, the practice of healthcare for pregnant women and their families during pregnancy, birth and the early months of parenthood.

Principles of Family-Centred Perinatal Care

Integrating the various concepts linked to a family-centred approach to care during pregnancy, birth and the first few months of parenthood reveals a number of principles. These principles form the basis of this text and are outlined in the Executive Summary. The principles are listed next together with the chapter in which they are discussed. Each chapter addresses one or more of the most central concepts included in these principles. The Appendix provides caregivers and healthcare facilities with measureable indicators of family-centredness as a starting point for self-assessment of their family-centredness, as well as a means of assessing women's perceptions of the family-centredness of their care. Using this 'question bank', caregivers and facilities are encouraged to customize their own self-assessment questionnaires to gain insight into how well they are achieving a truly family-centred approach to care during pregnancy, birth and the postpartum period.

The following principles apply to the care of women having either vaginal or caesarean births and to those experiencing optimal as well as adverse maternal or neonatal outcomes. The 10:10 Principles of Family-Centred Care are divided into 10 that focus on the needs of families and 10 that emphasize the caregivers' role.

The 10:10 Principles of Family-Centred Care

Family-Centred Principles

1. Care addresses the needs of women, their newborn(s) and their chosen family supports during pregnancy, birth and the postpartum period (Chapters 1, 2 and 14).
2. Care is sensitive to the individual psychological and social needs of women and their families – as perceived by them – including their needs for knowledge, emotional support and spiritual considerations (Chapter 7).
3. Care is culturally sensitive and informed (Chapters 10, 11 and 15).
4. Care is individualized to meet each family's needs (Chapter 11).
5. Families are cared for with respect and with concern for their dignity (Chapter 7).
6. Families are encouraged, prepared and supported to be actively involved in the care of their newborn, whether a healthy term infant or a sick or preterm baby requiring intensive clinical care (Chapters 4, 5and 8).
7. Families take an active role in decision–making about their care based on evidence-based information provided without either covert or overt coercion and with full knowledge about the potential adverse effects of any care procedure (Chapter 8).
8. Families are offered knowledgeable and appropriate care to support breastfeeding and, when needed, alternate feeding methods (Chapters 4 and 5).
9. Feedback from families is encouraged and facilitated and is then monitored and rigorously evaluated by caregivers and the healthcare facility (Chapter 13).
10. Information about mothers, partners and their infants is strictly confidential (Chapter 7).

Caregiver-Centred Principles

1. Care is based on the best available evidence-based information (Chapter 6).
2. Pregnancy and birth are regarded as healthy, normal life-events with caregivers remaining vigilant for deviations from normal (Chapter 3).

3. Interventions are used only when essential (Chapter 6).

4. Care is inter-disciplinary, requiring integration among caregivers (Chapters 9, 15 and 16).

5. A holistic approach to care is expected of all care providers regardless of disciplinary background (Chapter 2 and 3).

6. Professional education of caregivers should include the diverse principles of family-centred care as outlined in this book (Chapter 9).

7. Families are entitled to full, open and honest communication about all aspects of their care and are entitled to an apology in the event of avoidable negative outcomes (Chapter 7).

8. Care respects the reproductive and sexual rights of women and their families (Chapter 14).

9. Care is always non-abusive (Chapter 12).

10. Aggregated information about family-centred, psycho-social and clinical practices and outcomes is made publicly available and accessible regardless of socio-economic or educational background (Chapter 16).

Key Points

- 'Family-centred care' is defined as care offered to the woman and her supportive family members that is evidence-based, psycho-socially sensitive, multi-culturally adapted, inter- and multi-disciplinary and utilizing only essential and appropriate technology.
- Women, their babies and their partners are relegated to a peripheral role within the clinically focussed hierarchy of medical care. Reinstating women, babies and partners from the secondary role to which they are assigned to a central role within perinatal care services is the purpose of this book.
- There is increasing awareness of psycho-social issues in addition to biological concerns in the care of women during pregnancy, birth and the postpartum period.
- Family-centred care incorporates care for all those whom the woman regards as significant others.
- This book addresses family-centred, psycho-socio-cultural and clinical issues occurring primarily during pregnancy, birth and the first few months after birth. All healthcare, however – for example, cardiovascular, respiratory, neurological, endocrine, and others, and not only reproductive healthcare – should be family-centred.
- The 10:10 Principles of Family-Centred Perinatal Care apply to the care of women having either vaginal or caesarean births and to those experiencing optimal as well as adverse maternal or neonatal outcomes.

Part II

From Pregnancy to Parenthood

Chapter 3

Pregnancy and Birth Are Normal, Healthy Processes

Principles:

- Pregnancy and birth are regarded as healthy, normal life events with caregivers remaining vigilant for deviations from normal.
- A holistic approach to care is expected of all care providers regardless of disciplinary background.

Overview

For some, family-centred care has been limited to a – perhaps non-verbalized – assumption that it applies only to normal pregnancy and birth. In this view, once complications set in, clinical care becomes a priority, often at the expense of family-centred practices. In contrast, however, family-centred care is even more important when complications arise. Defining 'normal' pregnancy, labour and birth is, in any event, complex and is examined in depth in this chapter, revealing the extensive medicalization of all births in our modern world. Demedicalizing all stages of the pregnancy, birth and postpartum periods is discussed, and integrating the traditional medical model with a psycho-social approach is suggested and explored.

Outline

Defining Women as 'At Risk'
Defining 'Normal' Birth
Demedicalizing Birth
An Integrated Psycho-Social-Medical Model
   Before Pregnancy
   During Pregnancy
   In Labour and Birth
Immediate Postpartum Care
The Language of Birth
Challenges

Defining Women as 'At Risk'

Attempts to define normal pregnancy and birth have led, over decades, to various scales designed to attribute a 'risk score' to a woman with the intention of classifying women who are most likely to develop complications and need specialized care either during pregnancy or at birth. Nevertheless, as the World Health Organization (WHO) rightly notes, '[A]ccurately predicting which women will develop complications is not possible.'[1] Large-sample research into predicting obstetric complications on the basis of multiple obstetric indicators, a modified version of the Littman and Parmelee 'risk score', biological characteristics, as well as psychological and social factors, allows one to accurately predict complications of birth in fewer than 7% of women.[2] In theory, predicting risk may be helpful for the allocation of resources, as well as to ensure that women have appropriate levels of care available to them or their newborns at birth. In practice, such 'risk scores' have proved unreliable, and according to the United Kingdom's National Institute for Care Excellence (NICE) Antenatal Care guidelines,[3] there is no evidence to suggest that the use of antenatal risk-assessment tools improves maternal and neonatal outcomes.[4]

> My doctoral research, in the late 1970s, challenged the concept that adverse obstetric outcomes could be predicted based on classical obstetric risk indicators. I was curious as to the roles that psycho-social factors played in predicting these outcomes in addition to the traditionally used 'risk scores' based on obstetric variables. My large-sample research revealed that neither a standard risk score nor most of the multiple psychological or social factors, including life event stressors, that I assessed were reliable predictors of pregnancy complications. My attempts to publish these findings were rejected by obstetric journals as this finding was in stark contradiction to current knowledge and practice. Ten years later I was thrilled to listen to a presentation given by Professor Mahmoud Fathalla (past president of the International Federation of Obstetricians and Gynaecologists (FIGO) and former director of the United Nations Development Programme/ United Nations Family Planning Association/World Health Organization/World Bank Special Programme of Research, Development and Research Training in Human Reproduction) as a keynote address at the 13th FIGO conference in Singapore in 1991. He clearly rejected the notion that risk scoring tools could predict obstetric complications. I felt vindicated!

Risk scoring systems may also be misleading because most women may be at risk for specific problems or at various times during pregnancy, labour or birth, but not at all times or for all complications. In addition, the question of the effect on women of being labelled 'high risk' has been raised but not well studied. Classification of a woman as 'at risk' may well lead to more routine intervention than is appropriate or effective. In some cases, it can result in stigmatizing a woman (e.g. she's obese or is poor or uneducated), imposing a stereotypical adverse set of expectations on the woman which may or may not be true and clinical practices that might or might not be necessary in her individual case. From the woman's perspective, being classified as 'high risk' may have various psychological implications.[5] Anxiety may be increased, fear of unnecessary intervention or, in contrast, a wish for greater monitoring and intervention (to ensure that she and her baby are safe) may occur. Women may consider that they are 'abnormal'. They may anticipate their prenatal care appointments fearing that they will be treated as somehow 'less' than 'normal' women, that they may be lectured on their supposedly 'high risk' characteristics (such as obesity) and, as a result, may even delay prenatal visits. Worse, when complications arise, women may dismiss their symptoms as an expected part of their 'abnormal' pregnancy rather than seeking needed care. Perhaps even more concerning is that caregivers may dismiss their symptoms as readily, as being the result of their 'high risk' classification, rather than investigating them appropriately to be certain that the symptoms exhibited are indeed related to the obvious 'risk factors' and are not arising from a different cause. Clearly, also, complications occur in women who are not identified as 'high risk', whereas others, who are so classified, may well go on to have normal births. Every effort should therefore be made to ensure that all women have essential services available and accessible. More importantly, all women should be regarded as having normal pregnancies until proved otherwise, with caregivers remaining vigilant at all times for possible deviations from 'normal'.

Defining 'Normal' Birth

Similarly, definitions of what is a 'normal' or a 'complicated' birth should be dynamic rather than static. Yet, most available definitions of birth attempt to classify normal birth by means of specific interventions used, or not used, in labour and delivery. This approach leads to confusing and, at times, simply nonsensical definitions. There are a number of definitions of normal birth: a few are discussed here – those of the WHO, the WHO-Euro Bologna Score, Canada, and the United Kingdom. Only the WHO and the WHO-Euro Bologna Score approach the definition of normal birth as a dynamic process, with the remaining attempts being based on static classifications of interventions used or not used. Perhaps the simplest remains that of the WHO, which defines 'normal birth' as 'spontaneous in onset, low-risk at the start of labour and remaining so throughout labour and delivery. The infant is born spontaneously in the vertex position between 37 and 42 completed weeks of pregnancy. After birth the mother and baby are in good condition.'[6] The WHO-Euro Bologna Score develops this approach further, providing perhaps the most useful definition available today.

The WHO-Euro Bologna Score

The WHO-Euro Bologna Score is based on the assumption that no single indictor or set of indicators can assess whether labour is managed as 'normal birth'. The 'Bologna Score'[7] attempts to quantify, both in an individual labour and in a wider population, the extent to which labours in a hospital or a region are managed as normal as opposed to complicated. It incorporates the WHO definition of 'normal birth' as a pregnancy of more than 37 and less than 42 completed weeks' gestation with a singleton fetus, vertex presentation and spontaneous onset and requires that there is a skilled attendant at birth. This rating excludes women from classification as having normal births if they have induced labours or a caesarean birth (either planned or emergency). In addition, the more normal the management of labour, the more likely it is that women would (1) have a companion at birth, (2) be monitored by means of a partogram, (3) not have their labour augmented either pharmacologically or mechanically (including practices such as external pressure on the fundus), (4) use a non-supine position for birth and (5) have skin-to-skin contact of mother and baby for at least 30 minutes within the first hour after birth. The rationale for these inclusions and exclusions is as follows: having a companion at birth reflects evidence-based care, as well as the attitudes of professionals and the involvement of women (and their partners) in birth. It incorporates a family-centred approach to care recognizing psycho-social needs at birth. It is also indicative of flexibility in the delivery care system and may serve to indicate prenatal preparation of women for birth. The use of a partogram is an indicator of effective monitoring of progress of labour, providing guidance on the appropriateness of timing of this monitoring as well as clear warning signs as to when progress is deviating too far from normal and action or intervention is required. Absence of augmentation is indicative of persisting normal progress in labour as judged by professionals. Use of a non-supine position for delivery, as opposed to supine or lithotomy positions, reflects evidence-based care and the attitude of caregivers and will exclude almost all forceps or ventouse deliveries. Use of a non-supine position for delivery will also exclude epidural or spinal analgesia use, particularly if this creates an adverse effect on labour. Skin-to-skin care for at least 30 minutes within the first hour after birth is evidence-based practice and can serve as an indirect measure of both maternal and infant well-being and early initiation of breastfeeding. It is also indicative of caregiver attitude. The Bologna Score makes it possible to assess both attitudes and practices within a maternity service towards the dynamic management of normal labour.

Other definitions by professional organizations in both Canada and the United Kingdom, for example, are more complex and less helpful.

The Canadian Approach

A joint statement of the Society of Obstetricians and Gynaecologists of Canada and other Canadian professional organizations, including the College of Family Physicians Canada, the Canadian Association of Midwives, the Association of Women's Health, Obstetric and Neonatal Nurses, Canada, and the Society of Rural Physicians of Canada, distinguishes between 'normal' and 'natural' childbirth, with 'natural childbirth' involving little or no human intervention.[8] 'Normal birth' is defined as excluding elective induction before 41 weeks, spinal analgesia, general anaesthesia, forceps or vacuum, caesarean section, routine episiotomy, continuous electronic fetal monitoring for low-risk birth and fetal malpresentation. 'Normal delivery', however, may include interventions such as induction, augmentation, electronic fetal monitoring, artificial rupture of membranes and pharmacological pain relief such as nitrous oxide, opioids and/or epidural analgesia. 'Normal' pregnancy and labour may also include complications such as hypertension, ante-partum or postpartum haemorrhage, perineal trauma and repair as well as neonatal intensive care unit (NICU) admission. This complicated and confusing definition attempts to accept commonly used, current practices such as epidurals and inductions (i.e., the 'norm') as 'normal' in an attempt not to stigmatize the many women who experience these and other procedures or interventions as 'abnormal'. It is difficult to know whether women are truly 'fooled' by labelling their experiences of, for example, induction (after 41 weeks) or augmentation, epidural, haemorrhage, and NICU admission of their baby as normal birth, although it is unlikely that they are. It is even more difficult to think that caregivers consider these types of events as 'normal'.

The UK Definition

The Royal College of Obstetricians and Gynaecologists of the United Kingdom in its joint statement on making normal birth a reality[9] does not distinguish between 'natural' and 'normal' delivery; defines 'normal delivery' as 'without induction, without the use of instruments, not by caesarean section and without general, spinal or epidural anaesthetic before or during delivery' and would potentially also exclude augmentation of labour, use of opioid drugs, artificial rupture of membranes and managed third stage of labour from definitions of 'normal' birth if data were routinely available to monitor their usage.[10] This definition comes closest to the WHO-Euro Bologna Score but omits the dynamic assessment of labour progress in favour of attempting to classify some interventions as normal and others not – a potential quagmire. Fewer than half of all women in both Canada and the United Kingdom experience 'normal birth' as defined in their countries.

The development of definitions of normal birth based on types of interventions used or not used, as has occurred in the United Kingdom and Canada, has emerged from the increasing use of technology in birth over recent decades and the opposing approach that challenges birth to become demedicalized.[11]

Demedicalizing Birth

More use is being made of technology than ever before in medical care today. Because many of these technologies may be life-saving and beneficial, there has been a willingness to think that if they are good for some, they might be good for all. Fuelled by the (often legitimate) fear of litigation in the United States at least, these technologies are presented as the lawyers' redeeming feature: 'at least everything possible was done to prevent negative outcomes from occurring' is an easy defence even if not always justified by evidence. Belief in the infallibility of technology prevails subconsciously, if not consciously. The result has been an explosion in the routine use of such techniques as electronic fetal monitoring, ultrasound, epidural anaesthetic for vaginal delivery and caesarean section, among others. None of these is supported by evidence for their routine use, yet they are commonplace interventions. Almost every woman in pregnancy (in developed countries at least) has at least one ultrasound, and most have two, three or even more. In many parts of the world, caesarean section rates may range between 25 and 50% and in isolated centres may exceed this despite WHO recommendations to maintain this rate below about 15%.[12] In North America, epidural anaesthesia rates for vaginal deliveries may exceed 70%.[13] This might be regarded as absurd in some other parts of the industrialized world. For example, in the United Kingdom, epidural rates remain below 30%.[14] Reviews indicate that a range of commonly practiced interventions during labour, birth and the immediate postpartum period also affect the fetal to neonatal transition. For example, evidence does not support separation of mother and baby for some hours after delivery or in postpartum wards, routine supplementation of babies with water or breastmilk substitutes, routine suctioning of the newborn at birth, suctioning of meconium-stained liquor and intubation and suctioning of vigorous infants to prevent meconium aspiration.[15] As with maternal care in labour and birth, less intervention in newborn care is frequently better.

In their defence, physicians may quote women's choice, saying that women want this type of 'excellent, high-technology care'. Each birth has to 'be perfect', and every available technique possible may be used to achieve this. Sadly, available interventions are not always supported by sound research evidence as beneficial for either mother or baby when used on a routine basis. In reality, intervening in the normal physiological process of labour and birth in the absence of medical necessity increases the risk of complications for both mother and baby.[16] The challenge is determining just when interventions are beneficial for all or most women (e.g. taking folic acid before and in the first 3 months of pregnancy[17]) and when, or for which women, interventions might be harmful (e.g. shaving, enemas, pushing on the abdomen to help get the baby down in vaginal births and many episiotomies).

From a clinical perspective, a 'perfect birth' in this medicalized context is viewed as a healthy, live mother and baby with little else mattering. Over-reliance on medical care results in little concern for the emotional fulfilment that should accompany birth or the full experience of love and tenderness that should surround the birthing woman, the new mother and baby and her partner.

What has happened to consideration of the mother as an intelligent, emotional and sensitive being in achieving a 'perfect birth'? Giving birth is a psychologically profound experience. At hardly any other time in her life is a woman more psychologically sensitive or vulnerable, and yet, today, she may rely heavily on technology that regulates her biological functioning, although not obtaining optimal care for her emotional and intellectual needs. When experiencing the challenge of birthing, machines can never assess or relieve her anxiety, self-doubt, questioning, emotional need for comfort, safety and love, and perhaps not even all her physical needs. Findings that fear of childbirth results in prolonged labour clearly indicate that emotions and biological functioning are intimately integrated and that both levels of functioning need to be addressed in providing effective care during childbearing.[18] Pharmaceuticals can manipulate a woman's emotional and cognitive reactions to the events of birth and early infant contact so that she does not experience them in a normal, physiological way. Yet this solution to the challenge of birth – pharmacological pain management and technological intervention – is a commonly used first line of response. It is striking that in some Canadian research[19] 70% of women express a need to give birth naturally, without intervention, whereas the same number actually have considerable intervention in the process. What can explain this discrepancy? Is it that women cannot cope with the reality of birth despite their high hopes and good intentions prior to birth? Alternatively, is it that caregivers do not provide the type of support and care that women need to assist them to achieve their fullest psychological potential during labour and delivery?

> Caregivers sometimes manipulate women emotionally – intentionally or unintentionally – to make use of interventions. For example, I have heard anaesthetists asking women in labour, 'Would you like your epidural now dear, while I am still around? I may not be here later when you decide you want it.' Alternatively, caregivers may try a different approach: 'I recommend you have this ... you don't want to feel responsible for harming your baby by not doing this do you?' Also, few or no alternatives to pharmacological pain management may be offered, such as walking in labour, using showers or baths for relaxation, remaining mobile up to the moment of giving birth, adopting differing positions for pain relief and using breathing, relaxation and stress-reducing techniques[20] so that women's use of pharmacological pain management, in contradiction to their original 'natural birth' hopes, is easily understood. Giving birth is painful, and supporting a woman in managing this pain by using such time-consuming supportive processes may not be every caregiver's preference. Does this tell us that women are weak or that caregivers do not always offer appropriate support in birth?

Having a companion during labour is one of the most well-documented beneficial practices to emerge in perinatal care in recent decades. Remarkably, we think of this as an intervention even though this was standard care before hospitalization of births about a century ago. In addition to a supportive companion, optimal healthcare includes having one-to-one nursing care for women during labour and birth, although women are often left alone in labour between routine monitoring visits.[21] Most women in the developed and technologically sophisticated world, including Canada, for example, do not get the most appropriate support for maternal and child contact after birth or for the promotion of breastfeeding.[22] The Western world's and Canada's low breastfeeding rates within a week or two after birth are clear evidence of a lack of knowledge, skills and appropriate healthcare services regarding breastfeeding promotion. In some countries or in segments of societies, this may be accompanied by a belief that substitute technology – infant formula – is just as good, despite the abundant academic evidence supporting the value of breastfeeding and, in particular, exclusive breastfeeding for the first 6 months of life.[23] Hidden – emotional – losses also may occur: for some women, the sense of achievement in their ability to give birth or to breastfeed their baby is lost by their over-reliance on a technologically managed birth or postpartum experience.

The time has come to revise our understanding of birth. It is not simply a biological process. We need to experience birth in as emotionally and intellectually fulfilling a way as possible, as well as in a biologically safe way that uses only minimal, and essential, technology. These are not incompatible dreams. They simply require a change of approach on the part of caregivers and a change of heart among women. Both are achievable.

An Integrated Psycho-Social-Medical Model?

The move towards a medicalized model of care for pregnant women and their offspring has neglected the so-called softer sides of care. Women's feelings, hopes, wishes, expectations and needs are regarded as of less importance than their physical well-being. A holistic approach that encompasses both physical health and psychological and social health is preferable from before pregnancy, through pregnancy and birth, and well into the post-partum period.

Before Pregnancy

Recent trends have moved towards advocating a pre-conceptional programme for all women contemplating pregnancy, if not all women of reproductive age,[24] as about half of all pregnancies are unplanned.[25] At the very least, more effective pre-conceptional family planning is need. Most pre-conceptional programmes, however, routinely focus on clinical aspects of care in preparation for pregnancy, without serious consideration of their psychological consequences. For example, they advocate living healthy lifestyles and include advice regarding weight loss (or gain), exercise programmes, nutritious diet and avoidance of all alcohol (especially if pregnancy is potentially possible), smoking or substance abuse.[26] They do not often integrate care for the psycho-social implications of this advice on women. In addition, there are few, if any, data or evidence available supporting the efficacy of available programmes for many pregnancy outcomes, and a recent Cochrane review concludes that there is insufficient evidence to recommend widespread implementation of routine pre-pregnancy health promotion for women of childbearing age, either in the general population or between pregnancies.[27] Considering these programmes within a psycho-social-medical model requires consideration not only of their potential or real clinical benefit but also of their psycho-social implications.

Advising avoidance of medications or drugs during pregnancy is well founded and, perhaps with the exception of regular substance abusers, readily followed by women. In contrast, advocating weight loss in preparation for pregnancy among overweight women, while desirable, is unlikely to be either clinically or psychologically beneficial. Weight loss is exceptionally difficult, and a considerable dedication to exercise is needed in addition to reduced nutritional intake to achieve an optimal weight – often an overwhelming challenge for overweight women. It is also a slow process, taking many years for very obese women, if a safe rate of weight loss is planned. This is not always a feasible delay to encourage before conception. Instruction to reduce weight, although good advice for general health, may only serve to increase anxiety and create psychological distress in women who are unable to lose weight before embarking on pregnancy or who have unplanned pregnancies. Current approaches to reducing weight in pregnancy have also proved to be untenable and may lead to increased anxiety.[28] In addition, research now suggests that women achieve healthier pregnancy outcomes if they are fit and well and that being overweight per se might not be the determining factor of complications in birth when exercise and fitness are also considered.[29] Although the serious adverse consequences of severe obesity in pregnancy – including increased risk of pre-eclampsia, prenatal stillbirth, caesarean delivery, instrumental delivery, shoulder dystocia, meconium aspiration, fetal distress and early neonatal death – are fully acknowledged, advocating weight loss is a complex issue requiring sensitive and long-term attention.[30] Care must be taken in how 'good' medical messages are provided together with an understanding of their psychological or social consequences if successful pre-conceptional programmes are to be developed.

During Pregnancy

A 2015 WHO review of 85 prenatal care clinical guidelines, emanating primarily from the United States, the United Kingdom and Canada, revealed a wide disparity in both the number and types of interventions proposed for routine care.[31] Folic acid and iron supplementation, RhD diagnosis and management of nausea and vomiting were the only clinical interventions included in over 50% of the guidelines. For 33 of the 171 interventions highlighted across the guidelines, there were conflicting recommendations. For example, recommendations for vitamin or mineral supplementation, such as iron, calcium and vitamins A and D, were extremely diverse, with 50% of the guidelines recommending supplementing and the remaining half advising against it. Clearly, even considering only the clinical aspects of prenatal care raises questions of diversity and disagreement among professionals. This review examined traditional clinical assessments (not including psycho-social concerns during pregnancy), although advice and treatment included behavioural and emotional suggestions, such as offering advice regarding nutrition, exercise, smoking cessation, healthy lifestyles, self-care and emotional well-being.

Integrated medical and psycho-social models of care during pregnancy will likely be superior to a primarily clinically focussed approach – although possibly equally diverse across local, regional, national and international borders. Evidence in favour of a combined psychological and clinical focus is emerging in many areas. For example, a review of women's experiences of prenatal care in the United States found that psychological and social needs were as important as, if not more so than, obtaining good clinical care: some women reported respectful, comprehensive, individualized care; others experienced long waits, rushed visits and perceived prenatal care as mechanistic or harsh.[32] Women's preferences emphasised a more psychologically supportive approach, including reasonable wait times, unhurried visits, continuity of care and caregiver, flexibility, comprehensive care, meeting with other pregnant women in groups, developing meaningful relationships with professionals and becoming more active participants in care. Specific needs included preferring a single provider, counselling and education (which was lacking in the women studied), being involved in decision-making and being given information about physiological and emotional changes as well as common discomforts of pregnancy. A similar global review confirmed these American reports, indicating that women want a positive pregnancy experience that includes maintaining a healthy pregnancy, both physical and cultural normality and effective transition to positive labour, birth and motherhood. Simply offering routine, clinically focussed service provision is not sufficient: women need social, cultural and psychological support throughout, the provision of relevant and timely information, the detection and treatment of potential and actual pathology and the tailored (rather than routine) use of biomedical tests and interventions.[33]

Women need information regarding not only the 'common discomforts' of pregnancy but also about 'warning signs' indicating when caregiver advice should be sought. Knowing that, for example, nausea and vomiting in pregnancy are normal 'discomforts' or that many women experience pelvic pain is not sufficient: knowing when these symptoms become pathological, requiring referral to a caregiver for in-depth assessment, is of far more importance and more likely to assuage anxiety. For example, pelvic girdle pain is common in pregnancy but is by no means 'normal' and, according to physiotherapy guidelines, requires thorough investigation if reported by mothers.[34] There is a need to develop and implement evidence-based women- or family-centred guidelines regarding when a pregnancy might be becoming problematic so that anxiety can be reduced and essential care obtained.[35] Such guidelines are respectful of the significant role that mothers and families can play in monitoring their own healthcare and emphasize that care must be taken to 'listen carefully to mothers' as they are not professionals, will not use the terminology that is familiar to professionals but are often very much in touch with their bodies and their experiences.

One woman, in her second trimester of pregnancy, called her caregiver, between routine visits, to report that she had pelvic pain lasting for a week, resulting in her struggling to walk. She was reassured by telephone that pelvic pain is a 'normal discomfort of pregnancy'. Not wishing to be a 'complaining mother', she did not report this to her caregiver when it recurred closer to her due date, although she did frequently report ongoing difficulties in turning over in bed throughout the pregnancy – a classic sign of symphasis pubis dysfunction. Her case notes did not include this information, and at her birth, attended by different caregivers, this information was not known. A prolonged second-stage labour of 2 to 3 hours with virtually no progress, predominantly in a supine position with widely abducted legs, pressed against her caregivers' hips, followed by an epidural and forceps delivery, with abducted legs in stirrups, of a 9-pound, 13-ounce baby (with birth weight confirmed before birth at a 39-week ultrasound), left her with a clear symphasis pubis diastasis and displaced lower segments of her coccyx, as later revealed by x-ray. This, and her struggle to return to 'normal' in the years following her childbirth, might have been avoided if either she or her caregivers had been aware of the clear warning sign of pubic pain in pregnancy causing an inability to walk, coupled with the baby's size and her prolonged second-stage labour. Almost every position and procedure used during her second-stage of labour is contraindicated in the event of such prenatal pelvic girdle pain/symphasis pubis diastasis. Listening to the words that this mother used to describe her pelvic girdle pain (difficulty walking for a week and an inability to turn over in bed) might have led to a physiotherapy referral in pregnancy and avoidance of harmful labour and birth positions to help prevent her later complications.

While it is appropriate to regard most pregnancies as normal, it is always essential to remain alert to deviations from normal. Discounting a non-routine report of difficulty walking for a week as a 'normal discomfort of pregnancy' is an example of how this can easily go wrong.

Ensuring that pregnant women and their families receive psychological and social preparation for pregnancy, birth and the early months of parenthood is as important as providing good clinical care during pregnancy, yet this is not often regarded as a priority. In Canada, as many as one-third of all primiparous women do not attend prenatal education classes.[36] Fewer than a third of all women, primiparous and multiparous, regard their healthcare provider as their most useful source of information, and about one-fifth of women rate books as their most useful information source. Women value the Internet, family and friends even less often. Yet, in developed countries at least, almost all women attend prenatal clinical care.[37] Providing a balanced approach that considers clinical issues as well as psychological and social concerns is needed. A psycho-social-medical approach recognizes that women and their partners play an active role in their care and should be recognized as partners in care. Involving partners has been shown to be beneficial for encouraging healthy lifestyle choices among pregnant women, greater prenatal care usage, fewer low-birth-weight or small-for-gestational-age newborns and improved breastfeeding practices.[38]

As with prenatal weight concerns, monitoring weight gain during pregnancy is fraught with difficulties. This practice is a current popular focus given the global concern regarding obesity, and some countries still endorse weighing women at every prenatal visit regardless of the anxiety this might provoke. Others, with more level heads perhaps, such as the UK's globally respected NICE guidelines, do not advocate weighing mothers at any prenatal visit other than the first.[39] The WHO has also long advocated this.[40] Similarly, advocating a 'no alcohol during pregnancy' recommendation, as is the case in Canada, on the basis that we have not yet determined the optimal limit of alcohol intake that is safe in pregnancy, also leads to considerable anxiety among women – especially the many with unintended pregnancies – who may have had the occasional drink before learning of their pregnancy. Reduced alcohol intake and avoidance of binge drinking in pregnancy have known benefits, although careful thought is needed before continuing with such 'no risk' policies.[41] Such extreme policies, although intending to be biologically helpful, are not always evidence-based, may cause undue psychological concern and are unlikely to be beneficial.[42]

A further example of the importance of considering both beneficial clinical and psycho-social care arises with regard to giving women their own case notes to carry during pregnancy. This has long been endorsed by the WHO[43] and is supported by randomized trials[44] as resulting in increased maternal satisfaction as well as increased likelihood of a woman's records being accessible at the time of birth.[45] At the very least, women's records should be accessible either in hardcopy format or as electronic files whenever and wherever she gives birth. Mother-held electronic access cards or documents would facilitate this, although currently they are not frequently used.

In contrast, psycho-social considerations with regard to the mental health of women prenatally (and postnatally) are being recognized more often. Screening tests have been developed that help to identify women who have psycho-social family concerns (e.g. relationship difficulties, previous experience of abuse or emotional problems), allowing caregivers to 'red flag' them for increased attention and support. Two that can be used with some validity are the Canadian Antenatal Psycho-Social Health Assessment (ALPHA) scale and the Australian Antenatal Risk Questionnaire (ANRQ).[46] Life event scales that identify women with heightened stress levels in their lives are also useful in identifying which women are at increased risk of potential healthcare problems because of the increased life stresses they have experienced, particularly when these are undesirable events that have a greater impact on outcome.[47] The increasing attention being paid to psycho-social issues during pregnancy and their biological impact is a welcome development, especially as women with such concerns may not be able to offer optimal care and support for their offspring leading to a long-term cycle of challenging experiences for all concerned.

Perhaps the most stressful prenatal experience for families involves prenatal screening for anomalies. Strongly endorsed by most caregivers, prenatal screening is generally regarded as routine care. Yet the implications of this, both clinically and psychologically, may be enormous, and counselling for these consequences prior to testing or after confirmation of potential anomalies may be lacking. If families are unwilling to terminate an anomalous pregnancy under any circumstances, then careful consideration needs to be given to the value of the tests. Family understanding of the consequences, and their consent for the tests are important. If the family are willing to consider terminating the pregnancy, then pre-test counselling should also include the procedure that would follow a positive finding. In many cases, a confirmatory second screen may be undertaken prior to possible termination of the pregnancy. What information should be given to the family regarding the potential severity of the clinical problem to prepare them for potential loss of the pregnancy but at the same time to facilitate the seemingly endless wait time between tests and their results? Ready access to the Internet empowers families to explore their own potential clinical consequences with, perhaps, inappropriate fears and concerns being generated. The language used by caregivers may convey conflicting information to each parent, leading to emotionally challenging discussions of future plans of action in the event of an anomalous diagnosis. Decisions that must be faced may include termination of a clearly non-viable fetus (e.g. one with anencephaly), acceptance of a baby that might live but with disability and a potentially compromised lifestyle (e.g. one with a severe neural tube defect) or minimal disability (e.g. one with a cleft lip). Implications of each of these for each member of the family, including siblings, must be weighed and considered by the parents, ideally in collaboration with their caregiver. Emotional support following the diagnosis of a potential or actual severe anomaly is crucial, both prior to any further screening, after a termination or throughout the continuation of an anomalous pregnancy, following the birth and before any future pregnancy is undertaken.

A mother of two normal children was diagnosed with an anencephalic pregnancy. A dating ultrasound was conducted at 10 weeks showing a normal heartbeat and appropriate growth. At an 11-week scan, some potential skull anomalies were detected. A third scan 2 weeks later confirmed anencephaly, and termination of pregnancy was undertaken immediately.

The emotional trauma experienced by this mother and her family extended far beyond the clinical condition. Shock at the concept of producing a baby with severe brain damage, fear of repetition of the anomaly in any future pregnancy or future pregnancies of her own children, finding that regular intake of standard levels of folic acid prior to and during the first trimester of pregnancy had not protected her from this outcome, learning through Internet searches that increased doses of folic acid might have provided better protection and that other current research is exploring additional preventive treatments for the avoidance of neural tube defects (adding inositol – vitamin B_8 – to folic acid prophylaxis, although with insufficient evidence to date to require this to be standard care[48]) all contributed to immense emotional stress. Compounding this were the partner's interpretation of the caregiver's words following the 11-week ultrasound that 'I think your baby is okay, but we need to do further tests' led the partner to be reassured while she was not. Waiting for 2 weeks between ultrasounds was excruciatingly painful. Confirmation of the severity of the anomaly led to acceptance of the predicted problem and relief that there was no real decision to be taken for the mother but shock for the father who had anticipated that all was probably all right. Close emotional support for this family – like any family facing this type of event – was clearly important and is rarely available.

Even though the offer to talk further to caregivers in the period between the two ultrasounds might have been made, emotional distress, anxiety, tension and the belief that there was nothing they could do or say anyway until the diagnosis was finalized resulted in this family not seeking further consultation. Especially in situations of such severity and rarity, a follow-up call to this mother/family both in the intervening ultrasound period and following termination (when no contact or offer of contact was made in this case) would have facilitated this family (and others in similar situations) to avail themselves of helpful counselling or, at least, an opportunity to ask the many unanswered questions that they had.

In Labour and Birth

The clinical birth environment is stressful for many women and their families. Research has confirmed the beneficial outcomes of midwifery care that takes a more holistic, psycho-socially supportive approach.[49] In addition, explorations of the value of supportive companions in labour have shown with remarkable consistency and cross-cultural validity the power of this psycho-social intervention to modify any negative impact of the clinical birth environment.[50]

In 1991, Wendy-Lynne Wolman, a doctoral candidate working under my supervision at the University of the Witwatersrand in South Africa, completed a randomized trial showing the incredibly beneficial impact of providing companionship during labour on maternal-infant birth outcomes. This study, conducted in a hospital that traditionally did not allow partners to attend birth (Coronation Hospital), was the second trial – following Klaus and Kennell's pioneering research into support in labour – to show that social support in labour was the optimal route to follow. A Masters student under my supervision, Sylvia Csosz, in the following year, also successfully completed a similar randomized, controlled study at

Baragwanath Hospital in Soweto, South Africa, yielding similar findings but taking this one step further. This study showed that it was not simply a Hawthorne effect that was in operation (of knowing that one is in a research study and benefitting from the added attention this brings). Even women who did not know they were in the study until after all their birth data had been collected and who were then debriefed and retrospectively requested to grant permission for the data collected about them to be included in the analyses showed similar optimal outcomes. A number of additional studies all endorsing the same findings followed globally, changing the birth environment for families forever.

Maintaining a quiet, gentle, supportive, encouraging environment for birth is a given requirement in contrast to the common depiction of birth on TV and in film as a frantic, hurried and traumatic, albeit momentous, event. Caesarean sections can also be performed with more psychological sensitivity. Encouraging skin-to-skin care from the moment of delivery, not separating mother and baby, breastfeeding when the baby shows signs of readiness for a feed, in as quiet an environment as is possible in a surgical suite, can make the experience of caesarean section that much more psychologically satisfying for both mother and father/partner and can facilitate parent–infant attachment and breastfeeding. We included this approach in the WHO-Euro training programmes that were offered in the 1990s and 2000s in the former Soviet Union: it is now being termed 'gentle caesareans' in Western countries.[51]

The findings of meta-analyses of randomized, controlled trials on effective care in pregnancy and childbirth have questioned the routine use of many clinical interventions[52] and are welcome. Even when essential, however, the psychological implications of their use still require attention. The meanings of, for example, caesarean sections, forceps or vacuum extractions, inductions, augmentations of labour and a supine lithotomy position for the psychological experience of giving birth have still to be fully understood.

Encouraging siblings of the new baby to share the birth experience remains a controversial issue. Fears of infectious diseases such as the severe acute respiratory syndrome (SARS), which shocked the world in the last decade, have led to the exclusion of multiple family members from hospital births. During home births, siblings need careful preparation for birth if they are to attend, although in many settings designating a family member or caregiver to look after siblings during the long hours of labour and even for birth may be the optimal approach to follow until the new baby arrives.

Immediate Postpartum Care

Providing care for mother, father and baby together, in the immediate post-birth period is a central need in family-centred care. This applies to care of the family with a normal, term baby and to families whose newborn requires admission to a NICU. Applying the concept of rooming-in to include the father on a routine basis is needed.

Studies of the value of skin-to-skin contact for normal, term infants have revealed the considerable benefits of this approach.[53] Babies interact more with their mothers and cry less if held skin-to-skin. Mothers are also more likely to breastfeed in the first 1 to 4 months and tend to breastfeed for longer if they have early skin-to-skin contact with their babies.[54] Findings revealing the benefits of skin-to-skin care for newborns admitted to NICUs have revolutionized this bastion of high-tech care.[55] The growing rebirth of breastfeeding, driven by the WHO/UNICEF Baby Friendly Hospital Initiative (BFHI),[56] is restructuring maternity hospitals worldwide as well as reminding us that technology has not always been in the best interests of either mothers or their babies.

Postpartum Care of the Family

The primary focus of much care in the perinatal period is on the pregnancy, birth and the first few days after giving birth. Far less attention is given to the adjustment to parenthood, either physically, emotionally or mentally. Physically, the mother has experienced enormous demands on her body during both pregnancy and birth, whether by vaginal or caesarean delivery. She is likely to feel bruised and battered with discomforts – sometimes significant – arising from episiotomies, haemorrhoids, urinary or faecal dysfunction and painful breasts, combined with considerably disturbed sleep patterns. Hormonally, her body is undergoing rapid changes that often leave her with swirling emotional reactions that are compounded by insecurity regarding mothering abilities contrasting with the excitement and pride in new parenthood. Life for both mother and father certainly turns upside down when a new baby arrives. Few of our supportive care services address these changes and their resulting needs adequately, either in terms of providing adequate cognitive or emotional preparation for them or in assisting families to cope with them in the first months after giving birth.

Family planning is also an important consideration, although sexual intercourse is likely to be far from the mother's mind (if not the father's) in the immediate postpartum period. Advice that suits each individual family's needs regarding contraception is an essential component of care after giving birth. Given the high proportion of pregnancies that are unplanned, this advice (at least after the birth of each child, although preferably before any children are born) should be provided during pregnancy and reinforced after birth. Although it is often customary to advise mothers that contraception is not a serious concern in the first few weeks after childbirth, this is true only for about 98% of women up to 6 months after delivery who are breastfeeding exclusively, with no more than four (daytime) to six (night time) hourly gaps between feeds, and whose menstruation has not resumed.[57] Whatever the method of contraception chosen, the importance of including family planning advice prior to pregnancy, during pregnancy and after birth remains a central issue in family-centred perinatal care.

The Language of Birth

The terminology and language used by professionals regarding pregnancy, labour and birth reflect our approach to these events as 'normal' or 'complicated'. They also reflect our respect for and acceptance of a family-centred approach. A special roundtable discussion of this issue in the journal *Birth* acknowledged the increasing importance of the language we use when caring for pregnant women and their families.[58] We frequently substitute technological terminology for simple experiences, and a number of papers in this issue drew attention to the 'medicalization' of terminology used with regard to pregnancy and birth, in addition to practice. For example, we describe breastfeeding as 'lactation' (ignoring that the mother and not only her lactating breasts, as well as her newborn are involved in the process of breastfeeding) and caregivers who assist with breastfeeding as 'lactation consultants'. The term 'lactation' actually applies to the production of milk by the breasts: it does not include the transport of this milk to the baby, which is what breastfeeding is all about. One does not need a degree to breastfeed: every mother and baby can do it, so why do we need to invent technical terms for those who care for this simple process? We use 'non-nutritive sucking' for the need of a baby to suckle for comfort. We use 'non-clinical touch' to describe the comfort of a kind caress to support a woman in pain. It is as though we seek status and recognition for the importance of our work through official-sounding, medicalized titles. Using 'non-nutritive' and 'non-clinical' also implies a lesser worth to such actions: nutritive or clinical action is valuable; all other actions are not.

Furthermore, current trends towards referring to normal birth as a 'physiological' process (thereby minimizing psychological, social or spiritual components) reflects a clinical/medicalized approach that lacks recognition of normal psycho-social issues.[59] Language can also maintain doctor-patient power differentials in the childbirth setting (e.g. 'I am *just* going to examine you' instead of 'Please may I examine you now?' or 'What is she?', meaning how far dilated is the woman's cervix) and is used mindlessly and meaninglessly, without respect for the woman as anything more than a 'case' ('the section in room 22').[60] Language may be used imprecisely, such as 'trial of labour' (applied to women with previous caesarean-sections when all labours are, in reality, trials of labour) and 'failure to progress' (when this might mean 'failure to wait').[61] The word 'failure' is also denigrating to mothers: after all, other women whose labour progresses smoothly are successful, while they are failures. The excessive use of acronyms, including those used to reflect differing issues (e.g. IUD may be an 'intrauterine device' or an 'intrauterine death') also plagues our language of birth[62] but bolsters a medicalized/clinically focussed role rather than a sensitive, normalized interaction between caregiver and woman/family. Even the word 'sensitive' when applied to care (as occurs throughout this book) may be perceived negatively as meaning 'touchy-feely' or 'hippie-style' thinking rather than simply being the optimal and normal approach to care that combines clinical expertise with concern for the person's cognitions, emotions and social situation.

Use of acronyms is not only the domain of the medical profession. When I first joined the WHO Regional Office for Europe in Copenhagen in 1991, I was met with a welcome e-mail sent from a Canadian colleague. The entire message was a series of acronyms that took some time to decipher. In essence, it said welcome to the world of acronyms and the MCH, MPS, IMCI and FCH* programmes! I soon learned how apt this message was in the United Nations world.

* Maternal-child health; making pregnancy safer; integrated management of childhood illness, and family and child health.

A family-centred approach needs to retain constant consideration for how the terminology we use is perceived by women; it must remain respectful of both clinical and psychological needs. For example, describing an unwanted early pregnancy loss as an 'abortion' may be hurtful because this term is frequently associated with a deliberately induced pregnancy termination, with women preferring the term 'miscarriage' to describe unwanted pregnancy loss.[63] Caregivers often use terms such as 'failed pregnancy,' 'incompetent cervix,' 'inadequate germ plasm' and 'abnormal chromosomal material' to explain pregnancy loss, but these may be interpreted by women as reflecting their personal failure, incompetence, inadequacy and abnormality.[64] These terms reinforce women's common reactions to miscarriage as shame and feelings of failure, insecurity and depression. Early pregnancy loss is often referred to as loss of 'the products of conception' by caregivers and as a 'baby' by mothers or parents. These outcomes are usually 'disposed of' by sluicing or incineration rather than by burial, further denying the 'human' aspects of this difficult experience. As Freud would argue, our language sheds light on our true feelings and thoughts and thereby our degree of 'family-centredness'.

> When I made a brief comment on this language issue to a member of the editorial board of the *British Journal of Obstetrics and Gynaecology* in 1992, I was invited to publish a commentary on the psychological meaning of the language we use when talking about pregnancy loss. Some two decades later, I proposed that we again revisit this question, applied to the language we use regarding childbirth in general as a roundtable discussion for the US-based journal *Birth*. On both occasions, the issue was warmly welcomed as sorely needed, suggesting that little had changed over the two intervening decades.
>
> Two issues emerge from this: the first is that even after 20 years this issue is still of significance to academics, and the second is that we have yet to learn not to use 'family-unfriendly' jargon when caring for families.

Challenges

In an ideal world, the objective of care should be to protect the woman from emotional stress as much as possible. Incorporating psycho-social concerns together with a medicalized approach to perinatal care is challenging for clinically trained caregivers. The closer (or more approachable) one appears to be to the client psychologically and the greater the trust that is developed, the more likely it is for her to discuss her emotional concerns. Most caregivers are not trained to deal with such intimacies and feel threatened when they occur. Caregivers may, in fact, be encouraged to dissociate themselves from their patients' emotional states (e.g. by wearing white coats with the status-conveying stethoscope dangling around the neck) so as to allow them to provide (sometimes) painful clinical care or bad news. Revised preparation of caregivers is surely needed to help them to adopt a family-centred model and to feel competent in addressing psychological as well as biological considerations.

Key Points

- Family-centred care has been assumed to apply only to normal pregnancy and birth. In this view, once complications set in, clinical care becomes a priority, often at the expense of family-centred practice. In contrast, family-centred care is even more important when complications arise.
- All women should be regarded as having normal pregnancies until proved otherwise, with caregivers remaining vigilant at all times for possible deviations from 'normal'.
- Definitions of 'normal birth' vary widely across Canada, the United Kingdom and the WHO. Most women's births do not meet the criteria outlined as 'normal birth'.
- Most current pre-conceptional programmes routinely focus on clinical aspects of care without serious consideration of their psychological consequences.
- There is wide disparity globally in both the number and types of interventions proposed for routine prenatal care.

- Routine, clinically focussed prenatal care is not sufficient: women need social, cultural and psychological support, relevant and timely information, concern for potential pathology and an individualized approach to care.
- The clinical birth environment is stressful for many women and their families. Maintaining a quiet, gentle, supportive and encouraging environment for both vaginal and caesarean births is a requirement. Encouraging skin-to-skin care from the moment of delivery; not separating mother, partner and baby; and breastfeeding when the baby shows signs of readiness for a feed can make the experience of vaginal and caesarean birth that much more psychologically satisfying for mother, partner and baby.
- Terminology and language used must be respectful of both the clinical and psychological needs of families.

Care of Families after Normal Birth

Principles:
- Families are offered knowledgeable and appropriate care to support breastfeeding and, when needed, alternate feeding methods.
- Families are encouraged, prepared and supported to be actively involved in the care of their newborn, whether a healthy term infant or a sick or preterm baby requiring intensive clinical care.

Overview

Mother– and father/partner–infant contact after birth is examined in depth, with considerable attention being paid to family-centred approaches that closely integrate the father/partner. The Baby Friendly Hospital Initiative (BFHI) and breastfeeding are discussed with analysis of how well this is being implemented globally.

Outline

Family-Centred Rooming-In
Breastfeeding
Postpartum Care

Parent–infant attachment is facilitated by events occurring at the time of birth and in the ensuing months and is important for long-term development.[1] Uninterrupted skin-to-skin mother– and/or parent–infant contact, for the first hour or more after birth, is the goal to strive for in both vaginal and caesarean births to facilitate attachment. Most routine maternity and newborn care procedures, such as cord clamping, eye prophylaxis and clothing of the infant, can and should be delayed for at least an hour or more to allow for parent–infant time together, with both mother and baby covered to ensure warmth. Thereafter, rooming-in 24/7, care by parents and demand (baby-led or cue-based) breastfeeding constitute the optimal approach. At present, this is not always practiced, even in the best of maternity care services. In Canada, for example, 86% of women having vaginal births report holding their babies within five minutes of birth, although only 29% of mothers giving birth by caesarean section do so. Only 39% of women having vaginal births and 8% of those giving birth by caesarean hold their babies skin-to-skin at this time. Whereas 71% of women report 24-hour rooming-in after vaginal birth, only 47% of mothers giving birth by caesarean section do so. Only half of all mothers (50%) report baby-led breastfeeding.[2]

Family-Centred Rooming-In

It has long been recognized that healthy mothers and babies should room-in together after birth. Essential for effective breastfeeding, this practice also promotes mother–infant attachment and develops confidence regarding infant care. After 9 months of pregnancy, and probably a much longer period planning for and dreaming about having a baby, it is somewhat incomprehensible why mothers would wish to be separated from their newborns as soon as they are born. Yet many long-standing hospital practices encourage this. Some argue that mothers are tired after labour and need rest. Also, hospitals have, for so long, been organized with nursery-based care that physical layouts do not always facilitate rooming-in. In the immediate post-birth hours, however, sleep is likely the last thing that a mother can indulge in. She is hyper-alert at this time: tiredness will set in later. Her infant, too, is primed to be hyper-alert at birth (unless drugged by medications administered to the mother in labour). Such immediate post-birth alertness is probably an instinctive survival mechanism, ensuring the development of a mother–baby connection. Although maternal tiredness does ensue, sleep will be in short supply for a new mother due not only to the after-effects of labour but also to the need to breastfeed her infant every 2 to 3 hours for many days and weeks, continuing, with longer inter-feed intervals, for many months. This is the price of motherhood.

Healthcare providers need to assist this process not by separating the mother and baby but by assisting the woman to care for and feed her baby while obtaining as much sleep as possible between feeds. Whether or not she breastfeeds herself or a feed is given to the baby by someone else, her breasts will fill with milk within a few days, causing discomfort and wakefulness and potentially making latching more difficult if her breasts become too swollen and engorged with milk. Frequent suckling before the mother's milk comes in encourages milk supply and flow and allows the mother to position and latch her baby well, before her breasts fill with milk. Frequent feeding in these first few days will help to avoid excessive engorgement with its consequent difficulties and, in the long run, will probably be much less sleep disturbing than coping with breastfeeding difficulties. In the immediate post-birth period, practices such as disturbing mothers during a feed, or even frequently between feeds, to check on blood pressure, vaginal discharge, medication distribution, caregiver check-ups and meals need to be clustered and kept to a minimum. Although we have begun to recognize the importance of protecting infants' sleep patterns in neonatal intensive care units (NICUs), we have not yet realized that interfering with maternal sleep needs following the birth of a normal term baby by frequent interruptions is equally deleterious.

We have also not yet accepted that in nuclear families, involving the father or partner with the newborn and mother is probably just as important as including him or her at the birth. Encouraging a companion in labour and at birth is strongly endorsed by randomized, controlled trials,[3] although encouraging family support for women (and their babies) in the post-birth period is as important, if not more so. Isolating mothers from their partners or families in hospitals after birth is a product of the 'medicalization' of birth developed in the past century and is not a physiological need. On the contrary, it is counterproductive. If ever a mother needs assistance from others it is in the hours and days (and weeks!) after giving birth. Expecting nurses or midwives in the hospital setting to provide this is unrealistic and inappropriate: rather, family members and, in most cases, the partner are the optimal companions. Although nursing care is needed to care for the physical after-effects of birth, practical support with caring for the newborn is also needed. So too is time to share the joys and wonder of new parenthood together as a family. Providing rooming-in for families is clearly the next step to take in providing family-centred care. Although many hospitals do 'allow' partners to stay overnight with the new mother – usually if she is in a single room – little is done to accommodate them other than to provide an often extremely uncomfortable, extendable chair or perhaps a rollaway cot. This is, of course, far better than excluding partners altogether, and hospitals that do provide this option should be warmly praised and encouraged to continue working towards offering even greater comfort for partners. Meals are not usually available for partners, requiring alternate arrangements to be made. This provision could also be readily introduced into most maternity centres. Without these basic amenities, this is a far cry from a family-centred approach.

Providing postpartum family support is desperately needed for all mothers but is even more important for women who have given birth by caesarean section. Caesarean birth results in far less mother–infant contact, less skin-to-skin contact and less breastfeeding in the first 2 hours after birth, together with more pacifier use, more distribution of free formula samples and more schedule feeding than for mothers delivering vaginally, with subsequent poorer breastfeeding outcomes.[4] Some of the activities that support breastfeeding or that improve the postpartum experience of these mothers (and others with vaginal births and painful perineums!) could potentially be provided by partners or other family members.

We need innovative thinking to maximize the potential to improve the transition to parenthood experience of all new families, whether birth is by vaginal delivery or caesarean section. As a minimum, chosen support people for the mother should be encouraged to stay with her, to pick up the baby, change the diaper and carry the baby to the mother for feeding, in addition to helping her to move around. They can also offer emotional support and much-needed advice at this time and serve as maternal advocates. We cannot expect nursing staff to do all these tasks for all mothers: they are traditionally provided by family members but could also be provided by special postpartum supporters or 'doulas'. Yet healthcare facilities do not support this assistance from others, often limiting visiting hours or times as well as the number of visitors allowed. Developing systems that allow for extensive family – or postpartum doula – support in the hours and days following birth, while still in the hospital environment, can go a long way towards making this a truly family-centred experience. Facilities that are already changing in this direction are to be praised and encouraged to develop this approach to care as far as possible.

> Traditionally, the birthing woman's mother (or even mother-in-law) may offer extensive assistance to a new mother if she lives within a reasonable distance from the new family. For many, this is invaluable: for some, this is an uncomfortable experience depending on the relationships between mother (or mother-in-law) and daughter and, of course, with the son or son-in-law. While the practical help that this can offer the new family is wonderful, the differing experiences of the new grandmother regarding her own birthing and infant feeding and care practices can add additional tensions to this period of major change and adjustment. Ideally, grandmothers could be included in prenatal preparation classes to learn about newer approaches to infant and new-mother care prior to the birth of a new baby in the family. One of my valued colleagues, Shula Werner, always taught that grandmothers have to learn a new role: they cannot continue to play the mother role to which they are accustomed.

Breastfeeding

With the introduction of the World Health Organization (WHO) and the United Nations Children's Fund's (UNICEF) Baby Friendly Hospital Initiative (BFHI) and its associated Code of Marketing of Breastmilk Substitutes, an increasing awareness of the benefits of breastmilk for babies has been generated globally.[5] Initially emphasized in less developed parts of the world, where infant mortality is a common outcome of failure to breastfeed, the movement is infiltrating the technologically sophisticated world as well.[6] The WHO/UNICEF BFHI, supported by research evidence,[7] promotes exclusive breastfeeding (with no other liquids or solid food) for the first 6 months of life and continued breastfeeding, together with complementary foods, for 2 years or longer.[8] WHO and UNICEF together launched the BFHI in 1991 to promote, protect and support breastfeeding worldwide.

> In 1992, I was fortunate enough to be included in the launch of the BFHI in Eastern Europe that was held in St. Petersburg, Russian Federation, by the WHO and UNICEF. This launch, to which representatives of multiple countries of the former Soviet Union were invited, provided the starting point for a multi-year programme of training on the 18-hour course, on the two-week course, on the Code of Marketing of Breastmilk Substitutes and on accreditation assessments for Baby Friendly Hospitals throughout the region. This involved both training of international consultants (like myself, eventually becoming a Master Trainer) and consequent training of local trainers on programmes, in addition to training of staff at local maternity hospitals. These programmes were welcomed with open arms as breastfeeding was a valued process in the region. Some local practices – such as strict nursery-based baby care, schedule feeding and routine supplementation with glucose water or local herbal teas such as fennel tea – were routine practices and virtually sabotaged any attempt to breastfeed successfully.

The BFHI, developed in response to repeated resolutions of the United Nations World Health Assembly, endorsing the importance of breastfeeding, and approved by member states, is designed to create a favourable environment for breastfeeding in maternity hospitals and their associated institutions. The principles underlying the BFHI are summarized in the *Ten Steps to Successful Breastfeeding*, which outline the essential components for breastfeeding supportive practices in any healthcare facility caring for pregnant, birthing or new mothers.

> **The WHO/UNICEF BFHI 'Ten Steps'**
>
> Every facility providing maternity services and care for newborn infants should[9]
>
> 1. Have a written breastfeeding policy that is routinely communicated to all healthcare staff.
> 2. Train all healthcare staff in skills necessary to implement this policy.
> 3. Inform all pregnant women about the benefits and management of breastfeeding.
> 4. Help mothers initiate breastfeeding within half an hour of birth.
> 5. Show mothers how to breastfeed and how to maintain lactation even if they should be separated from their infants.

6. Give newborn infants no food or drink other than breastmilk, unless *medically* indicated.
7. Practice rooming-in-allow mothers and infants to remain together – for 24 hours a day.
8. Encourage breastfeeding on demand.
9. Give no artificial teats or pacifiers (also called dummies or soothers) to breastfeeding infants.
10. Foster the establishment of breastfeeding support groups and refer mothers to them on discharge from the hospital or clinic.

Although it is not included as one of the Ten Steps, a prerequisite for accreditation as a Baby Friendly Hospital (BFH) is adherence to the International Code of Marketing of Breastmilk Substitutes.[10] The United Nations has repeatedly endorsed this Code, initially adopted by the World Health Assembly as long ago as 1981. It aims to 'contribute to the provision of safe and adequate nutrition for infants, by the protection and promotion of breastfeeding, and by ensuring the proper use of breastmilk substitutes, when these are necessary, on the basis of adequate information and through appropriate marketing and distribution'. Infringements of the Code still occur globally. In North America, where the formula industry has a strong hold and is a lucrative enterprise, we disregard many contraventions of the Code. The Code and the BFHI call for hospitals to desist from accepting free or low-cost supplies of breastmilk substitutes or any other benefits that accompany the obligation to distribute such supplies to mothers within the facility or through its associated healthcare professionals. A small proportion of babies require breastmilk substitutes, but a BFH must purchase these supplies out of its own resources. In reality, in a BFH, most babies (at least 80% and usually closer to 95%) will breastfeed from birth until discharge and will never require bottles, teats or infant formula. A few will, but the associated costs of the formula needed for them will amount to only a few thousand dollars a year even in high-care facilities.[11]

The Code of Marketing of Breastmilk Substitutes
1. No advertising of breastmilk substitutes to families
2. No free samples or supplies in the health care system
3. No promotion of products through health care facilities, including no free or low-cost formula
4. No contact between marketing personnel and mothers
5. No gifts or personal samples to health workers
6. No words or pictures idealizing artificial feeding, including pictures of infants on the labels or the product
7. Information to health workers should be scientific and factual only
8. All information on artificial feeding, including labels, should explain the benefits of breastfeeding and the costs and hazards associated with artificial feeding
9. Unsuitable products should not be promoted for babies
10. All products should be of high quality and take account of the climate and storage conditions of the country where they are used

Even though substantial randomized, controlled evidence supports the BFHI,[12] very few hospitals in North America are accredited as BFHs and only some 20,000 to

30,000 worldwide. For example, at the time of this writing, only nine of Canada's approximately 350 maternity hospitals are accredited BFHs. Breastfeeding is becoming the cultural norm in Canada, with 90% of women intending to and initiating breastfeeding.[13] Significant challenges exist, however, with regard to exclusivity and duration rates. According to the Public Health Agency of Canada's Maternity Experiences Survey, only 14.4% of mothers giving birth in 2005–6 achieved the Canadian and global standard of breastfeeding exclusively at 6 months, although this figure is slowly increasing.[14] A little over half (52%) of Canadian women report exclusively breastfeeding their infants at 3 months of age. Any breastfeeding is reported by 68% of women at 3 months and 54% at 6 months. Within 1 week of birth, 21% of breastfeeding mothers add alternate liquids to their baby's diet, and by 14 days, 25% do so. Breastfeeding rates also vary widely across Canada, with rates being higher in the west than the east and among older mothers.[15]

> The Maternity Experiences Survey was a national survey of Canadian women's perceptions of their pregnancy, birth and postpartum experiences. Over 6,000 women, randomly selected from the Canadian National Census of Population, were interviewed by telephone at, on average, 7 months after giving birth. This survey was conducted by the Public Health Agency of Canada as part of its perinatal surveillance programme. Until this survey, this surveillance programme had monitored perinatal care practices by evaluating clinical records and hospital databases. As a member of this group, I asked why we were content to seek information about perinatal events from doctors' and hospitals' records only. I suggested that we should also be asking women how they viewed the care they received.
>
> As a result, I was asked to co-ordinate this survey, together with a Public Health Agency of Canada counterpart. I had no idea at the time that it would take 10 years to complete but remain appreciative that this mother-centred approach to perinatal surveillance was undertaken as a first step towards implementing even more family-centred assessments. Hopefully, this ground-breaking national survey will become standard surveillance practice.

Canada is not alone in its less than optimal breastfeeding practices. Many industrialized countries are aware of the BFHI and endorse its guidelines, although they are unable to implement them fully. While UK rates of breastfeeding initiation rose to 81% in 2010, only 55% of women were still breastfeeding at 6 weeks and just 34% at 6 months.[16] About 23% were breastfeeding exclusively at 6 weeks and only 1% at 6 months. This drop-off is not planned, with 80% of women who stopped breastfeeding in the first 6 months saying that they would have preferred to continue. Reasons for cessation are many but include a widespread lack of appropriate training for healthcare providers regarding the skills and techniques involved in effective positioning and latching of newborns to optimize breastmilk flow and to minimize nipple pain or damage.[17] We need a concerted effort to ensure that all caregivers including obstetricians and paediatricians, family doctors, nurses and midwives are trained on the basic and simple skills of breastfeeding that, judging from our less than ideal global outcomes, are lacking at present. Breastfeeding is not rocket science: almost any mother can do it. Skills in monitoring effective breastfeeding are lacking – many postpartum caregivers do not know what an effective latch looks like.

Even academic journal reviewers, who are supposedly 'experts in breastfeeding', are sometimes unable to recognize appropriate latching. When I submitted images of an effective newborn latch for publication in a prominent journal recently, they were rejected with the comment, 'Why are you trying to change breastfeeding practices?' Even 'expert reviewers' are swayed by the repeatedly published drawings of an effective latch showing the newborn baby's nose well clear of (about 1 cm away from) the mother's breast instead of – correctly – pressing in o the breast tissue.

In addition, contradictory advice is given to new mothers about breastfeeding concepts or practices. We are willing to – adamantly – advise mothers not to smoke, drink or use medications during pregnancy, but we hesitate to say that breastfeeding is best for fear of making mothers feel 'guilty'. We downplay the breastfeeding challenges faced by mothers who have caesarean sections. There is still much to do to promote, support and protect breastfeeding. It is not mothers who are failing to breastfeed their newborns but rather caregivers who are failing mothers.[18] Despite this, we often imply that mothers are somehow to blame for not attempting to breastfeed or not succeeding in breastfeeding, incurring feelings of guilt and, sometimes, anger towards the healthcare system that tends to equate breastfeeding with good mothering. While research clearly supports the importance and health benefits of breastfeeding for both mothers and babies, we must be careful to remember that good mothering comes from a multitude of actions taken to care for and provide a loving family for new babies and not only from breastfeeding.

Fortunately, in Canada and in many other countries globally, awareness of the benefits of breastfeeding for maternal and infant health and cognitive development of offspring is growing and is gaining some momentum. Rates of breastfeeding, and specifically exclusive breastfeeding for longer periods after birth, are increasing – and are welcomed. Many benefits – both maternal and infant – accrue from breastfeeding.[19] The Canadian-led Promotion of Breastfeeding Intervention Trial (PROBIT), the largest randomized trial ever conducted in the field of breastfeeding, provides strong evidence that the BFHI increases prolonged and exclusive breastfeeding, which, in turn, improves infant health in the first year of life and results in improved children's cognitive development at school-going age.[20] Other benefits, confirmed by meta-analyses, include protection against child infections, dental malocclusion and probably reductions in overweight and diabetes for children as well as protection against breast cancer and possibly ovarian cancer and type 2 diabetes in mothers.[21]

I was very much aware of the development of evidence-based perinatal medicine launched by Murray Enkin, Iain Chalmers and Mark Keirse in 1989, called – at that stage – 'effective care in pregnancy and childbirth'. I realized that a randomized trial of the effectiveness of the BFHI was needed. In Canada, I mentioned this idea to Ellen Hodnett, a colleague in my department.. She immediately introduced me to Michael Kramer, who was trying to launch such a study in Canada. Too many hospitals, however, were already implementing aspects of the BFHI to make the study feasible in this country. I offered to find a country where there was great willingness to introduce effective breastfeeding practices but where very few, if any, of the changes required by the Ten Steps had yet been introduced. Belarus, which was one of the countries I was working in at the time, proved to be the ideal venue. It did not take long before I was able to link Mike Kramer with the appropriate Belarusian counterparts to enable the Promotion of Breastfeeding Intervention Trial to be launched. I also managed to obtain seed finding from UNICEF to support the trial, which, in turn, assisted Mike in leveraging further funds. Thus began my involvement in a decade of research that contributed significantly to policies that have changed breastfeeding practices globally.

At first glance, the Ten Steps appear to be simplistic, although their implementation is difficult. Almost all of them require extensive revision of traditional maternal and infant healthcare practices that have been in place in modern hospitals for decades. Many also require substantive changes in prenatal, intra-partum and postpartum obstetric and neonatal care practices. As a package, their implementation has an impact on medical, psychological, social and economic assumptions underlying maternal and infant care. Dedication, commitment and conviction regarding the importance of breastfeeding are essential ingredients for successful implementation of this health promotional programme.[22]

The BFHI firmly established the importance and practice of breastfeeding newborns, particularly normal, term infants. Strongly supported by UN agencies such as WHO and UNICEF, this programme went far in creating awareness of optimal feeding methods and the importance of maternal–newborn contact and closeness from birth onwards. It was not, however, directly addressed towards the newborn requiring intensive care. In addition, its focus was on the importance of breastfeeding rather than on the inherent needs, and rights, of both the mother/family and the newborn to have psychologically sensitive and supportive pregnancy and birth care, evidence-based practice, as well as optimal infant feeding. I clearly voiced the BFHI's lack of attention to the NICU setting as well as its neglect of the rights of parents and newborns to both clinically and psychologically supportive obstetric and postpartum care in the *British Journal of Obstetrics and Gynaecology* in 2004.[23] The name 'Baby Friendly Hospital Initiative' has, in reality, been largely misleading. It is, in essence and as originally conceived, a 'Breastfeeding Friendly Hospital Initiative'. To be truly 'baby friendly' – or preferably 'family friendly' – hospitals need to incorporate breastfeeding support as well as 'friendly' or psycho-socially supportive evidence-based obstetric and neonatal care, which is respectful of the rights of babies as well as of their parents.

Postpartum Care

Many changes have occurred in maternity care settings in recent decades. Mother–infant contact was, in decades past, limited to regular 3-hourly feeding sessions, with nursery-based care for newborns between feeds being the norm. Fortunately, this has slowly evolved into encouraging rooming-in and mother–infant contact and care for many, but not all. Coming to grips with the concept that a new baby belongs to his or her mother and family and not to the birthing hospital – an old cliché – has yet to be fully assimilated into healthcare provider practice in many parts of the world.

We consider the care needs of the mother who has had a stillbirth or intra-uterine death and those of her partner and other family even less. Hospitalizing these families in standard postpartum wards surrounded by healthy newborns and their families is psychologically painful. Placing them in gynaecology units is probably more acceptable, although their obstetric needs must still be met. Discharging them from care as soon as possible may well leave them bereft of clinical explanation, as well as psycho-social and emotional discussion and support. Caregivers, and especially the obstetricians and paediatricians involved, need to spend as much time as needed with these families to assist them in dealing with their loss. Yet physicians are often not prepared to take on this role or to make the time to undertake it. Perinatal psychologists are clearly needed.

The first few postpartum weeks are one of the most neglected areas of family-centred care. Preparation for parenthood is rare, either in schools or during pregnancy, even though this is the one career that most people will undertake during their lives. For some mothers, their own baby may the first newborn they hold. Few first-time parents truly conceive of the enormous physical and emotional demands made by a new baby on the family. Early discharge from postpartum wards to home is a welcome recent development. Spurred on by financial issues (postpartum care in hospital is not lucrative for hospitals), it is also welcomed by many families who prefer the comfort of home compared to the sterile and impersonal hospital setting and the ability to minimize the time spent away from any other children. Early discharge has, however, also resulted in mothers having less time with professional assistance close at hand. Sufficient time was available when hospital stays lasted 5 to 10 days for healthcare providers to care for the physical health of the mother and newborn, to assist mothers to bathe and care for the baby, to establish breastfeeding, to discuss sexual behaviour and contraception/family planning, to advise families on immunization programmes, to consider safe infant sleeping practices, to warn against shaken babies, to plan maternal nutrition, to advise about symptoms of postpartum depression and to link the mother or family to appropriate peer and community support groups. With early discharge, these tasks are simply too overwhelming for nursing staff to implement adequately. In days gone by, mothers routinely underwent a six-week postpartum check-up, although this is no longer routinely required, and did not, in any event, meet any of the needs of new parents other than their clinical care. New families are simply left to their own devices, with family support (which is not always available) being their primary source of help. This may or may not be optimal.

New families experience uncertainty about their abilities and their activities. Companionship from family and friends – if not professionals – is welcomed and essential. Seeking alternate models of providing home-based support for new parents is a growing need for family-centred care. Exciting alternate models have been developed in some countries, such as maternity hotels, where families stay together for a few days in postpartum hotels adjacent to the maternity hospital, and the growing availability of postpartum doulas who provide mother–baby and home care for days or weeks after birth. Internet-based support can have mixed value: some sites are reputable, whereas others may offer misinformation. Mothers and families cannot readily judge which are more reliable. An evidence-based rating of pregnancy and birth websites (i.e. a 'family-friendly' website rating system) is sorely needed. Telemedicine networks or emergency nursing pools that mothers could draw on for daytime or night-time assistance when the going gets tough might well be valuable models to develop going forward that may complement the network of community clinics and home visiting or telephone contact services that currently exist.

In the 1990s, shortly after publishing an article in Canada outlining the principles involved in becoming a BFH and pointing out that no hospitals were accredited as such as yet, I received an angry letter admonishing me that all hospitals in Canada were baby friendly: after all, every hospital values good care for their babies. In similar vein, today, all maternity hospitals might claim to offer family-centred perinatal care as they no doubt do try to provide good care for families. Being polite to prospective or new parents and providing good clinical care are, however, simply not enough. As with the BFHI, specific practices and policies (as outlined in this book) have to be in place for a hospital to be acknowledged as either 'baby-friendly' or 'family-friendly'.

Key Points

- Uninterrupted skin-to-skin mother- and/or parent–infant contact for the first hour or more after birth is the goal to strive for in both vaginal and caesarean births.
- Mothers and babies should room-in together after birth. Ideally, fathers should also be able to room-in. Essential for effective breastfeeding, this practice promotes mother–infant (and father–infant) attachment and develops confidence regarding infant care.
- Encouraging a companion in labour and at birth is strongly endorsed by randomized, controlled trials, although encouraging family support for women (and their babies) in the post-birth period is as important, if not more so, and is lacking.
- The BFHI and the Code of Marketing of Breastmilk Substitutes are core components of family-centred care. To be truly 'baby-friendly,' however, hospitals need to incorporate breastfeeding support together with 'friendly' or psycho-socially supportive, evidence-based obstetric and neonatal care that is respectful of the rights of babies and their parents.
- We neglect postpartum care for families having normal-term babies or those experiencing pregnancy loss. Seeking alternate models of providing home-based support for new parents is a growing need for family-centred care in the first weeks and months of parenthood.

Care of Sick or Preterm Newborns and Their Families

Principles:

- Families are offered knowledgeable and appropriate care to support breastfeeding and, when needed, alternate feeding methods.
- Families are encouraged, prepared and supported to be actively involved in the care of their newborn, whether a healthy, term infant or a sick or preterm baby requiring intensive clinical care.

Overview

Whereas a family-centred approach to care of healthy mothers and newborns is more readily accepted, this need is even more important when newborns are preterm or sick. In most centres across the globe, mothers and preterm or sick newborns are separated. Highly specialized clinical care is viewed as a priority, with far less attention being paid to mothers', fathers' or newborns' psychological needs. This chapter, while not questioning the importance of specialized clinical care, does provide an alternate model that provides for a family-centred approach to neonatal intensive care unit (NICU) care.

Outline

Re-Visioning NICU Care
The Humane Neonatal Care Initiative
Mother–Baby Care in the NICU
Obstacles to this Approach
Psychological Support
Emotional Consequences of Family-Centred NICU Care
Stress
The Baby-Friendly Hospital Initiative in the NICU
Decision-Making about Care

The NICU environment is clinically essential but frequently psychologically isolationist. It is often characterized by separation of mother and baby, with minimal contact between them, and especially little skin-to-skin contact, as well as feeding with breastmilk substitutes either totally or in addition to breastmilk. In most of the industrialized world, these practices were accepted for some decades as essential means of providing optimal care for the sick or preterm newborn. As a rule, mothers do not stay with their babies in an NICU but are discharged from maternity units to home. During their stay in the maternity unit, mothers are generally encouraged to be with their babies at times during the day, but at night they are in their own rooms, apart from their babies. After discharge, mothers can spend the day with their babies in the NICU, but they usually leave the hospital for the night. In some progressive units, a few days before discharge of the infant, mothers may live in with their babies in a private room in order to learn how to care for their infants. Other family members can visit the baby in NICU care, although this practice (as with others) varies from country to country. These units have one thing in common: the infant is in constant contact with changing medical staff, is exposed to high-technology care and has limited contact with the parents. These conditions impede the mother's ability to attach emotionally to her baby, are detrimental to optimal recovery and growth and increase the risk of infection through exposure to multiple caregivers. Traditionally, the experience of having a baby in an NICU or special care baby unit (SCBU) is a traumatic one for parents and probably also for babies.

> Dr Adik Levin, an Estonian neonatologist who has challenged such care systems globally, calls this practice 'imprisoning'. He views babies held in isolation in incubators, away from their mothers or family members, as being 'in jail'.

Re-Visioning NICU Care

NICUs do not have to be organized this way.[1] It is possible for NICU care to result in both increased medical and psycho-social benefits. To achieve this, mothers (and fathers, when feasible) and babies need to be hospitalized together, remaining together 24/7. Mothers would become the predominant caregivers for the newborn (shared with professional caregivers), enabled and encouraged to offer extensive skin-to-skin contact (the latter often called 'Kangaroo Care'[2]). Infants would be breastfed or fed breastmilk with or without technological assistance as required. The care offered by both the mother and hospital staff would also need to be as de-medicalized as possible. Introducing this kind of approach does not question the current clinical care of sick or preterm babies but only the context in which it is provided.

Traditional Western models of NICUs provide stressful care regimens for sick and preterm babies. For example, during a 24-hour period, such infants are reported to be handled, on average, more than 200 times.[3] Not surprisingly, caregiving itself is associated with three-quarters of all hypoxic episodes[4] as well as increased levels of stress hormones.[5] Painful procedures are also commonplace in the NICU baby's life. Repeated heel pricks, for example, which may occur hundreds of times in a few weeks of care for the sick newborn, are currently well acknowledged to be perceived by them as painful and at times may even lead to iatrogenic anaemia.[6] We may choose not to heed their cries, but this does not mean that babies do not feel pain, discomfort or unhappiness. All the evidence points to the reality that they do.[7] I fully acknowledge the necessity of high-technology care and the life-saving procedures that are necessary for severely ill newborns, including their unpleasant and unavoidable side effects. It is the unnecessary interventions, regardless of how carefully administered or even theoretically painless they may be, that when taken together create a traumatic experience for the new family. All too often care becomes routine, and the evidence supporting continued repetitive tests and interventions becomes less reliable. The approach advocated here is specifically directed towards this aspect of care: do what is essential, and take deliberate steps to avoid what is not. In adult care, permission for every test performed must be obtained, and questions are asked regarding the necessity of any intervention. With neonatal care, and particularly in units where mothers are viewed as 'occasional guests', questions of this kind are not always asked. Even when such permission is asked of the new parents, the fear and worry that accompany having a sick baby may influence parents to give permission for more than what is strictly necessary. Coercion, even if unintended, is possible, for example, being asked to give permission for a series of tests with the caveat that 'you wouldn't want to take any risks with your baby.' The evidence suggests that it is not ethical to continue using the traditional approach. We cannot continue using painful, less effective and more costly treatments when more effective, less painful and less costly alternatives are available. Nor can we continue to deprive newborns and their mothers of contact with each other. We can no longer ignore the insensitive aspects of our current models of care.[8]

> Some decades ago, a young resident in the NICU at (the then-called) Baragwa-nath Hospital in South Africa recognized the importance of providing love and touch for the babies under his care. At the start of his rounds in the ward, he would lift a stable but tiny newborn to whom he had become attached and insert it into his lab coat pocket, where it would nestle, close to his body, for a consider-able period of time each day, before being returned to its incubator. The student's name is unknown, but he is to be credited as a forerunner of thinking about the importance of love, touch and caring for NICU babies.

Heidi Als and colleagues[9] developed a supportive approach for preterm newborn intensive care called the 'Newborn Individualised Developmental Care and Assessment Programme' (NIDCAP). Care is planned to be responsive to the infant's needs, while treatment and diagnostic procedures are timed to complement the baby's state. Detailed observations of the baby's behaviour are made so that care can be paced based on the infant's cues. It advocates individually appropriate infant positioning using comforting aids, individualized feeding support, opportunities for skin-to-skin holding and collaborative care for all procedures so that the parents can oversee the infant's comfort and well-being. The emphasis is on a quiet, soothing environment that supports the family's comfort and provides opportunities to feel close to, and affectionate with, the infant. Research findings indicate that this approach to care contributes to reduced morbidity, including lowered rates of intraventricular haemorrhage, reduced severity of chronic lung disease, less need for ventilator support and oxygen, earlier moving to oral feeds, better weight gain and signifi-cant cost savings due to earlier discharge and improved behavioural outcomes.[10]

The Humane Neonatal Care Initiative

Even more family-centred, and worthy of emulation globally, the Humane Neonatal Care Initiative (HNCI)[11] was first established in Estonia following a special request to the Soviet government by Dr. Adik Levin in 1979 to create an experimental unit, unique in that region. It involves the mother (and/or her partner) in a rooming-in neonatal intensive care service with direct parent care of the sick or preterm baby and close skin-to-skin mother- or father-baby contact with breastfeeding (or breastmilk feeding) from birth until discharge. Except for technical medical and nursing care, the mothers are taught and expected to provide *all* of the infant's care and to stay in the hospital until discharge. Nurses administer drugs and injections, supervise the infant's feeding program and assist with infant examinations. They also prepare mothers for caregiving and act as consultants. Generally, one nurse supervises 10 to 12 newborns and their mothers. The leading principles of care in this unit are 24-hour care provided by the mother with assistance from nurses and hospital staff as necessary; promotion of breastfeeding and skin-to-skin care whenever possible and from as soon as possible after birth; minimal use of technology and little contact between the baby and medical or nursing staff, who might expose the infant to pathology. This approach emphasizes the value of mother/parent care for NICU babies rather than primarily care by the neonatologist and nurses. Full-time psychologists, employed in the NICU, provide support for both parents and staff (who are not always provided with good preparation for dealing with death, loss and grief, all of which occur in NICUs[12]). The HNCI is endorsed by WHO-Euro, forms part of their perinatal teaching program and is being introduced in many other countries.

Dr Levin's initial motivation for initiating this system emerged from a nursing staff shortage that led to involving mothers in the care of their sick or preterm newborns in the NICU. Similar overloaded nursing responsibilities exist in many, if not most, hospital settings today. Continuous rooming-in (24/7) and significant primary care of the NICU baby by parents improves infant growth, facilitates earlier discharge, supports breastfeeding and creates maternal confidence and competence. In Levin's unit, mothers (and fathers) are encouraged to hold their babies skin-to-skin as much as they can and to 'bed-in' in special baby cots designed by Dr Levin that attach to the mother's bed. The encouragement of (almost) *continuous* skin-to-skin care is the norm. This practice should be carefully distinguished from the current regimens of relatively brief, *intermittent* skin-to-skin care often advocated in modern NICU settings. Care involving significant physical contact is very different from a few stretches of close contact at fairly regulated times during each day. In Levin's approach, close skin-to-skin contact with the sick or preterm baby is regarded as a normal expectation of caring for a baby. Benefits of continuous skin-to-skin care for babies in NICUs include lower mortality, optimal thermal regulation, improved mother–infant adjustment, improved immunological response, decreased risk of neonatal sepsis and need for antibiotics, reduced hospital readmissions and increased exclusive breastfeeding.[13]

Encouraging bedding-in is becoming more and more popular today for healthy term infants, although it raises concerns regarding smothering. To overcome this possibility, Dr Levin created a three-sided baby cot that could be easily attached to (and, for cleaning and linen changing, easily detached from) the mother's bed and which allowed mothers free and level access to their babies with no fear of lying over them. This novel mother–baby bed alone is a significant contribution to neonatal care for both normal and sick babies. Multiple suppliers are now providing mother–baby detachable cots around the world (called 'co-sleeper cots' or 'sidecars'), although care must be taken to ensure that these cannot allow for entrapment of the newborn between the mother's mattress and the cot. Having detachable but close-by sidecar cots may also prevent the difficulties that sometimes arise with encouraging infants that have become accustomed to bedding-in with their parents to sleep in their own beds as they get older.

In Levin's unit, mothers and fathers are taught to massage their infants daily, which gives them direction on a possible activity they can engage in with their infants regardless of any potential physiological benefits accruing from the massage itself. They are expected to keep notes of their infants' state of health with the hospital staff giving advice or assistance when needed. Two psychologists, who are permanent members of the staff, in addition to counselling families and staff, provide education classes for mothers and fathers on infant care, breastfeeding and relaxation. Almost all mothers breastfeed their babies on demand. When a preterm baby is too young to breastfeed, mothers express breastmilk and then feed it to the baby through a nasogastric tube. Nurses change the tubes daily, and the mothers administer the feed, usually while encouraging the infant to suckle at the breast simultaneously. The ultimate goal to work towards is a 50:50 split between the hospital and the mother in the care of the baby. In modern NICU settings, in contrast, care of sick infants has become super-specialized, and care of many different aspects of the infant's health is shared by a multitude of specialists. While a higher physician-responsibility load is needed with the smallest or sickest babies, the goal to strive for is to reverse this balance towards greater mother responsibility as the baby recovers and grows. Notwithstanding this changing responsibility load, a single, responsible contact person must be clearly designated to deal with all the parents' concerns and to prevent increasing unhappiness.

Mother–Baby Care in the NICU

Both Levin's and Als' approaches are innovative ways to care for sick and preterm newborns. Distinctive to Levin's approach and differing from Kangaroo Care's primary focus on skin-to-skin care and breastfeeding is the concept of predominantly mother/family-centred care in preference to nurse/physician-centred care. In Levin's system, if the infant is the most important person in the NICU, the mother and father are the next most significant. Systems of care prioritize meeting the needs of the family. It is this feature of predominantly parental care, together with its emphasis on skin-to-skin care and breastmilk feeding, which makes Levin's approach so appealing.

The practice of mother/father-care of NICU babies has multiple physiological benefits. Extensive skin-to-skin care of NICU babies leads to fewer severe infections or sepsis, less hypothermia, earlier discharge, improved breastfeeding initiation and duration and fewer severe illnesses at 6-months follow-up.[14] In Levin's unit, babies cared for in this way gain weight more rapidly, have enhanced immunological defences against infection, have infection durations reduced by three to five days, have reduced needs for antibiotics to treat infections, have three to five times fewer respiratory infections during the first year of life, have higher rates of physiological interferon and have improved neurological development and a stronger immunological barrier.[15] Levin's findings appear at first glance to sound almost magical, although readers who remain sceptical might recall the remarkable improvements that occurred in behaviour with the abolishment of institutionalization as a method of care for children some decades ago, as well as the classic, and dramatic, Harlow studies conducted on monkeys isolated from their mothers and provided with surrogate caretakers. What is remarkable is not that the babies in Levin's care unit thrive with tender, loving care but that we, in the twenty-first century, still enforce separation of babies and mothers as well as institutionalization of the neediest of our infants even in the best of our units.

Not surprisingly, benefits similar to those reported by Levin have been reported by participants in other programs that provide facilities for mothers to stay in the hospital and care for their babies in NICUs, such as in Chris Hani (formerly Baragwanath) Hospital in South Africa as well as in Ethiopia; Buenos Aires, Argentina; Santiago, Chile; and High Wycombe, United Kingdom.[16] Current research also indicates that at least with regard to abandonment of infants in hospitals in Thailand, the Philippines, Costa Rica and Russia, Levin's approach leads to fewer babies being abandoned by their mothers.[17] A large multi-centre randomized, controlled trial conducted in 25 level 3 NICU's in Canada and Australia, requiring at least eight hours of parent–infant contact a day, has examined the impact of Levin's approach to care for babies in NICUs.[18] Findings indicate that family-integrated care, or 'FiCare' – as it is called in this trial – results in greater weight gain over 21 days of enrolment in the trial and a significant decrease in stress and anxiety scores among parents compared to standard care.[19] The increasingly frequent indications for improved NICU outcomes following close mother–infant contact can no longer be ignored.

In the 1980s, an innovative neonatologist at Chris Hani (formerly Baragwanath) Hospital in South Africa, Keith Bolton, resolved to give preterm and sick babies back to their mothers and to encourage breastfeeding of these NICU-based babies by their mothers. His actions were in response to knowledge that many NICU babies were not being breastfed – as their mothers were discharged from hospital shortly after giving birth. These babies died shortly after their return home due to malnutrition and infection in the poor community that the hospital served. He created the ability to have what he called 'lodger mothers' – women who stayed in a special ward nearby their babies in the NICU and who breastfed them regularly throughout the newborn's hospital stay. Mortality and morbidity were, not surprisingly, reduced.

Although the family-centred, humane perinatal care initiative[20] approach has long been advocated, it is still to be extensively implemented globally. Mothers, fathers and siblings are now welcomed into many NICUs to observe, touch, hold and feed small and sick infants. In the FiCare trial, parents in numerous NICU care centres have, for about eight hours a day, been integrated into the care routinely offered by healthcare providers. It is time for all neonatologists to encourage the next logical step: of having mothers assume significant responsibility for all – except clinical – aspects of their baby's care, stay with their infants 24 hours a day with maximum skin-to-skin contact, provide breastmilk and breastfeeding as well as much of the direct care of the baby (under supervision) and participate in individualized baby appraisal and care programmes. Careful attention to the needs of the mother and partner/father for contact, rest, support, encouragement, counselling, attentive listening and close collaboration with their baby's caregivers will enhance parents' ability to meet the infants' needs. While first-time parents may be readily able to use such facilities, those with older children or other home or work responsibilities may find this more difficult to manage. Some countries are recognizing this need and have established or are moving towards formal provisions for both parents of a baby in an NICU to take maternity/paternity leave to at least allow for the father to stay home with older children while his partner stays with the newborn. Grandparents and other extended family, if available, can also contribute to support if needed. No doubt community support services will develop to meet this growing need in much the same way as doula care of women in labour is now extending to doula services for home care of the new mother and baby. Even if the mother of a sick or preterm newborn that requires constant NICU care cannot remain with her baby 24/7, whatever time she can stay with her baby should be unlimited and encouraged by healthcare facilities.

In addition, single-room family care, in contrast to large multi-baby NICU wards, is emerging as one potential model for the design of new NICUs. Benefits of single-room, family NICU care include reduced environmental noise, increased parent visiting, improved breastfeeding outcomes, reduced infections, shorter lengths of stay and increased staff satisfaction.[21] Further initiatives encouraging 24-hour rooming-in – of either or both parents – with a newborn requiring special care are to be strongly encouraged.

The survival of very-low-birth-weight (VLBW) ($<$1,500 g) infants has increased from 50 to over 80% since the initiation of NICU care in the early 1970s. A concomitant decrease in morbidity has not taken place.[22] For instance, the incidence of long-term pulmonary morbidity seems to have remained unchanged at 25 to 30%,[23] possibly because of the increasing number of surviving babies of extremely low birth weight ($<$1,000 g). Further-more, neurodevelopment outcome is associated with disability in 15 to 25% of all VLBW infants[24]; figures that have remained relatively unchanged over time. In addition, and as these children reach school age, more minor impairments, such as difficulties with atten-tion, behaviour, visual-motor integration, language performance and academic skills, are emerging and seem to occur in about 40% of the children.[25] It will be interesting to see whether Levin's and Als' innovative approaches to NICU care, offering more sensitive, family-centred care, lead to fewer long-term adverse outcomes as these outcomes are monitored more systematically in the future.

Obstacles to This Approach

The switch from a hospital/nursery system of care to a rooming-in approach for sick babies may well prove to be just as difficult to achieve as the change from a nursery-based system of care to a rooming-in approach for healthy term infants or the acceptance that paediatric hospitalizations should include the child and the mother/parent as well. Nevertheless, it is possible. The mother's presence and care are probably equally, if not even more so, justified in the care for sick and preterm babies. Staff may see caring for emotionally sensitive mothers as an added burden and may think that it is easier to send the mothers home and care only for the babies. Such fears have proved groundless in the Estonian unit, and although the staff felt, at first, that it was threatening to have mothers (and fathers) permanently 'observing' them, the care provided jointly by the mothers and staff has led to better outcomes. Having parental collaboration with overworked medical staff may also help to avoid accidental medical mismanagement, which is common in NICUs with particularly life-threatening consequences in this fragile patient population.[26] As much as caregivers may work to provide error-free care, and safeguards are in place to avoid mistakes, it is clear from the number of errors that do take place that existing precautions could be strengthened. Given that one-quarter of medication errors in the NICU are attributed to misidentification of the patient, having an adult present who is able to identify their child and assist caregivers to avoid such mistakes may be life-saving.[27]

Family-centred care may be difficult for families living far from hospitals and those having other home commitments. Parental leave conditions may also limit family-centred care and need amendment in legislation designed to support family-centred care of sick or preterm newborns. Parents tend to accept reassurances that it is the modern hospital equipment and care given by well-trained nurses and doctors that their babies in NICUs need most. Parents return home, perhaps unhappy about having relinquished their parental role to the hospital, but also somewhat relieved by being released from the responsibility of caring for their somewhat frightening newborn. These challenges have not proved to be a problem with regard to hospitalization of parents/mothers together with sick older children. It is time for the role of caring for her sick baby to return to the mother and her partner while at the same time providing them with the psychological support and appropriate technological aid they need to cope.

A further objection to mother-based NICU care is that caring for mothers/partners together with their babies will add expense for hospitals. The reverse has proved to be the case. Reduced costs of earlier discharge and less need for therapies quickly outweigh the minimally increased cost of lodging a parent with their baby. The NIDCAP system of care, for example, although continuing to incur the expense of highly trained NICU nurses, reduces costs by US$4,000 to US$120,000 per infant depending on severity of illness and initial birth weight.[28] It is likely that the Levin approach would reduce costs even further.

The greatest obstacle of all is overcoming the mind-set that imposes barriers to finding creative and innovative solutions to the challenges of facilitating family-centred care of sick and preterm newborns.

Psychological Support

Little is known about the psychological reactions of mothers or fathers who care for their sick and/or preterm babies, although Levin's observations on their adjustment are interesting.[29] Adjustment is different for mothers who have full-term but sick babies compared to those with preterm babies: full-term babies are easier for mothers to accept psychologically. Also, mothers of first-born babies admitted to an NICU find it easier to adapt to the NICU environment compared to those with a second or later child.

The most difficult contact time between parents and staff is in the first few days in the wards.[30] Most important is the mother's/family's first contact with the NICU. Being met by and introduced to the NICU setting by a very skilled staff member who makes good contact quickly is important. The family should be given written information about the unit and the care system as well as a notebook in which the mother can track her baby's progress and create a record for herself of her own experiences. At least the mother (if not the partner) should be present when examinations of the baby are done. This is not only for the benefit of the mother but also facilitates obtaining a record of events from her about her pregnancy and delivery. This also helps the mother to learn what issues are important to the staff and what she should observe on their behalf while caring for her baby.

Psychological support for mothers/families may be through individual counselling or in groups. Individual counselling is particularly important in the first hours and days after arrival in the unit. It is essential that mothers not be left alone at this time but be supported in their adaptation to their new situation. If this is not provided, mothers may well become aggressive and unhappy, making close contact between staff and mothers difficult. The more mothering that the mother can undertake herself, the quicker these feelings subside. In the Estonian unit, this process takes about five to six days, ranging from three to 10 days for most women. As the mother adapts to her new mothering role, she becomes less concerned about smaller irritants (such as the quality of food in the unit, room-mates, etc.) around her, starts to trust the staff and begins to feel that she is a member of the team that is caring for her baby. Support for mothers at this early stage includes midwifery care for her, breastfeeding or breastmilk expressing instruction and assistance, nursing support with handling the baby and psychological support for the father and family regarding their feelings and fears. It is most important to listen to the mother/parents and to assist them to emerge from their stressful situation and to adapt to their baby. Providing a comfortable space in the NICU for parents to meet with their own family members to share both their joys and concerns is important.

Teaching the mother/family about their stay in the NICU is crucial.[31] In particular, they need information about the importance of touch and skin-to-skin care. They need to learn how to express breastmilk and to feed this to the infant by nasogastric tube, if necessary. Initial fears regarding nasogastric feeding by mothers in the Levin unit (and in South Africa) proved groundless. Mothers do nasogastric feeding well. Mastering the tube feeding procedure is of much importance in facilitating the mother's acceptance and understanding of her baby and his or her needs. Mothers and their partners will also need education and assistance about general and health-specific baby care, breastfeeding (and particularly preterm or sick baby breastfeeding techniques) and the NICU environment and technology.

Group sessions for mothers/families assume increasing importance as days go by.[32] In these, the importance of continued contact between mothers/families and babies is explained, with the importance of 'listening to' the child's needs being the primary focus. Personal difficulties may be raised in the group and must be managed sensitively. Peer counselling also promotes breastfeeding of babies in NICUs.[33] In the immediate newborn period, babies and mothers are linked physiologically as well as psychologically through breastfeeding and skin-to-skin contact and will continue this connection until weaning. Levin calls this both a 'psychological and biological umbilical cord'.[34] Levin hypothesizes that by preserving the integrity of both physical and psychological closeness after birth, the infant's growth, nutrition and development, as well as mother–infant attachment, are enhanced, and parenting disorders such as abuse, abandonment and neglect with resulting failure to thrive – for which NICU babies are at increased risk[35] – can be prevented.

Emotional Consequences of Family-Centred Neonatal Intensive Care

Levin notes that the infant's growth may be affected by the mother's psychological adjustment.[36] Growth is slowed for as long as turmoil prevails, and once the emotional struggles subside, the infant benefits. The importance of good psychological counselling and sensitive care from the staff is obvious. Psychological care needs to be individually directed towards each mother/father. Mothers who are young, or old, having their first or a later baby, with or without previous experience of NICU care; mothers who are considering giving up their baby for adoption; and mothers who have struggled for years to give birth to a baby all require different psychological supports. There are few data available yet to support or dispute these observations. They are, however, founded on solid psychological counselling theory: they provide rich hypotheses for future investigation.

Adaptation and acceptance are facilitated through appropriate and sensitive communication with the mother (and partner) from the moment the baby's challenging situation is recognized through to explaining the baby's condition and his or her immediate and long-term care. In other settings, mothers of babies with anomalies have reported extremely disconcerting experiences regarding the way they learned about their babies' problems and the lack of honesty and consistency in the information, support and care they received for their infants.[37]

Parents' reports of the care they receive, on occasion, are sometimes scarcely credible. In my research into parents' experiences of giving birth to a baby with Down syndrome, limb defects or achondroplasia (dwarfism), parents added extensive qualitative comments to a predominantly quantitative survey.[38] Some of the negative comments were

'The doctor came to us on the waiting benches not even a waiting room; it was a passage and we had unknown people around us, and he told us, "Your child is abnormal and will not be able to walk or talk and will not go to a normal school and would need us to do things for him for the rest of his life."'

'When we asked if there was a possibility of having another achondroplastic [child], he said, "What are you worried about; you can always start a circus."'

On the more positive side, some comments included:

'The most amazing thing about having a child like this is the things he had learned to do that we never dreamed he would be capable of.'

'I had to be fairly accepting of the things I cannot change, and for me this is the only fatherhood that I know – and it's wonderful.'

Preparation of the mother/partner before arrival in the NICU is ideal.[39] Some of this preparation can take place through prenatal education programs. Although the hospitalization of a mother and baby in a NICU is usually unpredictable, general preparation for mothers would be appropriate, as many babies (ranging from 8 to 23% in differing regions of Canada, for example[40]) do require at least minimal observation in these units. Childbirth preparation programs do not usually include preparation for adverse pregnancy outcomes. While caesarean sections may be covered, pregnancy loss and NICU care do not have much presence in such courses. Hesitation about increasing women's anxiety about birth and babies may account for this neglect. It is not known whether mention of such issues would be welcomed by parents or whether most couples would prefer to only deal with these issues if or when they arise. Whether or not classes address these issues, almost all parents-to-be will experience concerns about potential adverse events at moments during the pregnancy period.

Establishing the importance of the mother and family as a member of the caregiving team right from the start is crucial. Creating a partnership is essential rather than developing a doctor (superior) to mother (inferior) relationship.

Stress

Stress is inevitable for mothers/parents with babies in the NICU.[41] In addition to having a sick or preterm baby – immensely stressful in its own right – multiple factors can aggravate this situation, including having a surgical delivery, a previous history of infertility and family concerns.

Calming the mother remains an important part of care. Sensitivity is needed not to deny the mother her feelings of worry and fear by only focussing on some positive aspects. Being immoderately optimistic is not advisable. Facilitating an acceptance of both positive and negative aspects of the situation simultaneously is important. Being truthful and cautious will be more difficult for the mother in the short term but more valuable in the end.

Major stress arises if the infant might die or remain with long-term disability.[42] If the baby's life is in danger and he or she is likely to die, staff cannot be clearly positive but must retain the mother's/families' trust in them while they remain open about potential outcomes. If the baby later dies, it then becomes easier to explain the situation to the family. Parents need to know exactly how much is being done for their baby and should be a central part of any decision-making processes. This collaborative approach between patients and staff facilitates caregiving policies for each child. Staff must be open to family interactions, must provide information regarding the child and need to maintain honesty at all times. This facilitates acceptance of outcomes. For babies who live, the growing trust between staff and family can be of assistance in encouraging the mother/family to cope with the seemingly slow growth of the newborn.

A second major stress situation arises with the baby who lives but might remain with a severely debilitating disability. Over many years of experience, the Tallinn group have learned to be most careful about recommending intensive treatment for such babies.[43] Instead, they follow a policy of providing oxygen, nutrition and warmth and minimizing pain for the infant. After that, it is up to these severely ill babies to survive if they will. When surveyed about this, most doctors and nurses in the Tallinn unit reported satisfaction with the approach. Parents play an integral role in making these decisions.

Caring for the baby who is likely to die, or live with severely debilitating disability, poses extremely difficult ethical dilemmas for parents and caregivers. It is time to reassess the moral and legal implications of caregiving decisions made in these circumstances to be sure that we are not doing more harm than good. In recent years, our attention has been focussed on saving smaller and smaller babies, and there is, perhaps only subconsciously in most instances, some sense of professional achievement or superior expertise in units that are able to save these extremely low-birth-weight babies, perhaps regardless of the long-term consequences. There is no argument with the need to provide the best possible care for these and other sick or preterm babies. There is, however, some question as to just what the most effective or appropriate care is and the potential place of 'heroic medicine' in these instances.

> I have sometimes challenged NICU caregivers around the world regarding their interest in and attempts to save all extremely low-birth-weight babies who have little or even no chance of a normal life. I have asked them also if they follow up on the progress of these babies if they do survive and are discharged from care, inquiring as to what health and developmental care services are available for both the babies and their parents. I have sometimes been told, in response, 'That's not our problem. Our job is to save them if we can.'

Possible reactions of mothers/parents include denial of the severity of the illness, mistrust of the doctor and/or hospital with subsequent seeking of alternate opinions, aggression expressed towards staff and transfer of aggression towards others, such as other people on the ward. The staff must exercise tolerance, acceptance and patience when helping the mothers to deal with these emotions. Such demands are difficult to meet and occasionally result in both staff and patient dissatisfaction. The psychologist plays a significant role in assisting both the family and the caregivers with these experiences. Resolving such difficulties as a team is part of the healing process for mothers and, in addition to supportive counselling, can include such actions as facilitating holding the baby, providing a remembrance pack and supporting rituals surrounding death and dying that are culturally and spiritually acceptable to the family.[44]

In Estonia, two psychologists care for staff and families in the NICU. One is Estonian, and the other is Russian speaking. Cultural differences and difficulties between these large population groups in this country require special consideration of the cultural identity of the supportive caregivers whom mothers/families will trust. Such differences in culture, language and/or religious practices occur in many countries, and it is important to provide caregivers who are suited to working within such social or cultural divides.

The BFHI in the NICU

Normal, term babies and mothers have been separated for years, without any good evidence to support this. Yet, even in the light of better knowledge, which strongly supports mother-infant care and exclusive breastfeeding, we sometimes continue this practice. Why should it be unacceptable to separate normal newborns whose mothers can arrange for private rooms but acceptable to separate women from their babies in general wards? It is equally unacceptable to separate sick or preterm newborns from their mothers as it is to separate babies who are well. Does not every baby, and particularly the sick or preterm baby, have a right to maternal care and breastmilk? How can we defend the standard NICU approach that separates mothers and babies any longer? Although it is gratifying to see major advances taking place in respecting the right to maternal care and breastmilk for the care of the normal, term infant, it is strongly and urgently suggested that this right be extended to sick and preterm babies who probably need these as much or even more. The WHO/UNICEF Baby Friendly Hospital Initiative (BFHI) gave mothers back their healthy, term babies by insisting on 24-hour-a-day rooming-in. The same is required for the care of sick and preterm babies.

My collaboration with Adik Levin on promoting the rights of the sick or preterm newborn extends over 20 years and began with a translational error. When local Russian Ministry of Health officials invited caregivers to attend the launch of the WHO/UNICEF Baby Friendly Hospital Initiative in St Petersburg, Russia, in 1992, they invited many neonatologists from sick children's hospitals. Adik Levin was one of those. Exposed to hours of lectures on caring for healthy newborns at the time of delivery, he expostulated loudly about what he was supposed to do about this when his healthcare services had nothing to do with birth. In the Russian Federation, NICUs were housed in separate hospitals from maternity homes, and their caregivers had little, if any, contact with mothers giving birth. The WHO/UNICEF co-ordinators of the meeting, not understanding the structure of the former Soviet healthcare system and Adik's role in it, thought Adik was being disruptive, and it was only after I met with Adik and his team for many hours late into that night that we could follow his arguments and his concerns. He was, in fact, already following most, if not all, of the BFHI's principles, but applying them to infants in NICUs, and had been doing so for decades, although he had little, if anything, to do with normal, term babies. He became a major ally of the BFHI in the region thereafter. The irony of this meeting was soon evident: in Russian, the formal name 'Baby Friendly Hospital' translates as 'The Hospital that Smiles on the Baby' – hence the invitation to neonatologists from sick children's hospitals to the meeting – and the start of our continuing, decades-long collaboration.

Although not originally applied to the NICU setting, we are increasingly often applying the BFHI to the care of sick and preterm infants with little question now being raised about the value of breastfeeding or breastmilk for these infants. Whether one has to add fortifiers to breastmilk for very-low-birth-weight babies is still being debated. Nevertheless, few would argue, on any grounds, that breastmilk is not good for these newborns. Systems that promote breastfeeding are beneficial. Rooming-in on a 24-hour-a-day basis is a basic tenet of the BFHI and a key to successful breastfeeding of normal, term babies. Without mother–infant contact, baby-led or cue-based feeding is extremely difficult, making it almost impossible to reach the target of exclusive breastmilk feeding for newborns that is one of the Ten Steps of the BFHI. Applying this principle to NICUs is simply logical. Most of the remaining Ten Steps of the BFHI can also be applied to NICU care, although some modifications and/or additions are needed. Levin's unit, for example, has adopted 11 steps to promoting breastfeeding in the NICU.[45] His model of humanistic neonatal intensive care makes promoting breastfeeding truly possible and is vastly superior to a system of care in which mothers express breastmilk for others to give to their infants. The practice of mothers feeding their babies themselves from the earliest possible time and providing skin-to-skin contact while feeding, even before the baby can suckle from the breast, offers additional essential aspects of care that cannot be provided by nursing staff dispensing bottles. One might ask whether this is really possible? In Levin's unit,[46] between 80 and 85% of all newborns are not only fed with breastmilk but they also are breastfed by their mothers.

Levin's proposals are compelling, although determining precisely how and why the approach appears to be beneficial will require further work. Newborn babies respond to various sensory stimuli from their mothers. For instance, they orientate to their mother's voices soon after birth, they select the breast that has not been washed compared to the one that has been washed for the first suckling and they appear to recognize the mother with other sensory systems.[47] When mothers are together with their babies, a cascade of interactions takes place which result in what has been called 'bonding' or 'attachment'.[48] Suckling releases at least 19 different gastrointestinal hormones such as oxytocin in both the mother and the infant that may contribute to their further close contact.[49] Breastfeeding facilitates this release, has a central role to play in the bonding process and may be even more important when the newborn is sick or preterm than it is in the normal newborn. If multiple caregivers are responsible for the infant's feeding, these beneficial processes are disrupted. Mother–infant attachment is a complex process made even more difficult by the birth of a sick or preterm infant. Providing behavioural changes that facilitate the process rather than hinder it is now called for.

There is now widespread and increasing interest in applying the principles of family-centred care and breastfeeding to the NICU setting,[50] following the impetus of Klaus and Kennell's ground-breaking work on the importance of early mother–infant contact,[51] Levin's Humane Neonatal Care Initiative, the promotion of 'Kangaroo Care' and the NIDCAP system. For example, recent developments such as the UNICEF-UK guidelines for neonatal units[52] and the BFHI in neonatal units[53] are most welcome. Such newly emerging guidelines, however, while endorsing the value of care by parents, are often tentative in their promotion of this concept due to our long-standing traditional attitude of the 'family as visitor in the NICU' that insidiously continues to dominate our thinking.

Decision-Making about Care

Making decisions regarding who will live and who will die is not easy but is a reality, at times, in the NICU. This decision is made every time one baby receives scarce resources and another does not. Even if resources are plentiful, should ill babies get heroic medical care to save their lives even when the prospect of survival, and particularly survival with any type of quality of life, is dismal? Who makes this decision and how? Must one save all lives at all costs? Is it appropriate to adopt this attitude solely to avoid litigation rather than for the benefit of the infant? Is it justified to charge a caregiver with murder when a severely abnormal baby with multiple neurological disorders and a clearly limited life span dies while being held, as has happened?[54] Who will love or comfort dying babies if they risk legal charges for doing so? Should the caregiver somehow set priorities over which babies will receive care and which not? Are some babies more 'special' than others? Such decisions occur in NICU settings. We cannot avoid them. Instead, we should openly confront them and develop ways of coping with them that are evidence-based and, at the same time, psychologically acceptable for each family and each child in question, as well as for their caregivers. All involved personnel and families may not always agree. While legal counsel remains the final step in the arbitration of differences between caregivers' and families' preferences for care, intermediate steps are taken to attempt to resolve such differences. These include seeking second opinions, involving ethics professionals and requesting transfer to an alternate caregiver, although each of these options may be difficult for parents to access in reality.

Key Points

- The experience of having a baby in an NICU or special care baby unit (SCBU) is a traumatic one for parents and probably also for babies. NICUs do not have to be organized this way.
- The Humane Neonatal Care Initiative (HNCI) includes the mother, her baby and her partner in a rooming-in neonatal intensive care service with direct parent care of the sick or preterm newborn and close skin-to-skin mother– and/or father–baby contact with breastfeeding (or breastmilk feeding) from birth until discharge. Except for technical medical and nursing care, mothers are taught and expected to provide all of the infant's care and to stay in the hospital until discharge.
- Distinctive to Levin's HNCI approach and differing from Kangaroo Care's primary focus on skin-to-skin care and breastfeeding is the concept of constant mother/family-centred care rather than nurse/physician-centred care.
- Most of the Ten Steps of the BFHI can apply to NICU care, although this may require some modification and/or additions.
- Caring for families whose babies are sick or preterm is psychologically challenging. As with all parents, information about their baby, the aetiology of its clinical needs, its treatment or prognosis and the parent's and caregivers' roles in the care of the infant should be handled with sensitivity to privacy needs and should remain strictly confidential.

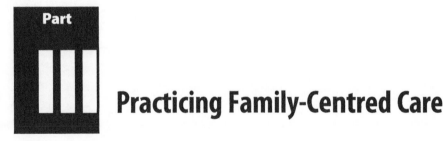

Part III

Practicing Family-Centred Care

Chapter 6

Clinical Care: Evidence-Based Family-Centred Care

Principles:
• Care is based on the best available evidence-based information.
• Interventions are used only when essential.
• Families are cared for with respect and with concern for their dignity.
• Information about mothers, partners and their infants is strictly confidential.

Overview

There has been evidence available since the late 1980s that many technologies used in perinatal care confer no clinical benefit and that some of them may indeed be harmful. Two resources have reached similar conclusions regarding the effectiveness of perinatal technology: World Health Organization (WHO) debate, deliberation and published recommendations,[1] as well as meta-analyses of randomized, controlled trials resulting in evidence-based guidelines.[2] Although over two decades have passed since this knowledge has been available, and although evidence-based perinatal care has become readily accepted in principle, inappropriate technology is still used in practice. These developments, and current clinical practice in a number of countries, are reviewed here.

Outline

WHO Activities
The Impact of the WHO Recommendations for Birth
Implementing the WHO Principles
Adoption of Evidence-Based Principles

WHO Activities

Concern over the increasing use of technology in perinatal care led WHO-Euro to undertake a survey of birth practices in the European region. In 1985, the WHO published the book *Having a Baby in Europe*,[3] as well as an article in *The Lancet* entitled 'Appropriate Technology for Birth'.[4] These publications were controversial as they challenged the existing emphasis on technological management of birth. They aroused debate throughout the European region and stimulated 43 'birth' conferences in 23 member states of the region as well as in Canada, the United States, Australia and China. Three inter-regional conferences (European and American) covering appropriate technology for care during pregnancy, birth and after birth were also held. Despite the underlying extensive research, debate and discussion, readers remained sceptical about the WHO recommendations for reduced intervention in childbirth. Questions were raised regarding their scientific basis, implying that these were simply the conclusions of left-wing, radical, or extremist 'natural birth' advocates.

It soon became possible to address the question of whether the WHO recommendations that emerged from discussion and debate at consensus conferences are supported by scientific 'evidence-based' research with the publication of *Effective Care in Pregnancy and Childbirth* and its accompanying *Guide* in 1989.[5] In reality, almost identical recommendations for a reduction in the use of many traditionally employed interventions in pregnancy and childbirth emerged in both the WHO recommendations for birth and the outcomes of randomized, controlled trials, leading me to conclude at that time, when comparing the two documents, that

> The WHO recommendations for appropriate technology for birth, as developed through survey research, discussion and debate, are strongly endorsed by the findings of carefully controlled, and critically evaluated, randomized, controlled trials.[6]

Since that time, numerous systematic reviews as well as national guidelines, including the respected National Institute for Health and Care Excellence (NICE) guidelines from the United Kingdom,[7] have confirmed these conclusions regarding using only appropriate and essential interventions during pregnancy and birth.

Impact of the WHO Recommendations for Birth

More than 20 years later, most countries could still benefit from an examination of their perinatal services in the light of evidence-based knowledge and the WHO recommendations for perinatal care. In 1998, this process of reassessment commenced in Europe with a Perinatal Care Workshop convened by the WHO Regional Office for Europe, which led to the development of principles that should underlie perinatal care in the future.[8]

Ten principles of perinatal care were listed by WHO.[9] These are

1. Care for normal pregnancy and birth should be de-medicalized, meaning that essential care should be provided with the minimum set of interventions necessary and that less rather than more technology be applied whenever possible.
2. Care should be based on the use of appropriate technology, which is defined as a complex of actions that includes methods, procedures, techniques, equipment and other tools, all applied to solve a specific problem.[10] This point is directed towards reducing the overuse of technology or the application of sophisticated or complex technology when simpler procedures may suffice or indeed be superior.
3. Care should be evidence-based, meaning supported by the best available research and by randomized, controlled trials where possible and appropriate.
4. Care should be regionalized and based on an efficient system of referral from primary care centres to tertiary levels of care.
5. Care should be multi-disciplinary, involving contributions from such professionals as midwives, obstetricians, neonatologists, nurses, childbirth and parenthood educators and social scientists.
6. Care should be holistic and should be concerned with intellectual, emotional, social and cultural needs of women, their babies and their families and not only with their biological care.
7. Care should be family-centred and should be directed towards meeting the needs of not only the woman and her newborn but also her partner and significant family or friends.

8. Care should be culturally appropriate and should consider and allow for cultural variations in meeting these expectations.
9. Care should involve women in decision-making.
10. Care should respect the privacy, dignity and confidentiality of women.

> I was integrally involved in the development of the WHO's 10 principles of perinatal care. At the time, I was serving a short-term contract at WHO-Euro and was asked to assist with the planning and implementing of two perinatal care workshops. At the first workshop, held in Venice in 1998, nine of the 10 principles were developed and formally approved. At the conclusion of this first workshop but after formal endorsement of the nine principles by the attending group, I suggested that the tenth principle be added. It was, but it was only formally endorsed by the group attending the second workshop, held in Bologna in 2000.

These principles strongly endorse the protection, promotion and support of effective family-centred perinatal care and were incorporated into the technical materials as well as the monitoring and evaluation tools of the European regional office of the WHO. The WHO developments reflect a growing acknowledgement of the need for a family-centred approach incorporating psycho-social and culturally sensitive perinatal care. Principles 5 to 10 clearly emphasize these aspects of pregnancy and birthing care, although evidence-based care remains a cornerstone of all 10.

Implementing the WHO Principles

To disseminate their ideas, two perinatal care courses were developed by the Child Health and Development Unit of the WHO Regional Office for Europe. One course is devoted primarily to obstetric care[11] and the second to neonatal care and breastfeeding.[12]

> At the first Perinatal Task Force Workshop, held in Venice, it was proposed that a training programme be developed by WHO's Regional Office for Europe to implement the nine principles of perinatal care that had been endorsed at that time. I was asked by the Regional Office for Europe to develop the obstetric component of this programme and to integrate evidence-based obstetrics with psycho-socially sensitive care into the course. I did so, and this course was then offered, from 1998 onwards throughout the European region. I remained a course trainer or team leader of this programme for many years and in many countries while also contributing to the neonatal care programme.

A unique feature of these courses is the adoption of a unitary approach to maternity and newborn care regardless of the professional background of the caregiver. Courses are not designed specifically for midwives, obstetricians, or family practitioners but for all caregivers involved in the care of women during pregnancy and birth. The Canada/WHO/St Petersburg Maternal-Child Health Program provided the model for this development.[13]

In 1996 and 1997, I ran a series of 10 one-week-long, training programmes in St Petersburg, Russian Federation, in partnership with the WHO's Regional Office for Europe and the Health Department of St Petersburg, funded by the Canadian International Development Agency. These were directed towards strengthening prenatal care, labour and birth care and the training of childbirth educators in all the hospitals in the city. My teaching team consisted of an obstetrician, a paediatrician/epidemiologist, a midwife, a nurse, and myself as a social scientist and breastfeeding consultant. Following an inter-professional teaching model, we also structured course participants to be multi-professional, with obstetricians, paediatricians, midwives and nurses all attending the same courses. The model proved to be so successful that I extended it into the WHO's Regional Office for Europe training programmes that followed in 1998 and onwards.

Both the WHO and the St Petersburg programmes are based on the philosophy that care should be rooted in the same principles of evidence-based practice together with a family-centred and respectful approach regardless of who the caregiver is. Courses are taught to mixed professional groups for this reason.

The WHO's courses have been offered in a number of countries of the European region. When offering these courses, as well as those provided by the Canada/WHO/St Petersburg Maternal-Child Health Program, participants initially divided themselves up by profession: obstetricians and neonatologist sat together on one side of the room and midwives and nurses on the other. By the final day of these 5-day programmes, participants mingled easily, with barriers to communication being shed through recognition of a shared approach to caregiving that was not congruent with their hitherto rigidly held, silo-based hierarchy that placed physicians at the apex and nurses at the base with mothers/parents not even considered as contributors.

An overriding philosophy of respect, support and care for the pregnant and birthing woman and her family pervades the WHO-Euro training programmes, together with endorsement for an evidence-based approach to care. In addition to effective perinatal care, WHO clearly regards psychologically sensitive, multi-disciplinary and culturally appropriate care as a priority. The WHO intends that this new approach will balance and combine with the past decades of technological development and emphasis in perinatal care to ensure not only good practice but also good care.

The WHO Regional Office for Europe's training programmes are often run by three trainers: an obstetrician, a midwife and a perinatal psychologist. When demonstrating alternative positions for women to adopt in birth, we would customarily role-play a birth situation, with the obstetrician playing the father and supporting the mother by sitting behind her and holding her in his arms while she gave birth in an upright, seated position, with her open legs bent and resting on the bed. The midwife on the team was always responsible for 'attending' the birth. The image created served to reinforce both the importance of midwifery care and the value of companionship in labour.

Adoption of Evidence-Based Practices

In 1989, the publication of *A Guide to Effective Care in Pregnancy and Childbirth* gave a major boost to the move to demedicalize perinatal care. In particular, the *Guide*'s strongly worded Appendix 4 recommended: 'Forms of care that should be abandoned in the light of available evidence.'[14] Subsequent editions have used less strident wording – 'Forms of care likely to be ineffective or harmful.' Nevertheless, its primary message was that evidence-based care required less routine use of interventions in perinatal care. Family-centred care acknowledges that optimal care during pregnancy and birth uses the minimum set of interventions regarded as necessary based on the best available evidence and that when a choice is possible, the more natural and less invasive option should be preferred.[15] Not only is the minimum use of interventions optimal but also the avoidance of the routine use of interventions: care needs to be individualized so that interventions are never routinely provided but only used on indication for each individual woman. Despite these recommendations, which should result in relatively similar levels of intervention based on actual clinical need, rates of intervention in pregnancy, birth and the postpartum period vary widely both between countries and within countries.

The globally rising caesarean section rate is indicative of the increasing use of intervention in childbirth, probably for non-clinical indications. The WHO continues to endorse its long-held statement that optimal care would allow for 5 to 15% of births by caesarean section.[16] The WHO's most recent statement reiterates that at the population level, caesarean section rates above 10% are not associated with lower maternal and newborn mortality rates, although there are insufficient data available to determine associations with alternate outcomes such as stillbirths, maternal or neonatal morbidity or psychosocial well-being.[17] In the future, the increasing use of the Robson classification of caesarean sections[18] might allow for more specific associations between rates and alternate outcomes, particularly at the hospital level. Two global reports on optimal caesarean section rates have found no reductions in maternal and neonatal mortality and morbidity when frequency of caesarean section was more than 15%.[19] One of these reports showed that an increased rate of intervention was associated with higher mortality and morbidity in mothers and neonates.[20] Many, if not most, technologically advanced societies have rates that far exceed this, such as Canada (28% in 2009–10),[21] the United States (33% in 2012)[22] and China (50% in 2010).[23] Some countries, however, have annual rates that are far too low, such as 1% of births or even less (in Ethiopia, Burkina Faso, Niger and Madagascar).[24] In a WHO survey, 54 countries reported caesarean section rates below 10%, and 69 had rates above 15%. These figures indicate that 3.2 million additional caesarean sections are needed in countries where rates are below 10% and 6.2 million unnecessary sections are performed in countries where rates are above 15%. The cost of the global 'excess' caesarean sections was estimated by the WHO to amount to approximately US$2.32 billion, whereas the cost of the global 'needed' caesarean sections was approximately US$432 million.[25]

As with caesarean section rates, there has been increasing recognition that despite evidence-based guidelines, childbirth practices and policies differ – sometimes widely – both between countries and across regions within countries. In 2010, rates of caesarean section across 31 European countries or regions ranged from 14.8 to 52.2% of all births.[26] Further data supporting this observation come from a number of national or large-scale regional surveys undertaken between 1997 and 2006 that explored women's perceptions of their maternity care in various countries.[27] These include surveys in the United States such as the Pregnancy Risk Assessment Monitoring System (PRAMS)[28] and the Listening to Mothers Surveys,[29] the Maternity Experiences Survey in Canada[30] and surveys in the United Kingdom,[31] Australia,[32] Sweden,[33] and a number of former Soviet countries, including the Russian Federation,[34] Lithuania,[35] the Republic of Moldova[36] and Azerbaijan.[37] These surveys indicate that intra-partum interventions, including caesarean section rates and epidural analgesia for vaginal births, were less frequent in the United Kingdom than in the United States and Canada but more so than in former Soviet Union countries.[38] One of the most striking differences in these surveys relates to the presence of the partner or husband in labour and/or birth. Whereas this is now almost standard practice in North America and the United Kingdom and well supported by evidence, only about half of all women reported having their partner with them in labour in Lithuania and fewer than 15% in Azerbaijan and St Petersburg, Russian Federation.

Epidemiological data have not always confirmed the value of a high-technology approach to obstetric and neonatal care, with countries adhering to this model sometimes reporting poorer maternal-child health outcomes than others who rely less on the use of technology.[39] For example, when comparing the United States and Canada, American mothers consistently reported higher levels of intervention.[40] Yet, maternal mortality in the United States in 2006 was more than twice as high (13.1/100,000) as in Canada (5.9/100,000), and infant health outcomes, such as perinatal and neonatal mortality, occur more often in the United States than in Canada.[41] Reasons underlying this discrepancy when making cross-cultural comparisons may vary widely, including differences in state-funded universal healthcare coverage versus private systems, or demographic differences. Finding the appropriate balance between effective use of technology as opposed to its routine use, given such variable contributing factors, is therefore one of the challenges facing this century – and family-centred care.

If evidence-based practices were advocated within a country (e.g. by that country's national guidelines), then one would expect rates to be similar across that country. This is not always the case. In Canada, a national survey revealed that rates of caesarean section, epidural analgesia for vaginal births, continuous electronic fetal monitoring, supine position for delivery, episiotomies and perineal stitching, among others, differ considerably across its 13 provinces and territories.[42] Similarly, a recent examination of regional variations in caesarean section rates among women in English National Health Service trusts revealed that maternal characteristics and clinical risk factors accounted for little of the variability that occurred across the country.[43] In Delhi, India, rates of intervention fall short of evidence-based guidelines, with relative overuse of interventions in private hospitals and deficiency of patient-centred practices such as labour support in public hospitals.[44] In South Africa, under the Apartheid regime, rates of caesarean section were almost twice as high in private (fee-for-service) hospitals than in state-supported (salaried staff) hospitals.[45] These wide variations suggest that the use of interventions is not only based on evidence or on medical need. Rather, a variety of other factors, including the types of healthcare providers in different regions, hospital size, availability of resources, maternal access to care, rural or urban residence, long-established ways of providing care, local cultural variations, medico-legal concerns, availability of technology and maternal demographic variables, influence practice. How maternity care is organized or reimbursed, how and where practitioners are trained and prevailing attitudes toward pregnant women and their families may affect practice.[46]

Evidence-based practice applies to all families regardless of socio-economic status or other discriminatory variables. Of some concern are the findings that some procedures for which there are no medical indications continue to be performed, sometimes in a discriminatory pattern.[47] In Canada, for example, socially disadvantaged women are more likely to have had enemas, lie in a supine position for birth, and have their legs in stirrups – all unproven, if not potentially harmful practices.[48] Among mothers having a vaginal or attempted vaginal birth, 19.1% had their perineal or pubic hair shaved, and 15% reported that someone 'pushed on the top of their abdomen to help push the baby down'.[49] Worse still, these procedures are performed more often in younger (teenage) mothers, poorly educated women and low-income women than in those who are older, better off and better educated. Discrimination based on other variables also occurs. For example, considerable evidence is emerging that many healthcare providers hold strong negative attitudes towards obese people and that these influence their judgement, interpersonal behaviour and decision-making and, consequently, the care that they provide.[50] For example, while it is acknowledged that obese women are at higher risk for stillbirth, thromboembolic and hypertensive complications of birth and larger babies, obese women may also be stigmatized to the extent that their management in labour differs from that of thinner women and leads to unnecessarily increased non-evidence-based caesarean section rates due to their body-mass index (BMI) rather than to clinical need.[51]

Best available evidence applies not only to labour and birth but also to prenatal and postpartum care as well.[52] There is still debate regarding some aspects of prenatal care, including the optimal number of prenatal visits needed (ranging from four or six to at least 10 or more), the value of routine first-trimester ultrasound when menstrual period dates are known, routine weighing of women at each prenatal visit, as well as the recommended weight gain advised for women at various levels of BMI, and routine iron supplementation in pregnancy, among others.[53] With regard to postpartum care, the adoption of the Baby Friendly Hospital Initiative (BFHI) in many Western countries is a clear example of the sometimes slow process of implementing evidence-based knowledge into practice: The BFHI was launched by WHO and UNICEF more than 20 years ago, yet – with a few exceptions such as Norway and Sweden – only a small proportion of maternity hospitals is accredited as a 'Baby Friendly Hospital' in most Western countries.

Evidence-based medicine is one response to emerge in reaction to the technological explosion in the developed world. The publication of *Effective Care in Pregnancy and Childbirth* and its accompanying *Guide*[54] and the subsequent development of the Cochrane Database have revolutionized perinatal care. Demanding that technology be applied when, and only when, it is necessary and ensuring that the strictest scientific rigour be applied to judge such effectiveness are leading the WHO,[55] as well as individual caregivers worldwide, to question the overuse of technology. Notwithstanding the preceding remaining challenges to the introduction of evidence-based care in technologically advanced centres, significant progress has been made in some respects. In general, the rates of episiotomy have plummeted in recent decades, and midwifery is rapidly gaining more widespread respect and endorsement. Home birth is being acknowledged in some countries, like Canada, as a safe site for childbirth, with the United Kingdom's NICE review concluding that healthy women with straightforward pregnancies are safer giving birth at home or in a midwife-led unit than in hospital under obstetric care.[56] Practices such as immersion in water during labour, offering non-pharmacological pain management techniques in labour and delayed cord clamping are being introduced; skin-to-skin care and breastfeeding are being increasingly supported as optimal policy and practice; single-room NICUs with rooming-in of the mother and/or partner are being created; and better facilities for fathers/partner's to stay with newly delivered mothers in hospitals are being pursued. In Canada, national guidelines for family-centred care are being revised to reflect these cutting-edge developments, whereas in the United Kingdom, the NICE guidelines are continually providing updated family-centred and evidence-based challenges to global perinatal care. It is clear, however, that much work and change are still needed.

Key Points

- Many technologies used in perinatal care confer no clinical benefit, and some may be harmful.
- The WHO recommendations for appropriate technology for birth, as developed through survey research, discussion and debate, are strongly endorsed by the findings of carefully controlled and critically evaluated randomized, controlled trials.
- Global reports of optimal caesarean section rates have found no reductions in maternal and neonatal mortality and morbidity when frequency of caesarean section was more than 15%. An increased rate of intervention is associated with higher mortality and morbidity in mothers and neonates.
- Despite evidence-based guidelines, childbirth practices and policies differ – sometimes widely – both between countries and across regions within countries.
- Countries adhering to a high-technology model of care sometimes report poorer maternal-child health outcomes than others that rely less on the use of technology.
- Evidence-based practice applies to all families regardless of socio-economic status or other discriminatory variables.

Psycho-Socially Sensitive Care

Principles:
- Care is sensitive to the psychological and social needs of women and their families, including their needs for knowledge, emotional support and spiritual considerations.
- Families are entitled to full, open and honest communication about all aspects of their care and are entitled to an apology in the event of avoidable negative outcomes.

Overview

Although the importance of psycho-social and cultural issues in obstetric care has been increasingly acknowledged in recent decades, there is still neglect and misunderstanding of what women (and men and siblings) want and need during pregnancy, birth and the postpartum period with regard to their care. There is a lack of acknowledgement that optimal biological care must incorporate psycho-social factors as these levels of functioning are integrally related. Excluding psycho-social concerns from perinatal care results in less optimal biological care.

Outline

Is Psycho-Socially Sensitive Care during Pregnancy and Birth Evidence-Based?
Supporting Women and Their Families through Obstetric and Gynaecological Procedures
Continuity of Care
Providing Respectful Care
Legal Issues in Healthcare
Listening to the Voices of Women
Stress during the Transition to Parenthood
Spiritual Needs
Principles and Values
Humanizing Care

In 2011, *The Lancet* published an editorial regarding its then recently published series on stillbirth.[1] The editorial expressed surprise at the worldwide emotional and heart-warming reaction the journal received in response to the series. What is remarkable about this is not the global response to the stillbirth papers but *The Lancet* editorial. When will the medical world realize that behind every stillbirth, miscarriage, birth of a baby with an anomaly and even difficult birth, unwanted caesarean section, failure to breastfeed successfully or similar, severe or less severe, negative outcome of childbearing lie real people with hopes, feelings, wishes, expectations and dreams. If they did, there would be no surprise at readers' emotional reactions to the stillbirth series.

A women giving birth is not just a uterus, vagina and perineum. This phrase has been reiterated – by others as well as by me – for at least the forty or more years that I have been active in promoting more sensitive care for women and their partners/ families during their transition to parenthood. Biological functioning is not the only level of functioning that characterizes a pregnant woman: her cognitions, emotions, interpersonal interactions, social setting and spiritual needs all require care. Sadly, our Western medical world neglects most additional levels of human functioning to concentrate almost exclusively on the biological when, in reality, the emphasis should also be on the psycho-social aspects rather than predominantly the biological events that contribute to this major life-changing transition. We have yet to learn from many of our neighbouring cultures that there is more to having a baby than the functioning of our biological selves.

Is Psycho-Socially Sensitive Care during Pregnancy and Birth Evidence-Based?

An examination of Tables 1 through 6 of *A Guide to Effective Care in Pregnancy and Childbirth*[2] from a psycho-social and cultural perspective is an interesting indication of the evidence available for the value of psycho-social interventions in pregnancy and birth. At least nine of the 39 interventions listed in Table 1 as beneficial forms of care address psycho-social concerns. These include assisting women to stop smoking during pregnancy; providing physical, emotional and psychological support for women in labour, as well as continuous support at this time; providing child care for disadvantaged women as well as for breastfeeding mothers; encouraging unrestricted breastfeeding and trusting women to carry their own case notes in pregnancy, among others. Approximately 34 of the 89 listed in Table 2 as likely to be beneficial forms of care refer to psycho-social issues and include prenatal classes, continuity of care, respecting women's choice of birth companion and place of birth, freedom of movement in labour and choice of labour and birth positions, non-pharmacological pain management tools, early mother–infant contact after birth, providing consistent advice to mothers, offering choice of length of stay in hospital, social and financial support, breastfeeding support, support for bereavement or misfortune and for postpartum depression and allowing women self-determination regarding aspects of their hospitalization and birth experiences. In contrast, virtually none of the interventions listed in the tables that include forms of care that are harmful or unlikely to be beneficial are psycho-social interventions. Although not a statistically sound or methodologically exact classification (and consequently not truly evidence-based!), this evaluation gives rise to much food for future psychological and obstetric thought.

Supporting Women and Their Families through Obstetric and Gynaecological Procedures

Meta-analyses of studies exploring the role of emotional support for women in labour[3] have shown the remarkable strength of this simple intervention in minimizing negative outcomes such as prolonged labour, the need for pain medication during delivery, less effective breastfeeding and postpartum depression, among others. Outcomes of these meta-analyses conclude that all women should have continuous support throughout labour and birth as this has clinically meaningful benefits for women and infants and no known harm.[4] The specific details of such issues as who is best able to offer support and what support entails, given cultural differences in these preferences, are still being debated, although the message is strikingly clear: women do better when their emotional concerns are cared for. If this intervention could be packed in tablet form, at no or little cost, every woman would be prescribed one.

Support for women, particularly by partners, is important. In addition, some have highlighted that men, in addition to their supportive spousal role, have needs of their own during labour and birth that require support during the transition to parenthood: these needs are not always considered fully.[5] Research into fathers' experiences is still needed.

Surprisingly, although for the most part the technologically developed world has agreed to admit partners or companions into the birth setting, they are routinely excluded from other aspects of care. 'Wait outside while we do this procedure, and then we'll call you in again' is not an unusual instruction for a companion. At the precise moment when the woman needs the support of a known and trusted person, this is removed. There is very little, if any, research on the value of a supportive companion during treatment procedures. Would encouraging (but not forcing) companions of the woman's choice to remain with her during procedures for which she is awake and aware reduce the fearfulness of these procedures and contribute to her acceptance and coping with them? Should companions be encouraged (and prepared) to sit at the mother's head during pelvic examinations, cervical biopsies or for dilatation and curettage procedures conducted under local anaesthetic? Would providing emotional support for women during these difficult moments reduce anticipatory fear or facilitate acceptance and recovery from the procedure? Such an approach allows laypersons to infringe on the traditionally defined 'medical territory' of the operating theatre or treatment room. However, this is precisely the same situation that prevailed some decades ago when encouraging fathers/partners to be present at vaginal birth was first broached, causing horrified reactions, yet now this is practiced in much of the developed world with beneficial outcomes. Considering encouraging partners to sit at the head of the woman's bed during a caesarean section under epidural or spinal anaesthetic is equally challenging today. 'Humanizing' the medical setting has become a clichéd term, yet it is still needed.

Continuity of Care

A significant variety of caregivers may look after a single woman even for a normal birth experience. Some studies report up to 16 different caregivers in a six-hour period.[6] Continuity of care hardly exists in this setting and may even be less possible when care extends over a longer period. Team approaches involving case conferences among caregivers are endorsed in theory but not always successfully implemented in practice. Women, in contrast, want continuity of care, and this need appears to be a significant contributory factor to women's positive evaluations of their perinatal experiences. It may also be one contributory factor to why women rate their pregnancy and birth care by midwives more positively than for any other category of healthcare provider.[7]

It is necessary to re-evaluate this component of care in obstetrics and gynaecology today. Obstetrics has recognized the importance of this earlier than gynaecology. There is, for example, significant evidence supporting the value of doulas, either in addition to or instead of partners, for labour and delivery, if not also for postpartum care.[8] Such companions provide continuity of care and offer an advocacy link between various caregivers who look after women and their families. In reality, however, women may find themselves referred from one specialist to another with remarkable discontinuity emerging through the experience. Concerned with their own areas of specialization, healthcare providers are not always aware of what the woman has been told or even what examinations have been performed before or are planned following their input. They may also not be empowered to inform women of their own findings but need to report these back to the referring caregiver, leaving the women wondering what was found for some days or even weeks following assessment. Moreover, communication between caregivers may resemble a game of broken telephone, with critical information being neglected, because its importance for one specialist is not recognized, although it may be crucial for another. For the woman, the extremely frustrating experience is one of falling through the cracks in the system.[9] To achieve continuity of care, the model offered by the doula might be a good one to explore. Providing a 'companion' for the woman to escort her through all components of her care will provide a continuous supporter as well as an advocate on her behalf. Companions can be trained hospital staff, volunteers or family members, although access to one trained healthcare provider as the primary responsible co-ordinator of care is needed.[10] Current research into this model of care is revealing positive outcomes, although some types of companions may be more effective than others.[11]

Providing Respectful Care

The lengthy delays often encountered when seeking consultations with specialists or when requiring diagnostic assessments, obtaining results or having treatments is a significant contributor to women's unease about both obstetric and gynaecological care and reflects a lack of respect for her.[12] Once a problem develops, anxiety levels are high, particularly when fear of severe illness (such as cancer), potential surgery (such as a caesarean section) or potential fetal anomaly becomes a possibility. Yet women and their partners frequently have to wait weeks or longer for simple diagnostic procedures such as an ultrasound and even longer for tests that are more sophisticated. Further delays before receiving the outcomes of these tests (such as following biopsies or screening procedures) then add to the women's anxiety and could potentially compound the clinical concern. In some systems of care women are only provided with adverse test outcomes, leaving them unnecessarily waiting anxiously for days, or even weeks, after a test. It is not surprising that feelings of frustration and helplessness arise in clients as a result, together with irritation, anger and suspicion of the healthcare services.

In some industrialized countries, such delays may be due to financial restraints, although better management of resources might well improve care despite any perceived or actual financial restrictions. If reorganization of systems of care is undertaken, the primary goal should be to re-think the processes in place from the perspective of the woman/family.

A lack of respect for the client is evidenced by providing impersonal care, continuing conversations with colleagues while administering routine procedures such as blood collection, failing to provide privacy for a client by drawing curtains, or to provide privacy for clients while they move from one treatment area to another and not preserving the dignity of clients while undergoing procedures. Respectful treatment requires avoiding such actions and is an essential and elementary component of care.[13]

> For example, in Canada, a woman who had undergone a dilatation and curettage under local anaesthesia was told that she could personally fetch her husband from the waiting room to join her in her post-operative recovery room. She learned, much to her dismay, and only after entering the room still dressed in surgical gown, hat and boots, en route from the operating room to the recovery room, that the waiting room was filled to the brim with family members of all patients receiving care that morning. Embarrassed, and still shocked by her recent clinical experience, she rapidly withdrew from the waiting room, asking her caregivers to call her husband for her. Although probably well intentioned, such advice from caregivers is insensitive to the needs for privacy, dignity and confidentiality of patients.

We frequently use the term 'consumers' to describe healthcare clients. If commercial stores treat shoppers with similar delays in service and impersonal attention, customers will simply shop elsewhere. Within the healthcare service, with its more threatening and intimate experiences for clients and its lack of real alternatives from which to choose in most instances, there is reluctance to apply a similar model. The fact that clients stay on, however, does not mean that all is well in the state of healthcare. That dissatisfaction exists is evident in the increasing reality of litigation and the low ratings of satisfaction with care that are common.[14]

Vast differences in respect for women in childbearing do occur across countries. For example, the following story would be shocking to most caregivers in industrialized countries, but this type of action is not all that uncommon in countries with less sensitivity to psycho-social concerns.

> As an international health consultant visiting a hospital in Eastern Europe, I recall being taken to meet a mother in the recovery room shortly after she had given birth. I had recently asked my host – the obstetrician in charge – whether the hospital routinely shaved women's pubic hair before vaginal birth. We entered her room, and without any introduction or, in fact, even speaking to her, my host simply pulled her covering sheet off showing me that she was shaved. I apologized profusely and left the room as quickly as I could. Respectful care was clearly not yet in evidence.

Legal Issues in Healthcare

Litigation and fear of litigation strongly influence healthcare, particularly in the United States.[15] The benefits that might be gained from discussing healthcare with women and in understanding areas of neglect outweigh the risk of receiving negative feedback. Fear that this might encourage litigation proceedings when care has been unsatisfactory is possibly unfounded: seeking discussion of difficult experiences might do more to prevent litigation than to precipitate it. Litigation may be more likely to occur when there has been minimal or inadequate communication between doctor and client than when the communication channels have remained open and supportive despite unwanted outcomes of care occurring.[16] The development of 'apology law', which is not a legal admission of fault but is a means of apologizing to patients for errors and non-optimal care, provides a means of clarifying 'what went wrong' for patients and offering – hopefully – heartfelt concern.[17] By requiring caregivers to be fully transparent and to disclose safety breaches and caregiver errors, this law holds the promise of a means of meeting patients' overwhelming needs for explanations of adverse outcomes and psychological 'validation' of their experiences.

Perceptions of professional incompetence may well contribute to the likelihood of taking legal action. In the Canadian Maternity Experiences Survey, three-quarters of the women rated their caregiver's competence most positively, whereas as many as 25% rated this as less than ideal.[18] More than half (52%) of Canadian women with previous experience of female genital mutilation rated the doctor who assisted their delivery as not competent to do so.[19] Such ratings of perceived caregiver in/competence by women following birth suggest that clarifying potential misunderstandings about their care might be valued.

It is, however, unacceptable that questions of law should determine appropriate medical practice as, for example, may currently be the case regarding the excessively high caesarean section rate (to cover oneself in case of negative outcomes) in some countries. Whether a legal system based on trial by jury as opposed to trial by judge is more, or less, persuaded by clinical or pharmaceutical argument is also unknown. Resolution of the conflicting needs of legal, financial, psychological and healthcare issues is needed urgently to prevent the further direction of, and in some instances misdirection of, medical care arising from legal concerns.[20]

Listening to the Voices of Women

In perinatal care, the voices of all women and their families should be heeded.[21] Ongoing quality assurance assessments based on asking women and men about the care they wish to and/or have received should be a normal and routine part of healthcare services. The concept of feedback regarding educational programmes is well recognized, integrated and accepted in technologically sophisticated societies. No conference or educational course ends without delegates completing an evaluation form. Why is this, similarly, not integrated into healthcare services? Is it because women's (and men's) voices are still not acknowledged as an integral part of the healing process and are weighted as of far less significance than the biological basis of their illness or their clinical outcomes? Becoming partners in care, rather than simply clients, is still a challenge for the future

In many parts of the world, women's voices regarding their perinatal or general healthcare are disregarded completely.[22] Surveys of women's perceptions of their perinatal care are conducted more often in Western countries such as Australia, Canada, the United States and the United Kingdom.[23]

I completed large-scale surveys of women's and, occasionally, their partner's perceptions of their pregnancy, birth and postpartum care in many countries. In South Africa, I explored black women's perceptions of their care followed by those of women of mixed cultural origin – the so-called 'coloured' people – as well as views of Muslim and Hindu women and Caucasian mothers. I was fortunate to be able expand this research to examine women's experiences of their perinatal care in Russia (in St Petersburg, as well as in Arkhangelsk and Murmansk, compared to Norwegian mother's experiences) and in Moldova, Azerbaijan and Lithuania, providing a model for future healthcare service assessment in those countries. In Canada, this experience led to my involvement as Co-Chair of the national Maternity Experiences Survey conducted by the Public Health Agency of Canada. Such surveys exposed areas in need of strengthening in perinatal healthcare services.

Although reactions to the use of specific practices in pregnancy and birth care are the usual focus of these surveys, perhaps the most overarching outcome is women's ratings of their satisfaction with their care. Satisfaction is, however, difficult to assess and is only a partial step towards evaluating cognitive and emotional contentedness. Numerous issues contribute to satisfaction ratings, including a positive birth outcome; congruence between expectations and reality regarding pregnancy, labour and birth; the number and nature of medical interventions used; postpartum care; type of caregiver and continuity of caregiver; place of birth; social support in pregnancy, labour, birth and the postpartum period from the partner and other family members; previous birth experiences and the newborn itself, among others. Despite the difficulties of measuring satisfaction, surveys of this kind can reveal telling information: for example, that a little over half of Canadian women (54%) were 'very positive' and a further (26%) 'somewhat positive' about their overall experience of labour and birth. Satisfaction levels among the 4% of Canadian mothers who were attended in labour and birth by midwives averaged 71% with ratings of 'very positive' compared with those of obstetricians (52%) and family doctors (58%)[24] This situation is not unique to Canada: only 35% of women in the United States rated the quality of their maternity care system as 'excellent'.[25] Viewed in a different context, any business where one out of every two or three customers is not fully satisfied with their service would soon cease to exist. Notwithstanding the difficulties inherent in assessing satisfaction with birth, there is clearly room for improvement with regard to this indicator across all the surveys evaluated here.

Ideally, a very positive rating should be the goal to achieve for all women, regardless of birth outcome. Women with adverse pregnancy outcomes might give lower ratings, although, in an ideal world, well-managed and supported pregnancy distress could be rated reasonably well by women whose psychological as well as physical needs at birth are supported.[26]

In some countries – where women's rights for independence have not been seriously considered – conducting surveys may require the approval of their partners. Although such patterns of conduct may seem strange and unacceptable in the Western world, these practices are common in many societies. Researchers need to be respectful of these differences and take care when seeking women's opinions.

In Eastern Europe, caregivers never sought women's opinions of their care. Even when visiting mothers in their postpartum wards in the 1990s and 2000s (for at least 10 years after the collapse of the Soviet Union), I would ask mothers questions about their birth experiences only to have my escort, the chief of Obstetrics and Gynaecology or similar, move to stand between me and the mother and answer for her. These officials clearly thought that their thoughts on the woman's birth experiences were more important than were hers. As far as I am aware, no surveys of women's experiences of birth were undertaken under Soviet rule prior to my own.

Why would some mothers – in countries such as Canada where (predominantly hospital-based) birth outcomes are very good – choose to give birth at home with midwives in attendance? Why do some women in Canada and the United States even consider, or actually choose, to give birth at home without *any* skilled birth attendants? In 2006, 36% of 24,970 US home births were not attended by a physician or midwife according to the US Centers for Disease Control and Prevention.[27] About two-thirds of these were reported as 'planned'.[28] Although comparable Canadian figures do not exist, Vogel reported that on April 5, 2011, about fifteen thousand active discussions on unassisted childbirth appeared on a popular website.[29]

The blame for the current state of over-medicalized and under-sensitive perinatal care can be attributed to many factors.[30] We readily blame mothers for not listening to their doctors' advice when it results in their baby's death, thus justifying a medicalized approach to birth. We also blame mothers for increasing the rates of caesarean sections and other interventions when they comply with our endorsement of medicalized care by requesting caesareans, epidurals, inductions or even nursery-based infant care. We can even blame current evidence-based medicine that emphasizes a 'scientific' or technologically biased approach.

We avoid blaming ourselves – the caregivers – for what might actually be the underlying reasons why some mothers are so dissatisfied with their care that they even choose unassisted home births.[31] Caregivers are comfortable with a medicalized approach: we are taught that is how births should occur. We also view technology as more important than sensitive care. Good intervention is seen as good medicine. Yet, mothers in the Canadian Maternity Experiences Survey clearly showed that for vaginal births the more interventions they experienced, the lower were their ratings of satisfaction with their birth experiences.[32] Caregivers may view being emotionally supportive and empathetic as unimportant, time-consuming or not authoritative. Only two-thirds (65%) of Canadian women in the Maternity Experiences Survey gave 'very positive' ratings of their caregivers' compassion and understanding.[33] Many women who have had caesarean sections choose to have a vaginal birth (VBAC) for their next birth: some report such negative and traumatic experiences of impersonal and disrespectful care during their in-hospital birth care that they opt for a home birth after caesarean section (HBAC) for their next birth.[34]

Of great concern, and only recently receiving the attention it deserves, is the premise that women may regard over-medicalization of perinatal care as abusive, exemplified in the recent Society of Obstetricians and Gynaecologists of Canada publication entitled, *Improving Sexual and Reproductive Health: Integrating Women's Empowerment and Reproductive Rights.*[35] This document lists the right to health, free from non-consensual medical treatment, from violence and from harmful practices, as second only to the right to life.[36]

Researchers have pointed to serious shortcomings in current maternity care and to some guidelines that have encouraged caregivers to use possibly unsafe interventions and practices.[37] In addition, even when fully informed choice may be feasible, caregivers may disregard women's preferences for less intervention and adhere to these guidelines.

Caregivers should heed the messages from these authors and others[38] who value women's feedback and take greater responsibility themselves rather than blaming a multitude of other sources, including women or guidelines, for the excessive use of many obstetric practices. They need to explore an evidence-based, less interventionist, more considered, normalized and sensitive basis for how they teach and practice if they want to improve both the safety and satisfaction of women's birth experiences.

Care providers are not always, or everywhere, insensitive to women's concerns about interventions. In 1990, a Masters student (Joyce Hayward), working under my supervision in the School of Psychology, University of the Witwatersrand, examined both obstetricians' and mothers' views of the same obstetric interventions. At the time of this research, it was commonly believed in some circles that doctors were frequently insensitive to the psycho-social experiences and needs of women during birth. In contrast, this research revealed a considerable understanding by doctors of women's fears and feelings during birth, to the extent that doctors rated many of the interventions experienced by women during childbirth as more difficult to adjust to than women themselves rated them. Needless to say, the findings of this research raised considerable controversy when presented at international conferences. For example, at one of these conferences, a line-up of audience members wishing to question me began even before I had completed my presentation of our work. Each of the dozen or so participants challenged me on the issue of doctors being even more sensitive to the fears and feelings of the women for whom they cared. Fortunately, Murray Enkin (of evidence-based obstetrics fame) joined the end of the line and resoundingly opposed these speakers, endorsing my findings. I was most grateful!

That physicians were becoming increasingly responsive to psycho-social concerns surrounding childbirth issues is reflected by a review of presentations made to the first 10 'Priorities in Perinatal Care Conferences' held annually in South Africa in the 1980s. Trends over the years indicated a growing concern with psycho-social issues relating to reproductive health being raised in this respected forum. Of interest, but not surprising, was that the number of papers incorporating psycho-social components increased as the years passed. Of more significance was the finding that, unlike in earlier years, physicians presented more of these papers than social scientists, indicating a growing concern among physicians themselves for the psycho-social well-being of their patients.

Stress during the Transition to Parenthood

Psychological concerns or stresses arise during pregnancy and birth and in the days and months after birth, even when this is a normal, healthy experience, and mothers and partners could benefit from debriefing some time after the birth. The Maternity Experiences Survey examined the stress experienced by Canadian women in the year before giving birth. About one-fifth (17%) of women reported experiencing three or more stressful life events during this period. Almost 13% reported that most days were very stressful. The majority (87%) did have support available to them all or most of the time during their pregnancy which assisted in coping with such stresses.[39] For many pregnant women, birth itself looms large on the horizon, and imagining the newborn or contemplating caring for the newborn is difficult. Although prenatal preparation programmes do offer classes for women and their partners on breastfeeding and newborn care, the reality of looking after a new baby may only become apparent once the newborn arrives. On top of this is the need for women and their partners to deal with the events of birth, especially if those were difficult, traumatic or disappointing experiences.[40] For many, consequently, new parenthood is stressful. Emotional distress such as postpartum blues, affecting up to 80% of women, or depression, emerging in approximately 10 to 20% of new mothers, or, more severely and rarely, psychosis (in fewer than 1% of women) can be most difficult to manage.[41] Fathers, too, may experience pregnancy- and postpartum-related depression.[42] Most significant in this respect is the importance of coming to terms with a pregnancy loss or birth of a baby with special needs. Pre-existing psychological or psychiatric concerns including severe depression or addictions to alcohol, drugs or other substances make adjustment even more challenging. Physical, emotional or sexual abuse before, during or after pregnancy also makes the transition to parenthood more difficult. The Maternity Experiences Survey revealed that 11% of Canadian women reported physical or sexual abuse in the years before and after giving birth, with younger, less educated and lower-income women reporting abuse more often.[43]

Women – and their partners – may benefit from debriefing emotionally regarding their experiences. Caring for families facing any of these challenges is central to ensuring the emotional health of mother, father/partner and newborn. Supporting families emotionally during the pre-conception, pregnancy, birth and early postpartum months is central to promoting infant mental health as well as parental mental health. Parental stress and mental health pathologies during the perinatal period can adversely affect the parent–infant relationship, leading to later infant mental health development concerns.[44] In the absence of any specific professionals dedicated to caring for psychological concerns during pregnancy, at birth and in the postpartum period, these concerns become the responsibility of any or all professionals (and/or family members) caring for new families during their transition to parenthood, with more debilitating disturbances requiring referral to specialist caregivers.

In all cases, discussing the birth and its outcomes with a mother and encouraging – but not forcing – her and/or her partner to talk about their birth experiences can go a long way towards relieving anxiety and releasing pent-up emotions. Psychological and psycho-social forms of postpartum care are helpful in reducing the severity of these emotional experiences.[45] Accepting what happened compared to what was hoped for is a major psychological milestone that must be achieved to allow the couple to move on with their lives. Reassurance that she, personally, was not able to control her body's largely involuntary activities during birth or her baby's development, size or positioning, or the routines in place in the institution in which she gave birth, or indeed the preferences and practices of her caregivers can serve to ease the (often inappropriate) personal responsibility that women may assume (and are encouraged to undertake by many) when they are pregnant or give birth. Offering an opportunity to debrief after giving birth, with a chance to discuss what happened and how this compared with her expectations for birth, may contribute to her ability to reconcile her prior hopes with possible feelings of disappointment. She requires validation that her thoughts and feelings are normal and justified. Perinatal psychologists can play an immensely important role in providing this supportive care. Sometimes these discussions are best held shortly after birth. In other situations, and particularly with a pregnancy loss or when women are upset by their experiences, discussions may be needed on a number of occasions in the weeks or months after birth.[46] Such discussions need to occur when the woman is ready for them: for some this might be soon after the birth, while for others the need may arise some weeks or even months later. As with any aspect of clinical care, mental health concerns need to be treated in the strictest confidence.

Society can help families to move into parenthood with happiness. Encouraging women and their families to avail themselves of community-based social networks can be immensely helpful. Some prenatal classes continue to meet and share parenting experiences for years after their first meeting. Extended families can provide much of this support – if they are close by – but many families in today's highly mobile world may not have such traditional support systems in place. Even if they do, local community support networks provide extensive opportunities to learn from and share with other families facing similar experiences.[47]

Spiritual Needs

Spiritual needs require consideration with regard to both normal pregnancy and pregnancies with adverse outcomes. For some this might involve support from religious personnel in times of need, such as when a pregnancy loss occurs. For others this need may manifest as wearing or maintaining contact with some symbol of spiritual importance or the following of traditional rituals or practices. Whatever spiritual needs women have should be encouraged and supported, particularly when they may contribute to enhanced emotional adjustment.

Principles and Values

The preceding issues are not exhaustive of the psycho-social concerns of families experiencing obstetric and gynaecological care today. Nor do they necessarily reflect the current interests of researchers as published in journals such as *Birth*, the *Journal of Reproductive and Infant Psychology* or the *Journal of the International Society of Psychosomatic Obstetrics and Gynaecology*, all of which tend to focus on more specific questions regarding reproductive healthcare practices and women's or families' experiences. In contrast, this chapter highlights some of the critical issues surfacing in healthcare services of both the developed and developing world. It also highlights some of the underlying principles regarding offering psychologically sensitive but also evidence-based care that pervade our work in this field.

Long-held values underscore the importance of these issues, such as concern for the whole person and not only the body, respect for women and their families and for their perceptions and needs when undergoing medical care and a sincerely gentle and concerned approach to care, with sensitivity rather than routine politeness being the order of the day, all combined with evidence-based clinical practice. It is apparent that although we have long recognized the importance of providing respectful care and have gone far in introducing systems that encourage such approaches, we are still grappling with the effective application of this fundamental tenet in many parts of the world, both developed and developing. At the very least, the integration of this approach into educational programmes for caregivers is a first step.

The inclusion of psycho-socially sensitive concepts into the United Nations agencies for health recommendations will do much to raise awareness of these issues in medical circles. Recognition of their importance in health has emerged in the publications of UN agencies in recent years. Concerns with issues such as women's and children's reproductive healthcare rights; violence against children and in families; bullying in teenagers; child employment; trafficking of women and children; the reproductive health plight of immigrants, refugees and displaced persons; and the dilemmas of street kids are now given equal, if not even greater, weight than the traditional healthcare indicators of morbidity and mortality. The academic and professional world would do well to follow their direction.

Humanizing Care

Why are we so surprised that well-designed studies confirm what we have known for decades: that women wish to be cared for with sensitivity; respect for their dignity; concern for their cultural, religious or ethnic needs; and with gentleness as well as with evidence-based care? Have we become so engrossed in science that we have separated it from humanity? As a scientist, I am aware of the importance of randomization, reducing bias, testing hypotheses and checking beliefs. As a psychologist, I know that emotional integrity is central to well-being. As a woman, I realize that when I am afraid, I want to be with those I love and trust, who understand me and who will protect me from harm or at least look out for my interests. As Maslow said many decades ago, safety and love needs are primary, especially when they are threatened.[48] Why do we continue to ignore or neglect these messages?

Why are we so awed by the medicalization of birth that we have lost the ability to accept that psychological sensitivity during pregnancy and birth is just as important as techno-logical advances, if not more so? Why are we afraid to *not* intervene? In the modern North American hospital, most women cannot give birth spontaneously without multiple medical and/or surgical interventions. Although some are essential at times, none is routinely required.[49] It is time to seriously rethink aspects of perinatal care.

Key Points

- A women giving birth is not just a uterus, vagina and perineum.
- Behind every stillbirth, miscarriage, birth of a baby with an anomaly, a difficult birth, unwanted caesarean section, failure to breastfeed successfully or similar, severe or less severe, adverse outcome of childbearing lie real people with hopes, feelings, wishes, expectations and dreams.
- Excluding psycho-social concerns from perinatal care results in less optimal biological care.
- All women should have continuous support throughout labour and birth.
- Men's needs during labour and birth require support.
- Women want continuity of care.
- Discussion of difficult experiences might do more to prevent litigation than to precipitate it.
- All aspects of clinical and psychological care must remain strictly confidential.
- We need to heed the voices of women and their families.
- The more positively women rate their caregiver interactions, the higher are their ratings of satisfaction with their labour and birth experience.
- Women – and their partners – may benefit from debriefing regarding their pregnancy and birth experiences.
- Perinatal psychologists can play an important role in providing supportive care.
- Spiritual needs require consideration with regard to both normal pregnancy and pregnancies with adverse outcomes.
- Women and their families wish to be cared for with sensitivity; respect for their dignity; concern for their cultural, religious or ethnic needs; and with gentleness as well as with evidence-based care.

Including Families in Care

Principles:

- Families take an active role in decision-making about their care, based on evidence-based information, provided without either covert or overt coercion and with full knowledge about the potential adverse effects of any care procedure.
- Families are encouraged, prepared and supported to be actively involved in the care of their newborn, whether a healthy, term infant or a sick or preterm baby requiring intensive clinical care.

Overview

Obtaining information about their transition to parenthood and making decisions about these events are central issues for all childbearing families. The importance of preparation not just for birth (e.g. pregnancy care, labour, birth, mother–infant contact and feeding, and partners' needs, roles and support) but also for parenthood (e.g. early child development, infant nutrition, discipline, marital adjustment, motherhood, conflict resolution, employment and parenthood) cannot be underestimated. Providing information about pregnancy, birth and parenthood prior to pregnancy, during pregnancy and after birth is an integral component of family-centred care and is central if families are to be included in decision-making about their care.

Outline

Preparation for Childbirth and Parenthood

Empowering Women and Their Families to Make Decisions

Preparation for Childbirth and Parenthood

Families rely on a number of resources – both formal and informal – to assist them in learning about this experience, including healthcare providers, family and friends, the Internet, books, prenatal preparation classes and, for families having their second or later babies, their previous pregnancy experiences. Childbirth and parenthood educators are a major source of information, support and knowledge for families during pregnancy and sometimes following birth.[1] Childbirth educators focus primarily on preparing women and their partners or family members for birth, although there is an enormous need for them to extend this care into the postpartum period.[2] Preparation for parenthood is possibly even more important than preparation for birth and is a sadly neglected part of education globally. Although almost everyone enters the profession of parenting, there is no preparation for it other than the example set by one's own family. This may or may not be a satisfactory model.

In most countries, there is no specific training provided for prenatal educators and little or no standardization of the content of programs. Classes became popular at a time when childbirth moved from the home environment to the less emotionally supportive hospital setting. They also achieved prominence as families moved from an extended to a nuclear structure, depriving women of the benefit of family members' own experiences of pregnancy, birth and parenthood. Classes initially promised some relief from pain as well as some preparation for the unknown and more fearful hospital setting. Later, classes added further goals of increasing knowledge about pregnancy and birth; physical preparation for the event; techniques to assist women to cope with labour, such as relaxation, controlled breathing or even hypnosis; knowledge about baby care and breastfeeding; and psychological adjustment to parenthood. Programs were initially directed towards women and later included their partners and, sometimes, additional family members or friends. They are offered by professionals with varying qualifications as well as by those without any tertiary-level training. Some are offered by mothers without training but with experience (good or bad) of birth. They may be offered by hospitals, public health units or private educators; may be short or long; and may be accompanied by exercise programs, baby care meetings and postpartum get-togethers. Gaps in preparation programs exist, such as a paucity of preparation for unexpected outcomes, including caesarean sections and pregnancy loss, despite a considerable number of women in technologically advanced societies experiencing surgical delivery and many infants requiring a period of neonatal intensive care unit (NICU) care, if not experiencing morbidity or, more rarely, mortality. Monitoring of the outcomes and effectiveness of courses may not always confirm their value[3] and is hampered by the wide variability among them regarding content, objectives, format and trainers.[4] Evaluation of their effectiveness may also be masked by a focus on physiological outcomes of the research such as reduced length of labour or type of birth rather than psychological and social outcomes such as mothers' and fathers' increased satisfaction with the pregnancy-birth experience or their adjustment to parenthood.

> For many women in a nuclear family setting, the first baby they hold may be their own, especially if they were the youngest of their own family network. Unless they have siblings or cousins who have had babies before them – and with whom they have extensive contact – becoming a parent can be a frightening, even though exciting experience.

Given the wide variety of subjects that could, and probably should, be included in such courses, it is unlikely that educators with only one professional training background could do justice to these expectations. What is needed is a specialized expert, well trained and capable of guiding new couples and their families through their multi-faceted transition to parenthood.[5] Lamaze International, the National Childbirth Trust in the United Kingdom and the International Childbirth Education Association of the United States go some way towards meeting this need by offering extensive training for childbirth educators. These are not, typically, university-level programs. Shifting them to the level of higher education, however, might be a major step towards standardizing the level of knowledge required and providing some level of quality assurance for prospective participants. At present, there is little in the way of global, standardized content, teaching approach or evaluation of such courses or their proponents.

A graduate diploma in childbirth education was developed at the University of the Witwatersrand in South Africa in 1989 and was approved by the Medical/Health Faculty of that university but never implemented due to funding restrictions.[6] This program would have facilitated students from a variety of disciplines, including medicine, nursing, midwifery, physiotherapy, psychology, social work and others, to undertake the program. It allowed course credits to be granted, exempting students from further study in the subject of their undergraduate training but allowing them to develop expertise in subjects of importance for childbirth education to which they had not yet been exposed. The worthwhile intention was to provide a standard of excellence for childbirth educators and their course contents: still a goal worthy of pursuit.

Prenatal preparation classes for families provide an additional value beyond the specific information conveyed in them. The emotional support that can be derived from sharing their pregnancy and birth experiences with others – often friends or neighbours going through the transition to parenthood – can be both reassuring (if these confirm the couple's own doubts or concerns) and disheartening (if they provoke previously unconsidered fears). Yet, for most, the ongoing benefit of sharing both the vicissitudes of becoming a parent before birth and, for some groups, for many years after birth probably outweigh any potential negative moments.

Sources of information about pregnancy, birth and parenthood extend beyond childbirth preparation programs. These include healthcare providers, books, previous pregnancies, families and friends, the media and the Internet. To date, there is insufficient evidence available to indicate which of these sources provides the most effective preparation for women and their families. In all likelihood, there is some benefit (and likely misinformation as well) to be gained from most, if not all, of them, although the websites of most professional organizations are likely to prove more trustworthy than others, at least regarding clinical components if not psycho-social ones. Health and healthcare have become enmeshed in the web, so medical information and knowledge are moving more readily into the hands of laypeople than ever before. Medical practitioners are now expected to share their knowledge with their clients, raising issues such as shared decision-making, collaborative care, information exchange, confidentiality and informed choice by recipients of care. In our increasingly web-based world, these avenues provide exciting opportunities to explore.

There is an explosion of information available on the Internet for families embarking on parenthood. Similarly, there are hundreds of books on pregnancy, birth, babies and parenting. Many of these provide good information, and some provide misinformation. In addition, caregivers may differ in the advice they provide, and all of this may differ from what the woman's mother or other family members tell her. It is frequently difficult to decide what information is best to believe. These contradictions probably arise because of the passionate feelings that birth and babies evoke in us all – professional and non-professional. They also reflect the facts that every mother, father and baby is different and that parents differ each time they have another baby because of increased learning and experience. So too is every caregiver different. Knowledge is changing day by day as new research is undertaken and new findings emerge, some taking many years to disseminate across all caregivers. Parents are best advised about these contradictions and to choose caregivers, websites and family and friends whose opinions they respect and trust and to listen most closely to these. In addition, they need to consider that one of the basic principles of perinatal care is that of 'individualized care', meaning that what is best is what suits each mother, baby and family during each pregnancy and that there is no universal 'right' way to give birth or be a parent.

Empowering Women and Their Families to Make Decisions

Regardless of their sources of knowledge, decision–making by women and their families regarding their care during pregnancy, birth and the postpartum period – as is encouraged – needs to be based on unbiased information and evidence. Facilitating 'informed choice' has long been a basic component of family-centred care. Care choices should be offered to the woman/family in an objective manner based on the best available evidence and should be devoid of coercion or 'informed coercion'. Despite its appealing face value, this goal may be difficult to implement because information provided by a caregiver will be influenced by his or her personal approaches, practices or biases. Ideally, objective information should also be available from sources other than the woman's primary caregiver, with the primary caregiver available to respond to questions and supplement the evidence-based information. Information preferably should be offered in writing, allowing women the opportunity to consider, research and thoroughly evaluate it before making decisions about their care.

Involvement in decision-making incorporates the concept that a woman and her family have a right to refuse consent for care. In most cases, this right is respected, although at times a conflict of interest between the rights of the mother, the baby, the partner or the family arises. In family-centred care, the needs and expectations of the mother are a priority with respect to her care. Once the baby is born, the needs of the newborn become a priority with regard to the baby's care. Individualized care advocates that 'each childbearing woman and her family should be treated as if they are extraordinary.'[7] Although professional guidelines and the best available evidence can indicate what approach to care is generally best, each individual woman's and family's needs may well require that alternative practices be followed.

Conflicts may also occur between a woman's decision or request for a particular form of care and her caregiver's own professional, philosophical or religious commitments. Giving priority to the mother's needs and expectations may give rise to issues of crucial importance in questions of life or death but also applies to less crucial or non-life-threatening situations such as facilitating skin-to-skin care at birth or not using stirrups to support the woman's legs. In emergencies, the hierarchy of needs may change so as to give priority to a caregiver's needs in order to provide optimal care for the mother and newborn. Although there has long been a value on individualized care, the meaning of this – and how this value is implemented – is worthy of renewed attention.

Women's decisions regarding their perinatal care are not limited to their own pregnancy, labour and birth experiences. Their voices need to be heard by maternity care services, including organizations and the professionals who work within those organizations.[8] Some maternity and newborn centres are increasingly including women and parent advocates in their decision-making processes, with a few national centres such as the UK's National Institute for Health and Care Excellence (NICE)[9] involving women directly in their globally respected national policy and standard-setting programs. Ideally, an overarching national organization including one branch that represents families' perspectives in the process of becoming parents and another that represents inter-professional viewpoints is needed to ensure widespread dissemination of family-centred concepts to both. Close collaboration – if not full integration – between these branches is optimal. The lack of implementation of such an organization in most places, and especially in the industrialized world, reflects the considerable gap that still exists between current systems and truly family-centred approaches.

> In South Africa, in 1984, I was fortunate to be included in the initiation and development of a national association for childbirth and parenthood and to later become its president. This organization was inter-professional and multi-cultural, incorporating all professional groups linked to childbearing in any way. In addition to holding national conferences, it organized a monthly speaker series on topics of current interest and facilitated problem-solving meetings between, for example, childbirth educators and labour ward caregivers to facilitate congruent preparation for labour and birth as well as to influence labour and birth care. A sister organization directed at families provided similar information dissemination to parents and worked collaboratively with the professional association, sharing many events and activities. Even during the Apartheid era, the constitution of the professional organization stipulated its multi-cultural membership, earning it formal approval, recognition and membership of the International Society of Psychosomatic Obstetrics and Gynaecology prior to the collapse of Apartheid.

Attending to the needs of parents for appropriate and evidence-based information about their pregnancy and birth experiences and facilitating their participation in decision-making about their own or their baby's care are central to meeting the family's needs for knowledge about their transition to parenthood.

Key Points

- Making decisions about their transition to parenthood is a central issue for all childbearing families.
- Providing information about pregnancy, birth and parenthood prior to pregnancy, during pregnancy and after birth is essential if families are to make informed decisions.
- Prenatal preparation classes for families provide emotional support.
- In most countries, no specific training is provided for prenatal educators and there is little or no standardization of the content of programs.
- There is insufficient evidence available to indicate which of the multitude of sources of information about childbearing provides the most effective preparation for women and their families; in all likelihood, there is some benefit (and likely misinformation!) to be gained from most, if not all, of them.
- Facilitating 'informed choice' has long been a basic tenet of family-centred care. Care choices should be offered to the woman/family in an objective manner based on the best available evidence and should be devoid of coercion, or 'informed coercion'.
- A woman and her family have a right to refuse consent for care. In family-centred care, the needs and expectations of the mother are a priority with respect to her care. Once the baby is born, the needs of the newborn become a priority with regard to the baby's care.
- 'Individualized care' is crucial: what is best is what suits each mother, baby and family during each pregnancy. There is no universal 'right' way to give birth or be a parent.

Inter- and Multi-Professional Care

Overview

It is best to choose the caregiver(s) with the most appropriate skills needed for the level of care required.[1] Primary care practitioners such as midwives or family physicians ideally care for normal pregnancies and births: the development of complications requires referral to specialists. Choice of caregiver is affected by the availability of types of caregivers and maternity care centres, geographical limitations, transport facilities in case of need and families' personal choices. Whatever option is decided upon by the woman and her family, inter-professional collaboration is needed to facilitate optimal maternal and newborn safety, particularly as care is transferred to or shared with alternate professional caregivers. The sometimes conflicting roles of obstetricians and midwives and the emerging roles of psychologists, as well as family and community members, are discussed in this chapter.

Outline

Midwives and Obstetricians

Psychologists

Inter- and Multi-Professional Education, Teaching, Practice, Associations and Policy

The growing contribution to family-centred healthcare by family and community members is being increasingly recognized.[2] Research highlights the importance of non-professional, supportive companions in enhancing childbirth outcomes.[3] Lay health workers also promote immunization uptake and breastfeeding and reduce child morbidity and mortality when compared with usual care.[4]

An emerging issue relates to the rapidly growing use of alternative/complementary/natural or herbal therapies in both everyday life and maternity care.[5] A recent literature review identified the need for greater respect and co-operation between conventional and alternative practitioners as well as communication between all maternity care practitioners and their patients about the use of complementary and alternative medicines.[6]

I served as a member of the Health Science Research Ethics Board for many years at the University of the Witwatersrand, South Africa. Occasionally, proposed research projects sparked heated debate among our approximately 20-member group. One of these was a proposal to study the value of alternative remedies such as the use of cabbage leaves to reduce breast engorgement after birth.[7] Some members of the board believed that conducting research into such topics would grant them validity as potential treatment methods. Others argued that unless we test them we will never know if they are, in fact, helpful or not. Ultimately, the Ethics Committee granted permission to undertake such studies. A randomized trial revealed that women who used cabbage leaves tended to report less engorgement, but not significantly so. These women were, however, more likely to be breastfeeding at 6 weeks after birth and to breastfeed for longer. Their greater breastfeeding success may have been due to the use of cabbage leaves or may have been secondary to the reassurance and confidence they gained by this intervention. Regardless of outcome, this study did much to legitimize the importance of studying less conventional practices.

Midwives and Obstetricians

For some decades, there has been overt and covert conflict between midwives and obstetricians regarding their value or place in maternity care, with family doctors providing an intermediate role offering some elements of both professions.[8] In some parts of the world, the midwife's role is well recognized, and they are responsible, as the World Health Organization (WHO) advocates, for the care of normal birth. Obstetricians in this context provide specialized care for complications – an entirely appropriate use of resources. Yet, in other parts of the world, particularly in North America, battles have long raged over the place of midwifery in perinatal care.[9] Midwives have been excluded and, some would say, persecuted at times for their approach to care. Yet midwives are welcomed by most mothers who use them as they provide continuity of caregiver and holistic, supportive care. In Canada, for example, almost three-quarters of women cared for by midwives rated their overall pregnancy and birth experience as 'very positive' compared to a little over half cared for by obstetricians, family doctors or nurses.[10]

Midwives offer a personal and holistic approach to perinatal care, regarding themselves as responsible for preparing the woman and her family both emotionally and intellectually for all aspects of birth and parenting in addition to providing clinical care, whereas physicians do so to a much lesser extent. Family doctors provide continuity of caregiver, particularly if they offer care at birth and after birth as well as during pregnancy, but may take a less holistic approach to care than midwives. Obstetricians (57%) and family doctors (36%) are most likely to regard birth as dangerous, although few midwives agree (4%).[11] Randomized trials have clearly shown that intervention rates for similar kinds of mothers and levels of risk/complication are far higher among physicians than among their midwifery colleagues. Not surprisingly, outcomes of such midwifery-managed births tend to be better than outcomes of physicians.[12] Despite this, in many countries, including Canada and the United States, fewer than about 10% of women are able to access midwifery care.[13]

The conclusion to be reached is not necessarily that midwives should care for all normal births but that *the quality of care that is needed by women is the same, no matter who the caregiver is.*[14] Holistic, sensitive, caring support, together with respectful treatment that is considerate of biological, emotional and intellectual needs of women and their family members, should be offered by all caregivers for all pregnant and birthing women regardless of the normality of their birth experiences or the degree of complications they develop. There is no theoretical or practical justification for condoning differences in this regard.

Psychologists

In addition to preparation for birth and parenthood through prenatal education classes, psychological support may be needed at many stages of the perinatal and parenting period, although this is not often acknowledged or provided.[15] Difficulties regarding adjustment to pregnancy (e.g. in families experiencing pregnancy following infertility treatments, previous pregnancy loss, among teenage mothers, unmarried women with unplanned and unwanted pregnancies and women with previously traumatic birth experiences) could be assisted with appropriate psychological support. In addition, women experiencing a pregnancy loss in their current pregnancy, or the birth of a preterm or stillborn baby, or a baby with special needs may benefit from counselling. Ideally, every maternity care setting should have access to trained perinatal psychologists to provide support and care for women, their families and their healthcare providers in the event of adverse pregnancy progress.[16] Even when all goes well, adjusting to pregnancy, the events surrounding birth and the postpartum period creates demands on women and their families that are not always well met without professional support. The many women experiencing postpartum depression (about 10 to 20% of all women) are ample testimony to this need.

It is not only women and their families who could benefit from the support of psychologists, but healthcare providers as well.[17] In particular, those caring regularly for babies or parents in difficulty, such as in NICUs, may value assistance. The difficulties inherent in working in this environment, with its emotional pressures, naturally create significant stress. Psychologists can play an important role in easing the pressures on these healthcare providers. Although this need is often recognized, it has not always led to the creation of positions for perinatal psychologists, although it is standard practice in Levin's Estonian neonatal care centre.

The normal concerns of adjusting to parenthood are not generally regarded as the purview of healthcare providers but are considered to be the responsibility of parents or their family members. Whereas, in an ideal world, healthcare providers would alleviate emotional concerns related to any biological events, this is not, and probably never will be, reality. Consequently, some other resource is needed to assist parents emotionally. Perinatal psychologists can fill this gap.[18]

As can be expected, due to the lack of recognition of their importance, little formal training is available for perinatal psychologists.[19] Psychologists with an interest in healthcare can, and do, choose to specialize in one or another aspect of medical practice, including perinatal care. Traditionally, these caregivers focus on theoretical aspects of psychology with a particular emphasis on counselling for more extreme cases of emotional distress such as postpartum depression. They are rarely integral members of the perinatal team, as is advocated here, but are used as specialist referral agencies in case of crisis. Psychologists with a thorough knowledge of perinatal practices, who are a part of the perinatal care team and who focus on the emotional, intellectual and spiritual challenges faced by couples when negotiating through the present-day medicalized experience of a normal transition to parenthood are rare.

Inter- and Multi-Professional Education, Teaching, Practice, Associations and Policies

Education to prepare for a multi-cultural, psycho-social and evidence-based approach to health should be a prerequisite. Traditionally, the teaching of obstetrics, neonatology, nursing, psychology and other disciplines involved in childbirth in medical schools has been separated along disciplinary lines.[20] Some components of care are not included at all, particularly those relating to social science issues such as social work, psychology and childbirth education. More importantly, a concentration on pathology may overshadow the care of a woman with a normal birth and normal newborn.[21] We do not train perinatal caregivers to be sensitive to the emotional, cognitive or spiritual aspects of perinatal care – or if we do, the training is insufficient.[22] We do little to encourage medical students to take courses in the humanities applied to medicine or in psycho-social-cultural issues. Banaszek recently reported that only 69 of 133 accredited medical schools in the United States required students to take courses in the medical humanities.[23] Few, if any, of the 17 medical schools in Canada require a similar course, although a few offer an elective option.[24] Many of these programmes, particularly if they are based in psycho-social or behavioural science departments rather than medical schools, or if they are limited to pre-clinical years and focus on theory rather than application, have failed or are likely to fail. They may be perceived by students as programmes to be endured or which are undemanding 'bird courses' (so named because one 'flies' right through them) and not central to their ability as future doctors. When offered at a graduate level, within the medical curriculum, as students face the challenge of caring for people in clinical practice, they are perceived as more valuable.

Inter-professional, psycho-social and cultural issues involved in clinical practice should be integrated into mainstream medical teaching programmes. For example, when clinical management of a fetal death is taught, both the psychological impact of the experience and the appropriate diagnostic and treatment procedures should be considered. Teaching should be shared by physician and social scientist (and/or other professionals involved) concurrently. Joint teaching programmes of this nature, when tried, have shown promise of a new and better model for educational success.[25]

Schools of psychology do not provide training for perinatal psychologists frequently enough, resulting in a dearth of trained professionals able to fill this void. Such obstacles to inter-professional collaboration in perinatal care are, however, being identified, and methods of overcoming these barriers are being postulated.[26] Exploratory steps towards inter-professional perinatal education are in place at some universities, showing some success.[27] Fortunately, those involved in education for healthcare providers are increasingly receptive to new inter-professional developments.[28] The WHO has recently taken up the challenge of directing attention to inter-professional models of education, practice and policy across healthcare specializations and has developed a framework within which to consider local initiatives for greater and more successful inter-professional practice.[29] New developments along these lines, with particular focus on perinatal care, are to be encouraged and welcomed.

> The University of the Witwatersrand, Johannesburg, initiated an early model of integrated education as early as the 1970s. Medical students generally scorned taking courses in human behavioural science that were offered as options.

Disillusioned with offering curses for only a handful of students, I recommended that the school allocate this teaching time to courses that faculty obviously valued highly, such as anatomy and physiology, rather than pay lip service to the idea that they were teaching medical students about the social sciences. In response, the school decided that students would be required to take, and pass, the medical school's human behavioural science course before being allowed to progress to their fourth year of study and the start of their clinical training. This requirement was implemented, to the mortification of a few students.

Problem-based learning models require that the somewhat artificial distinctions between disciplines be minimized. Instead of teaching obstetrics separately from neonatology, the care of the mother during birth as well as the baby immediately after delivery and the interaction between the two requires a more closely integrated teaching model. The traditional distinctions between these disciplines in the classroom allowed for the customary separation of mother and baby into postpartum wards for mothers and nurseries for the babies. The need to integrate these disciplines academically has made itself clear in the clinical setting. Combined care requires combined teaching models. Changed healthcare services today encourage rooming-in for all mothers as well as early, if not immediate, contact between mother and baby at delivery without separation from this moment on. To achieve this goal, close co-operation between obstetricians (or other delivery assistants) and neonatologists is required. It seems logical that the teaching of these disciplines likewise should be closely associated as it is in the model followed by WHO training programmes.

As an international health consultant, I have visited hundreds of hospitals around the world, particularly in developing countries. In many, the structural layout of delivery rooms includes a separate area to which the baby is removed almost immediately after birth and cared for by a neonatologist or neonatal nurse rather than an obstetrician, obstetric nurse or the mother. Often this is in a completely separate room adjacent to the birthing room. The separate teaching model followed for obstetric and paediatric education has, in these settings, become formalized into the physical layout of the maternity hospital. In Eastern European settings, this structural divide was taken even further: 'women's consultations' (women's hospitals) cared for mothers after delivery, whereas infants were cared for in separate buildings by totally different caregivers (children's polyclinics).

Hospitals may address the complexities of inter-professional care in different ways, including through education and quality assurance programmes. Many hospitals (in Canada 67%) regularly schedule inter-disciplinary meetings (which may include mortality and morbidity rounds) that include multiple professionals such as nurses, midwives and physicians. In Canada, many hospitals (75%) have also established systems for resolving problems among nurses, midwives, obstetricians and family doctors that might arise.[30] Although these may represent the major categories of maternity healthcare providers, they do not often examine the full array of professionals – beyond midwives, family physicians, obstetricians and nurses – who contribute to maternity and newborn care. Adopting an integrated, multi-disciplinary approach to teaching about perinatal care would, in all likelihood, prevent many of these problems from arising in clinical practice rather than trying to resolve them after they have emerged.

Key Points

- Primary care practitioners such as midwives and family physicians ideally care for normal pregnancies and births: the development of complications requires referral to specialists.
- Midwifery care is rated more highly than care by other providers.
- Holistic, sensitive, caring support together with respectful treatment that is considerate of biological, emotional and intellectual needs of women and their family members should be offered by all caregivers for all pregnant and birthing women regardless of the normality of their birth experiences or the degree of complications they develop.
- Psychological support may be needed at many stages of the perinatal and parenting periods.
- Every maternity care setting should have access to trained perinatal psychologists to provide support and care for women, their families and their healthcare providers.
- Little formal training is available for perinatal psychologists. Psychologists with a thorough knowledge of perinatal practices, who are a part of the perinatal care team and who focus on the emotional and intellectual challenges faced by couples are urgently needed.
- Inter-professional, psycho-social and cultural issues involved in clinical practice should be integrated into mainstream medical teaching programmes.
- Instead of teaching obstetrics separately from neonatology, the care of the mother and baby and the interaction between the two requires a more closely integrated teaching model. Combined care requires combined teaching.

Culturally Appropriate Care

Principle:
- Care is culturally sensitive and informed.

Overview

The world is increasingly multi-cultural, revealing diversity of ethnic origin, religion, race and language. Global population movements have allowed for, and even encouraged, the intermingling of cultures through migration, and political upheavals and war in multiple countries have resulted in major demands for refugee relief.[1] Perinatal care must meet the needs of this changing cultural mosaic.

Cultures differ significantly in their beliefs regarding health and illness, as well as in their attitudes and practices regarding childbearing.[2] Biological functioning is considered to be paramount in Western societies. In contrast, significant sections of the global village regard this level of functioning as of least importance, with spiritual, social and psychological concerns playing a primary role in illness aetiology, treatment and prognosis.[3] It is as unacceptable in these cultures to neglect spiritual rites as it is to omit checking blood pressure in pregnancy in the West. Examples of these variations in five differing cultures from four continents are provided here. These include the Aboriginal peoples of Canada, women giving birth in Canada but who had experienced female genital mutilation earlier in their lives performed predominantly in central African countries, South African Black women, Hindu and Muslim Indian women and women giving birth in Central and Eastern Europe in medical systems inspired by Communism. Their differences highlight the importance of understanding the psychological, social and cultural background of women in addition to caring for their physiological well-being when providing family-centred care.

Outline

Cultural Differences and Similarities in Perinatal Care
Cross-Cultural Terminology
Variations in childbearing practices in five differing cultures from four continents.

Cultural Differences and Similarities in Perinatal Care

The lowliest woman in the poorest country gives birth in the same way as royalty. Childbirth is the greatest leveller we have; we are all equal in this experience.[4] There are, however, significant variations in birth practices based on cultural, economic, social, religious or medical factors. These include, for example, choice of caregiver as midwife, obstetrician, family physician or traditional birth attendant; position adopted for birth, ranging from lithotomy to a supported, standing position; place of delivery as hospital, birth unit or home; presence or absence of a partner/companion during delivery; and breast or bottle feeding practices, to name only some. Variations in approaches are evident worldwide.[5] There are variations in childbirth practices from place to place, from hospital to hospital within the same city and from doctor to doctor within the same hospital.[6] In many places, there is no doctor at birth, and it does not take place in a hospital: the mother, in her home, attended by the midwife, is the central focus. There is enormous variability in the world, and people differ widely in knowledge, attitudes, values, expectations, beliefs, societal conditions and economic levels. The birth experience can vary within the same mother from birth to birth just as it varies for different mothers with different social, cultural, and psychological backgrounds.

Cross-Cultural Terminology

The terms used to distinguish culturally divergent groups require some clarification. For example, the term 'African', as used here, does not apply to all the peoples of the continent of Africa. It is intended to refer to Black people of the Southern African continent who share a philosophy of life termed 'African' as opposed to, for example, 'Western' or 'Eastern'. It is understood that the term 'African' is further compounded by the complexities of the peoples to which it refers. It is acknowledged that there is remarkable variability within the Southern African peoples included in this term.

Similarly, the clustering of peoples from the various countries of Central and Eastern Europe into a single group labelled 'Eastern European' is an artificial categorization that, while being geographically based, ignores the distinctive and varied practices occurring within each culture and country. The term 'Eastern European' is used to capture the overriding influence of the former Soviet Union in this geographical region.

While distinctions accorded to cultural groups, such as are embodied in the terms 'African', 'Caucasian', 'Indian', 'mixed cultural origin' and 'Eastern European', are theoretically unacceptable, the reality of differing expectations and experiences of birth among the various peoples and cultures reported necessitates the use of such terminology for the sake of academic understanding.

Aboriginal Peoples of Canada

Socio-economic marginalization and poor health status characterize many First Nations, Inuit and Métis women in Canada, if not in many countries where Aboriginal women live. First Nations, Métis and Inuit people continue to be adversely affected by a long history of residential schools and colonization.[7] Such schools were first established in 1879,[8] with the last only being closed in 1997 (Muscowequan School in Saskatchewan).[9] Schools imposed forced separation of children from their families together with suppression of their traditional language, religion, diet, dress and traditions, coupled with unbearably harsh conditions including physical, sexual and emotional abuse. Re-introduction of these children as adults into their former societies and families proved to be almost impossible, with unemployment, disillusion and depression being common responses, resulting in alcohol and substance abuse among many. Even more deleterious was the absence of any acceptable family life experience with a consequent inability to maintain marital harmony or stability as these children moved into adulthood. The lasting effects of this brutal history of colonization, including the practice of residential schooling, are mistrust in the Western medical and educational system, as well as a cycle of violence and disrupted parenting in the community.[10] Healthcare providers, when working with Aboriginal women and their communities, must be aware of and sensitive to these issues, making respect, information sharing, partnership and collaboration key actions to take.

The abuses experienced by children in the residential schools, together with the breakdown of traditional family life resulting from their forced assimilation, have left their mark on many Aboriginal families of today and include disruption of traditional pregnancy- and birth-related events. There is tension because relocating women from their homes to give birth in technologically based and interventionist hospitals has been widespread in past decades due to less sophisticated healthcare facilities closer to home,[11] a problem exacerbated by Canada's vast geographical spread and sparse Aboriginal populations. Evacuation of women for childbirth, usually without any supportive family member, to hospitals far from their homes has deleterious psychological, social and cultural effects. A growing pride in their various cultures in recent years has resurfaced, calling for particular respect for Aboriginal traditions and needs, including issues relating to childbearing. There is now considerable support for the establishment of traditional community birthing centres combined with biomedical techniques and technology closer to home.[12] Hospital- or clinic-based maternity care programmes for these women and their families need to achieve a balance of clinical safety and culturally respectful practices.[13] Outcomes are better with less travel to outside communities, but where travel is necessary due to the vast geographical expanses involved in the regions where many Aboriginal women live, social, emotional and financial support to allow for supportive companions for women to accompany them – not currently allowed – should be provided.[14]

Community-based Aboriginal midwives, integrating both traditional and modern approaches to care and education, are viewed as the ideal model to follow regarding caregiver choice. This idea is integrally linked to community development, cultural revival and healing from the impact of colonization and involves effective teamwork among midwives, physicians and nurses working in the remote villages and at the regional and tertiary referral centres.

The *Report of the Royal Commission on Aboriginal People* stated: 'Aboriginal women who are pregnant need culture-based prenatal outreach and support programmes designed to address their particular situation and vulnerabilities.'[15] A culturally safe model of family-centred perinatal care that is designed to empower the expectant mother, family and community needs to consider obstacles such as the lack of transportation, inadequate or absent prenatal care or postpartum childcare, a fear of being judged for lifestyle choices and fear of the healthcare system due to historical legacies. It is necessary to develop a holistic care model for the mother, father and family that connects with the teachings of the 'Medicine Wheel' to support a balance among mental, emotional, spiritual and physical wellness.[16] A family-centred approach to care that emphasises the interaction and importance of physical, emotional, mental and spiritual aspects of care – as encouraged in this book – is congruent with the fundamental principles long established in Aboriginal conceptualizations of health and well-being. Childbearing practices that include respect for and appreciation of these long-established cultures and their historical childbearing experiences are to be actively encouraged and welcomed.[17]

Giving Birth in Canada Following Earlier Female Genital Mutilation (FGM)

Soon after moving to Canada, I gave a presentation on my previous work on African women's birth experiences. Following this talk, Kowser Omer-Hashi, a Somali midwife living and working in Canada and an advocate against FGM, approached me. She appreciated the respectful way that I spoke about traditional African birthing customs and, in consequence, asked me to work with her on the subject of FGM. I agreed and expressed a preference to explore the experiences of women with previous FGM who had moved to Canada and given birth there. Our research into Canadian immigrant women's experiences of giving birth with previous experience of genital cutting revealed a disconcerting dearth of knowledge among caregivers regarding the meaning of this long-established practice or how to care for women with FGM during either pregnancy or birth. Our research also revealed a shocking level of disrespect for, and emotionally abusive care of, women with this experience.[18]

FGM (also referred to as 'circumcision' or 'cutting') involves the 'total or partial removal of the female external genitalia or other injuries to the female genital organs'.[19] Four types of FGM are described.[20] The first type refers to a number of procedures that usually involve the clitoral area, including partial or total removal of the clitoris (clitoridectomy) and/or the foreskin (prepuce). The second form, called 'excision', refers to the removal of a part of or the entire clitoris itself plus a part or all of the labia minora. 'Infibulation,' also known as 'pharaonic circumcision' (because its practice has been recorded as far back as the time of the Pharaohs), is the third and most extensive form and involves not only excision but the removal of the medial parts of the labia majora and the joining of the two sides of the vulva with thorns, silk or catgut sutures. A small opening is preserved, by the insertion of a foreign body, to allow the passage of urine and menstrual blood. As the skin of the remaining labia majora heals, a bridge of scar tissue forms over the vagina, leaving only a small hole to allow the slow passage of urine or menstrual flow. The legs are bound together for several weeks to allow scar tissue to form. Since a physical barrier is created, during sexual intercourse, the infibulated woman may have to undergo gradual dilation by her husband over a period of days, weeks or even months. This painful process does not always result in successful vaginal penetration, and the scar tissue may have to be cut. At childbirth, the woman will have to be cut once more to allow the passage of the baby. After birth, the raw edges are re-sutured. This form of mutilation is practiced in about 15% of all women exposed to genital mutilation.[21] A fourth form of circumcision involves any other type of genital mutilation such as the insertion of corrosive substances into the vagina to facilitate 'dry' sexual intercourse.

The procedure is valued in societies that practice it as a guarantee of marriage and subsequent economic security,[22] among other perceived benefits. Not having the procedure may be psychologically more disturbing in these cultures than having it. Notable too is that the procedure is implemented by women/mothers on their daughters out of love and a need to provide the best possible chance for their daughters for a normal married life – for which genital cutting is required.

Although some forms are more problematic than others, all may lead to various problems, some of which are highly debilitating and lifelong. Reproductive health is compromised through infection, sterility, coital difficulty, pregnancy loss and complications during child-birth. The impact on psycho-sexual and psychological development can be severe.

About 130 million women worldwide have been circumcised,[23] and 2 million or even as many as 3 million girls experience this procedure each year. Most of these women live in 26 African countries, a few in Asian countries and increasingly, as a result of immigration, in Europe, Canada, Australia and the United States.[24] The practice is still widespread in some countries and is primarily, but not exclusively, practiced among Muslims. Not all Muslim groups perform genital mutilation.

A Canadian study of over 400 women's experiences of childbirth following previous experience of FGM shows women's dissatisfaction with care and a perceived lack of knowledge and ability by health practitioners to care for them appropriately during birth.[25]

> Kowser Omer-Hashi conducted interviews with women who had previously experienced FGM for our study. Kowser has come under considerable pressure from those within her community not to continue her opposition to FGM, as she is seen as betraying her community by speaking out against its traditions. She and her family members received numerous critical and/or threatening telephone calls pressuring her to stop 'betraying' her culture.

Striking in the reports from women are the comments regarding the lack of cultural sensitivity shown to women concerning their cultural practice. Abhorrent though this practice might be to caregivers, the care of any individual woman in pregnancy and childbirth requires sensitivity and respect, which, according to women's reports, was often lacking. Most women (88%) participating in the Canadian survey reported hurtful com-ments being made at some stage during their care.[26] Women indicated that doctors did not provide the kind of birth procedures (such as vaginal delivery rather than caesarean section) that they would have preferred. The caesarean section rate of over 50% for this sample is excessively high compared to the national average of less than half this figure at the time of the survey.[27] While the perineal area of women with FGM does require special care during birthing (e.g. either or both anterior and lateral episiotomies), the vaginal canal and uterus are no different from those of women without FGM and should therefore be at no greater risk for caesarean section. At least half the women felt pressured to have their partner with them in labour and delivery when a female companion would be far more culturally acceptable than a male. Women reported insensitivity regarding pain management for their ultra-sensitive perineums (a consequence of multiple cuttings) in prenatal examinations, labour and delivery and in their postpartum care. The women were not afforded privacy during examinations, and gentleness of touch was not always in evidence. It appears from women's reports that little attempt was made to discuss birth practices and care manage-ment with them, specifically, caesarean section options or pain management needs. Women did not perceive their caregivers – doctors or nurses – as knowledgeable enough to look after them, and most would choose a different caregiver or birthplace for a future preg-nancy. It is clear that healthcare services for women with this experience still leave much to be desired and that education for both women and providers needs to be strengthened.[28] Even when cultural differences are valued and respected in society, as in Canada, ignorance and prejudice still appear to play a disconcertingly large role.[29]

Based on women's perceptions, it appears that women who have previously experienced FGM need changed practices. Better preparation of care providers regarding the needs of women with female mutilation and particularly concerning issues of cultural difference may lead to more sensitive treatment and respectful care. Care that is more sensitive may be facilitated by clinical practice guidelines regarding appropriate care. These have, fortunately, recently been released in Canada, and although some aspects of these guidelines remain controversial, they go some way towards meeting women's clinical needs during their perinatal care.[30]

In general, women in the Canadian survey gave very mixed reports regarding both their experiences of FGM in childhood or of giving birth in Canada. Greater attention needs to be paid to preparing caregivers to attend to the needs for communication and understanding of women with previous FGM if standards of care are to reach customary medical and psycho-social expectations.

Traditional African Birth in South Africa

Ancestral spirits blessed my research into African birthing traditions and how these changed with rural to urban migration.[31] When seeking research assistants, two African midwives were referred to me by the matron of Baragwanath Hospital (now Chris Hani Hospital). They were initially polite but non-committal about working with me. Two weeks later, they contacted me, excited and enthusiastic to begin work. My inquiries as to why their attitude had changed so dramatically in this short time period was answered by the information that they had consulted the spirits, through their traditional healer, and that the spirits had informed them that the work was blessed and that they should assist me in every way they could. Our relationship continued for another decade or more, and in all honesty, I can say that this research was the smoothest undertaking I have ever encountered in over four decades of academic study. I will be forever grateful to the spirits, to Mama Mona, the midwives' spiritual healer, whom I later met, and to these midwives.

Traditional African birth takes place in a supportive, secure environment that is provided by the grandmother's hut. Here the woman is surrounded by the people she knows and trusts. The ancestral spirits protect her here, and she is free from 'polluting contacts' such as menstruating women.[32] As women move from rural to urban environments, all this is exchanged for the promise of medical security offered by hospitals. There can be little argument that this promise will be fulfilled in complicated deliveries. However, it is not so certain that the hospital environment is of equal benefit for routine, normal deliveries. In this situation, the psychological safety and medical well-being of the mother take equal precedence.

One of the most striking changes to take place in the move from home to hospital delivery in Southern Africa is the position adopted for delivery. Traditionally, African women are encouraged to remain ambulant and active during the first stage of labour.[33] A kneeling position is adopted for birth with the knees held apart and the heels together, supporting the perineal area. In hospitals and clinics, however, a supine position is usually adopted for delivery, as is customary in the West, although the Western world today is moving away from the supine delivery position. In contrast, the African woman is willingly adopting this position, probably in response to caregiver influence. It is ironic that Western women are currently struggling to attain what African women are so readily relinquishing! Although some traditional practices regarding childbirth may well be harmful, for example, vulval bloodletting,[34] it is a pity that those that are apparently beneficial, for example, an upright delivery position, are also being discarded in the process of cultural transition. This is truly an instance of throwing out the baby with the bathwater!

A characteristic of traditional rural births among Southern African women is the presence of abundant social support.[35] During birth, the woman is accompanied by a traditional birth attendant and a trusted woman of her family – a value learned in Western cultures only relatively recently. In addition, in some cases, a number of younger women are present to share the experience and act as 'messengers' if needed. These birth assistants give physical as well as emotional support to the labouring woman while at the same time learning about birth themselves. Abundant social support is also available in both the prenatal and postpartum periods. [36] Prenatally, the woman can turn to trusted family members or older women of the group for advice about her changing state. The older women enforce many traditional behaviours expected of pregnant women, such as sitting up straight to allow the embryo to position itself correctly. In addition, others supervise the performance of traditional, and sometimes questionable, customs such as the wearing of the first maternity covering, vulval bloodletting, particularly when oedema occurs, and the taking of *isihlambezo* – a herbal medicine believed to 'open the way' or stimulate contractions. Postpartum women also receive a great deal of social support, albeit intensive and restrictive. For example, women are isolated after birth together with an older, trusted relative, such as the mother-in-law. This close relative is responsible for caring for the new mother, instructing her about breast care and infant feeding, caring for the newborn and performing traditional rites. Although this may be ideal, it can sometimes prove emotionally traumatic, particularly if relations between the older woman and her younger charge are troubled.[37]

Most reports of traditional African birth customs confirm that it is customary to exclude the husband from procedures associated with birth and the postpartum period.[38] Reasons advanced for this are, firstly, that the blood of childbirth is believed to be able to 'weaken' a man's spirit so that he would be likely to die in his next battle. Secondly, on a more socio-political level, it is suggested that the primary source of power or status for women in the tribal community lies in her ability to give birth, and women, consequently, are reluctant to relinquish this power to their men folk. This is not altogether clear, since women's status in the rural community stems from her ability to give birth, and no amount of husband involvement in the process of birth can alter this. Whether it is women who have excluded men from birth or men who have excluded themselves, the reality is that in both the traditional and current settings, little support is available from men at birth. In addition, hospitals and clinics fail to provide alternate sources of social support for black labouring women.[39] In contrast to traditional custom, mothers or other family or friends are not allowed to attend births. Nurses serve as the primary, if not only, birth companions, and shortages of staff, as well as customary expectations for women to be strong in labour and not to express pain, often deter them from providing support.

The need to exclude the husband from delivery will, hopefully, change. Some women probably do want to share the emotional experience of birth together with their husbands, as is the frequently expressed desire of Western mothers. Other women express a need for husbands to be present 'to see how difficult it is, so that he too won't want any more babies' or 'to see for himself if things go wrong, so that he won't blame me if they do', as often occurs. As family sizes are customarily larger than in developed societies, and as economic pressures and social custom make the woman's role of rearing her offspring difficult, these motives are understandable.[40]

Alternatively, and most importantly, cultural and language differences may result in health professionals being unaware of either the women's lack of knowledge of, or of her reluctance to comply with, some Western medical procedures.[41] Women may, for instance, refuse caesarean sections as providing their partners with 'evidence' of their unfaithfulness during pregnancy, which, according to traditional belief, results in a difficult delivery. Misunderstandings between the healthcare providers and women will result unless they understand such traditional beliefs.

> While the study of Western approaches to birth raised fascinating questions regarding the ongoing medicalization of birth in the Western world, my work explored, in addition, the rich diversity of cultural experience of birth in South Africa. Underlying this exploration was a number of questions: how could differing worldviews regarding health and illness, and particularly regarding birth and parenthood, be integrated across traditional Western and African (and other) groups in healthcare practice? What was happening in those hospitals and clinics designated (under the then Apartheid regime) to serve people of colour, and particularly African women, during pregnancy and birth? Did doctors serving these women understand traditional practices, beliefs and knowledge? Was there any attempt to conserve traditional practices, to understand them or at least to respect them during the care of pregnant and birthing women in the health facilities available in South Africa? Did African women, living in both rural and urban settings, wish to preserve their traditional birth and infant care practices? What impact had Apartheid had on the maternal and child healthcare services available?
>
> At the time this research commenced (in the early 1980s, a decade before the breakdown of Apartheid), little was being done to examine these issues. In essence, my research indicated that the rich customs reported in rural anthropological research were being lost in urban centres. Many women, and particularly urban women, were no longer aware of such customs, and virtually nothing was being done from the healthcare professionals' perspective to respect traditions if some women wanted them. This applied, primarily, to practices surrounding birth itself, which generally took place in hospitals or clinics in urban areas. Traditional practices that occurred outside the healthcare facility (such as at home) tended to continue.

Of most interest was the differing worldview regarding health and illness in general and pregnancy and birth in particular among Black women. Western approaches emphasized the biological role in health and illness almost to the exclusion of other levels of functioning. In contrast, African viewpoints placed a predominant value on spiritual, social and psychological levels of functioning rather than on the biological component of health and illness. For example, maintaining good relations within the family, community and ancestral world is more important in maintaining one's health and well-being, with biological concerns playing a lesser role in contributing to ill-health. Integrating these in the provision of healthcare services without losing the benefits inherent in each approach was the challenge to combining African and Western views of health in South Africa.

Pregnancy- and Birth-Related Customs among Indian Women

Inspired by the challenge of grasping for an understanding of or at the least an appreciation for cross-cultural birthing diversity, I embarked on a series of large-scale surveys that examined similar issues among Indian (Hindu and Muslim) and mixed-cultural-origin women living in South Africa. These groups appeared to share similar worldviews (regarding assumptions about health and illness, pregnancy and birth) with each other and with Western approaches as compared to an African standpoint. My research therefore examined these three groups (Caucasian, Indian and mixed-cultural-origin women) for comparative purposes. Topics explored included infant feeding practices, miscarriage, traditional Indian customs, experiences of birth, sexuality and contraception in pregnancy and afterwards and preparation of women for pregnancy and birth.

Of the 16 to 18 notable Hindu *sanskara* (sacraments) of the *Grhya Sutra* (laws governing behaviour), 11 relate to conception, pregnancy, birth and early infancy. One rite – *Garbhadhana* – is performed to favour conception of a healthy child. A second – *Pumsavana* – is performed at about 3 months' gestation to assist the child's nourishment in the womb. Some regard this ritual as determining the baby's sex – preferably a boy. During the seventh month of pregnancy, *Anavalobhan* is performed to ensure the baby's growth, whereas *Simantonnayan* is carried out in the eighth month to ensure a perfect, whole child that is mentally healthy. Many beliefs about conception and pregnancy are common to both Hindu and Muslim women, including the belief that conception involves the mingling of substances from both parents, although the degree to which each contributes is debated. *In utero*, the fetus is believed to be nourished by direct blood transfusion from the mother via the fontanelle, the 'soft spot' on the baby's skull. The umbilical cord is thought to develop only during the last month of pregnancy. Dietary restriction, in terms of both quantity and quality is practiced. Too much food is believed to be harmful, although the mother is encouraged to satisfy food cravings lest the child develop birthmarks. 'Cooling' foods are avoided as well as eruptive or windy foods, all of which may threaten the fetus. Women are cautioned not to catch 'cold touch' during pregnancy or for 40 days after birth as this can cause miscarriage, fever or madness. Women are advised to remain tranquil during pregnancy. Superstitious beliefs are common, and everyday objects may be perceived as omens; for example, women are believed to be susceptible to cosmic changes such as eclipses, and intercourse is forbidden at these times.

Traditionally, both Hindu and Muslim women return to their mother's home about a month before birth and have their baby in an isolated part of the house attended by a traditional birth attendant of a lower caste who is able to dispose of the polluting by-products of birth. The mother and experienced family members or friends also attend the pregnant woman, providing support and empathy. If birth is attended by a doctor or takes place in a hospital, the traditional birth attendant will provide assistance in the postpartum period. During the time of birth, men are banished from the household.

Women labour in a supported seated position. It is important to note the exact time of birth, which is defined as the moment the head can first be seen because the birth horoscope must later be calculated. *Jarkarem* or the *Chattie* ceremony is a further sacramental rite associated with the birth. Among Muslims, it is important that someone close to the child whispers the name 'Allah' into the child's ear. It is also important not to draw the attention of malevolent spirits to the child at birth and before the cord is cut and tied so the father is notified of the birth indirectly by a messenger. A child born in a breech position is said to have special powers of healing, particularly for those having cramps, sprains or muscular injury. Explanations of anomalies are either spiritual (it is God's will), psychological or philosophical (it is one's karma).

The new mother is isolated in a dimly lit part of the house after birth and drinks warm foods such as coffee or hot water rather than cooling liquids such as tea. Milk and yoghourt are believed to inhibit the healing of wounds and are forbidden. Colostrum is believed to be dirty and to cause infant diarrhoea. It is also regarded as a weak and impure form of milk not suited for a new baby's digestion. The mother may not nurse her baby until the third day after birth, during which time the baby may have a wet-nurse or be given sugar water or condensed milk mixed with water. The new mother is regarded as physically and ritually unclean and is given a ritual bath on the third day after birth as part of the cleansing process. Contact with the woman's breasts or with breastmilk is a ritual danger to men, and intimacy during lactation is frowned upon. Ritual pollution from birth lasts for 31 days among Hindus and 40 days among Muslims.

In the days after birth, an oil-based liquid mixed with ingredients that are believed to make it wither quickly is rubbed into the umbilicus. The afterbirth is kept safely – tradition-ally for 9 days but for less time after hospital birth – before being buried in a deep hole. If an evil person or spirit accidentally took it, it is believed that the mother would become infertile or the child harmed. The baby must be cleansed of the 'dirt and heat' collected while in the womb, and to this end, from the first day after birth, the mother is given small quantities of castor oil mixed with honey. Throughout pregnancy, the mother also takes small amounts of castor oil so that the food she eats does not make the layer of 'dirt' on the child difficult to remove.

Of major significance is the rite associated with naming the child – called *Namakara* – that takes place about 12 days after birth. Religious and secular ideas are incorporated into the choice of the name. For Indian Muslims, numerological concepts are also incorporated. Five further purification rites are performed for the baby during its infant years. A great fear is of the 'evil eye'. For this reason, the mother must be careful not to breastfeed with her breasts visible or, if bottle feeding, must wrap the bottle in a cloth. The baby is weaned at about 9 months.

Infertile women are regarded as personally unfulfilled and ritually inauspicious. Barrenness is probably the worst affliction that a woman can bear. Even the woman who only has daughters is frowned upon: her status is little higher than an infertile woman. The father who has no sons is pitied, although his wife is blamed: occasionally, supernatural influences may be regarded as causative. Spiritual components clearly play a significant role in traditional Indian customs. Although these differ somewhat between Muslim and Hindu, the various ceremonies are similarly directed towards protecting the mother and baby and cleansing both of the pollution arising during pregnancy, birth and the postpartum period.

I have been fortunate enough to collaborate on perinatal care issues with Muslim women in South Africa, Canada and Central Asia. In the latter countries, I had opportunities to work with secular women as well as with women belonging to fundamentalist – and occasionally revolutionary – groups. When ideological differences that are difficult to accept emerged, I was faced with the question of whether I felt comfortable assisting women whose value systems were so vastly different from my own. I quickly realized that women giving birth are all equal and that every woman may need, and value, assistance at this time. Although I occasionally feared for my safety, especially when working in war-torn areas such as in Tajikistan or in Southern Sudan before it attained independence, I did not hesitate to offer whatever assistance I could. Nevertheless, such moments were disconcerting, such as when I was boarding our *Médecins Sans Frontières* vehicle for a trip to an unsafe part of Tajikistan and was told that the previous car going on the same route had been hijacked and all its passengers killed.

Giving Birth in Central and Eastern Europe and Central Asia

My work in Eastern Europe was stimulated by such questions as, how would these cultures adapt and change their maternal and child health services while experiencing the enormous upheaval in cultural, social, economic, religious and political systems following the fall of the Union of Soviet Socialist Republics? Would traditional ways be preserved? Would these be respected? Would there be any attempt to integrate the 'old' and the 'new' ways, or would both the 'good' and the 'bad' of the previous system be discarded in favour of the 'new' models to which they were being exposed? Would women's perceptions be regarded as important? Would the medical regimes of the 'West' be transplanted without regard for whatever richness or diversity existed in the countries of Central and Eastern Europe? The answers to some of these questions are included here.

The review provided here highlights key features of maternity services in the region of the former Soviet Union.[42] Maternity care in Central and Eastern Europe under Soviet rule until 1989, as well as in the decades following, was largely based on experience, case studies, local knowledge and tradition.[43] Prenatal and perinatal procedures followed 'edicts' issued by the Ministry of Health in Moscow, with no deviation from these being allowed without punishment. These edicts – and particularly 'Edict 55', directed towards maternity hospital care – were enforced through the powerful Ministerial Division of Sanitary and Epidemiological Control that regularly inspected all healthcare facilities and covered every aspect of care from medical procedures to the timing of airing of rooms each day and the hours of sleep, meals or infant feeds. Unable to have access to Western information, these systems of care lacked the benefits gained from developments in maternal-child healthcare worldwide. For example, the value of randomized, controlled trials in assessing the benefits of interventions was not evident in the former Soviet Union healthcare system. Nor was there concern for family-centred care, except in rare 'experimental settings' which were given special permission to try alternate forms of care, such as in Adik Levin's neonatal intensive care unit (NICU) in Estonia. The relatively high maternal and infant mortality that existed in these regions is evidence that the Soviet system of care was less than optimal. Intervention programmes were concerned with updating existing knowledge, introducing appropriate technology and altering attitudes to incorporate a more humanitarian concern for healthcare recipients than had been the custom.

In Eastern Europe, maternity care was and still is in many places divided into care of women during pregnancy and after birth (offered by 'women's consultations'), intra-partum care (offered in 'maternity houses') and postpartum care of the baby (provided at 'children's polyclinics'). Continuity of caregivers was not a prevalent concept. Infection control was, justifiably, one of the primary concerns of the edicts as little in the way of antibiotics or even reliable cleaning materials were available, making infection a significant source of mortality as well as morbidity.[44] Traditional methods of infection control were based on outdated beliefs regarding the sources of infection. For example, mothers were viewed as the prime sources of infection and were separated from their newborns from birth, with limited contact being allowed, even during scheduled feeding times. During feeds, protective clothing was to be worn by the mother (hats, masks and gowns) with plastic sheeting placed between the baby and mother or between the baby and the bed to prevent the spread of infection from mother to baby. In contrast, staff hand-washing, between contacts with different mothers or babies, was not strictly monitored or enforced, even though the wearing of hats, gowns and shoe coverings by staff was required. Maternity care facilities were routinely closed for disinfecting for about one month, two or three times a year, with walls, floors and all equipment being disinfected and tested for bacteria.

> International health consultants may take different approaches to influencing change in local practices. Marsden Wagner (then the World Health Organization's Regional Advisor for Maternal and Infant Health in Europe) took delight in nonchalantly draping the white coat given to him to wear before a ward round over his shoulder instead of putting it on. Others, like myself, used to always take the opportunity the white coat offered to discuss appropriate infection control – a less dramatic but sometimes more acceptable – approach. I am not sure, how-ever, which method was more effective. Certainly, Marty made his point very clearly, while my less confrontational way was easier for locals to ignore.

Maternity Care

Under Soviet rule, clinical care during pregnancy involved regular and frequent check-ups following much the same protocol as is found internationally, although as many as 30 prenatal visits and hospitalizations for weeks or even months for hypertension or urinary tract infections, for example, were not unusual.[45] Women were admitted alone to the maternity house for their labour, delivery and postpartum care: family members were excluded at all times.[46] Women stayed in hospital for 7 days following vaginal births and for 10 days after caesarean sections.

Women were examined on admission to hospital to assess the progress of labour and were then showered and given a hospital gown. Such niceties as privacy and dignity during perinatal care (e.g. adequate gowning) received little attention primarily because this was not a priority. Women were hospitalized together with other women in a labour ward. Although this was usually one or two women per room, in some hospitals as many as 20 beds for women in labour were grouped in one large ward. The mother moved from her bed to a centrally positioned examination table where she received her routine internal monitoring examinations in full view of the others in the room. Walking around and eating or drinking in labour were not allowed. Instead, women were confined to bed and given intravenous (IV) fluids, often leaving them with severe bruising. Staff contact with women was limited to routine assessments of progress until close to full cervical dilation.

Shaving, both pubic and perineal, administration of enemas and artificial rupture of membranes were routine for all labouring women.[47] A 'cocktail' of drugs was also given to women, commonly reported as containing some, or all, of a spasmolytic to reduce muscle tension, a sedative to quiet the mother and an oxytocic agent to speed up labour. Mothers were often admonished not to cry out or express anxiety or strong emotion in labour and were chastised as potentially (negatively) affecting their baby by doing so. In general, staff valued an 'efficient', 'authoritative' and 'disciplinary' approach to care.[48]

Women moved to the delivery room in the second stage of labour.[49] This too usually had beds for at least one or two other mothers to labour side by side, without any curtain between them. All mothers delivered in a supine position with their legs in stirrups. The 'Rachmanov' delivery bed (a surgical, split delivery bed with stirrup supports) was standard equipment across the region, and delivery in any other position was, and still is, largely unthinkable. Iodine was spread from the abdomen to mid-thigh for infection control. Episiotomy or perineotomy was routine for all primiparas and for most multiparas. The vaginal opening was manually swept/stretched during the second stage, often repeatedly, before an episiotomy. Routine examination of the mother's cervix after birth was aided by the insertion of a speculum, together with the grasping and visualization of the cervix with forceps to check for tears or bleeding. Repair of the episiotomy was often performed without anaesthetic, as this was not in abundant supply. An ice pack was placed on the mother's lower abdomen to encourage uterine contraction after delivery.

At birth, the baby was delivered onto the delivery bed, suctioned, the cord clamped and then dried.[50] The baby was shown to the mother, by being held up in the air, and then removed to an adjacent room. The baby was cleaned – usually with oil but in many places by being held under running tap water – given eye-drops, the baby's navel and breasts were swabbed with 'green brilliant' – an antiseptic mixture – swaddled and then left under a warmer until transferred to the neonatal ward apart from its mother. The baby was not returned to the mother before transfer, except for a few minutes in some places. Mothers did not usually hold or even touch their babies, let alone breastfeed them, until some hours (for normal vaginal births) or even days (for caesarean sections) after delivery.[51] Mothers lay alone in the delivery room or nearby it once the necessary birthing procedures had been completed for one to two hours of observation until transfer to the postpartum wards. During this time, their babies lay nearby, but apart, in the neonatal area. Postpartum, mothers were cared for in maternity postpartum units by maternity nurses, and babies were cared for in separate newborn nurseries by neonatal nurses. As immediate postpartum contact of mother and baby was encouraged with the introduction of the Baby Friendly Hospital Initiative (from 1992 onwards), wrapped babies (and later unwrapped babies) were given to mothers to hold after neonatal examination and washing in the hour following birth. Rooming-in was slowly adopted in postpartum wards.

With introduction of the Baby Friendly Hospital Initiative (BFHI) in the region in 1992, pressure was exerted on maternity units to introduce rooming-in in postpartum wards and to replace the separate responsibilities for care of mothers and babies with a combined-care approach. This was implemented relatively quickly despite objections that this would increase infection rates, that mothers were too tired (or unskilled) to care for their babies, that there was not enough space for babies to be placed in the same room as the mother and that such an arrangement was not allowed in terms of the 'edicts' governing postpartum care. At first, only those brave enough to defy the edicts implemented the changes. I much admired these pioneers, who were often senior healthcare providers who felt somewhat 'immune' from the consequences of their actions due to their proximity to retirement. Later, the Ministry of Health in Moscow was encouraged to revise the edicts to incorporate new approaches to care that sanctioned such perinatal practices as rooming-in and combined care as well as additional procedures advocated by the BFHI. Today, many hospitals in a number of Eastern European countries have become formally accredited by the World Health Organization (WHO) and the United Nations Children's Fund (UNICEF) as Baby Friendly Hospitals – even more so than has occurred in North America and Canada.

Breastfeeding

Breastfeeding, although fully endorsed in the traditional Soviet setting and initiated by almost every mother after delivery, was, nonetheless, often unsuccessful, with mothers being commonly reported as not having enough milk.[52] Mothers introduced alternate liquid feeds shortly after delivery and solid foods within the first month of birth in accordance with edicts governing infant nutrition. Routine supplementation of all newborns with water, glucose or locally produced breastmilk substitutes (from cow's milk) inevitably contributed to the decline in breastmilk production. This decline was, however, interpreted as being due to the poor social, nutritional and physical condition of virtually all mothers (regarded as mothers of 'low culture') rather than to the oversupply of substitute liquids and the under-use of breastmilk.[53]

A rigidly enforced set of practices regarding breastfeeding was based on caregivers' (understandable) concern with infection and their (often inappropriate) assumptions underlying its cause.[54] Mothers did not have access to their babies except during strictly scheduled and limited feeding times. Mothers were advised to feed for only a few minutes on each breast on the first day and to increase this time slowly over the ensuing week. Any maternal or infant deviation from 'normality' was usually regarded as a contraindication to breastfeeding. These contraindications included caesarean section, forceps or vacuum extractions, episiotomies, prolonged labour, any signs of asphyxia in the neonate, an Apgar score below 7 at 5 minutes, or even the mother having a mild cold.[55] Physicians estimated that at least 80% of women giving birth have some pathology of pregnancy, and at least 80% of their infants also show signs of pathology.[56]

Knowledge about appropriate positioning and latching of babies at the breast was scarce before the introduction of the BFHI.[57] With the excessive swaddling (including the baby's head and neck) that was the custom (practiced because 'it is cold in our homes,' 'babies are more comfortable like that' or 'it reduces crying'), good positioning of the baby at the breast was difficult. Use of bottles for supplemental feedings resulted in high rates of oral thrush in newborn nurseries. The widespread introduction of the BFHI resulted in dramatic increases in the duration of breastfeeding and, in particular, exclusive breastfeeding, as well as the sudden virtual elimination of infant thrush in postpartum units.[58]

Neonatal Intensive Care

Babies requiring intensive or special care were stabilized and then transferred to a separate 'sick children's hospital'.[59] Sanitary control regulations were even more strictly enforced in these units, and mothers were not transferred with their babies. Mothers could visit their babies at set hours and for limited times but were provided with few comforts or freedoms (such as chairs to sit on in the newborn nurseries or opportunities to pick up and hold their babies or to even feed them by bottle or breast). Mothers were encouraged to bring expressed breastmilk for their babies, but little assistance was given on how, or how often, to express this milk. Few were expected or were indeed able to successfully develop or maintain an adequate milk supply, and most NICU babies were fed locally produced cow's milk–based substitutes prepared by milk kitchens in the hospital or local community. Information about their baby's progress was reputedly difficult to obtain, with contact between the mother and her infant's neonatologist being limited to a fixed-time appointment each week.

Changes

Many changes are being introduced following the reform programmes initiated by international aid agencies such as UNICEF and WHO.

> Although change occurred slowly across the region after the collapse of the former Soviet Union in 1989, some changes happened so quickly as to be breathtaking. Sometimes, in our training programmes, we would discuss alternate approaches to delivery, such as using an upright position of the mother for delivery or delivery in a hands and knees position. It was not uncommon to find that caregivers had tried the new approach overnight when returning to class the following day. We quickly learned to be careful about what changes we advocated, knowing that these might be applied immediately, without further training or forethought.

These five examples of culturally diverse perinatal practices among the Aboriginal peoples of Canada, women with experience of FGM, South African Black women, Hindu and Muslim Indian women and women giving birth in Central and Eastern Europe or Central Asia highlight the importance of recognizing cultural diversity. They are by no means representative of varying cultural practices or exhaustive of them. They emphasize the importance of understanding and exploring the background and cultural practices of women that caregivers may encounter in their practices. They also emphasize the value of understanding women's knowledge, expectations and perceptions when providing perinatal care so as to incorporate a truly family-centred approach.

Key Points

- The world is increasingly multi-cultural, revealing diversity of ethnic origin, religion, race and language. Cultures differ significantly in their beliefs regarding health and illness, as well as in their attitudes and practices regarding childbearing.
- Childbirth is the greatest leveller we have; we are all equal in this experience.
- There are significant variations in birth practices based on cultural, economic, social, religious and medical factors. Examples of these variations in five differing cultures from four continents are provided. Their differences highlight the importance of understanding the psychological, social and cultural background of women in addition to caring for their physiological needs.

Is There a 'Universally Ideal Birth'?

Principles:
- Care is culturally sensitive and informed.
- Care is individualized to meet each family's needs.

Overview

Sensitivity is called for when caring for multi-cultural differences within any one society as well as when working in countries or cultures beyond one's own borders. This chapter challenges the concept of seeking a universal 'best' approach to perinatal care and proposes advocating instead that we should acknowledge the universal needs of women that may require differing but culturally appropriate perinatal practices to satisfy them.[1]

Outline

Maslow's Hierarchy Applied to Birth

Challenges to Working with Childbearing in Different Cultures

Many writers have sought to determine an ideal approach to birth for all women.[2] The assumption that their way is the best way is implicit in any country's educational system regarding maternity care and every caregiver's practice. What, then, is the 'right' way to `do' birth? Until recently, Eastern European doctors and mothers were convinced that their doctor-centred, highly medicalized approach offered the best deal. Their Northern European counterparts regard midwifery attendance as superior, whereas rural African women respect traditional birth attendants. Who has the right to say which approach is best? Does a supposedly universal approach to birth apply equally in rural settings as it does in urban homes and modern tertiary care centres?

The variable nature of the birth experience makes seeking a universal formula for birth meaningless. Nevertheless, it may be possible to highlight *universal needs of women* in childbirth rather than *universal means of satisfying them*.[3] By using a framework of need hierarchies, such as that proposed by Maslow,[4] we can pinpoint universal needs of women in birth.

Maslow's Hierarchy Applied to Birth

It has been many decades since Maslow proposed his five levels of human motivation and their hierarchical nature. Since then, they have been enthusiastically debated, and although remaining controversial, they provide an interesting framework within which to consider women's needs in childbearing. These needs – physiological, safety, love/belonging, self-esteem and self-actualisation – are discussed in turn in relation to pregnancy, birth and parenthood.

Application of Maslow's theory suggests that, firstly, physiological and safety needs are universal.[5] In Africa, these needs may be perceived by women to be met by birth in the grandmother's hut under the protection of the spirits who reside in the thatched eaves and with the assistance of a traditional midwife. In North America and Europe, most families and their caregivers believe that these needs will be met within a hospital setting assisted by physicians. For others, the safest birthplace may be at home, attended by a midwife. Within each of these cultural groups, maternity care is directly focussed on ensuring the woman's (and her baby's) physiological survival needs within the context of her particular surroundings. Caregivers need to be aware of what factors will contribute to the woman's and family's psychological and emotional needs for safety during birth and must explore this issue with their clients long before birth.

Maslow's next level of need involves emotional needs for love and support. These too are universal, but what is seen as supportive varies from culture to culture and woman to woman.[6] Among some African women, the traditional birth attendant is valued, although the husband is not; for many Western women, the husband is essential; and for women in Eastern Europe, the medical professional is regarded as appropriate, with husbands usually excluded from birth – although this is changing. Sensitive and supportive care from caregivers contributes to meeting this need. Caregivers need to explore whom the woman would choose to have with her in childbirth and to fulfil this need as far as possible. Companions and caregivers at birth need to provide reassurance, praise and support for women throughout the process of giving birth.

> When conducting one of the earliest randomized, controlled trials of the value of a supportive companion during labour, we asked laywomen with no special training in childbirth but who liked the idea of sitting with a woman in labour to stay with a randomly allocated woman continuously during labour and until the first hour after delivery. Their only role was to provide comfort, reassurance and praise for women through touch and speech. The outcomes of this study were stunning, with supported women experiencing less anxiety during labour and better adjustment to parenthood and infant feeding.[7]

The need for self-esteem is also universal.[8] Motherhood confers status and esteem on most women. Sometimes motherhood is the exclusive means for achieving status in society, as in many places in Africa or India. At other times, motherhood is only one of the means of gaining esteem, as in most Western countries. How well women believe that they have accomplished pregnancy, birth and parenthood is partly determined by societal or cultural role expectations, for example, having a male baby as is often preferred among Indian and Chinese women, giving birth without pain relief among natural birth advocates or, alternatively, with a high degree of pharmacological pain management in other circles. The woman's self-esteem is influenced by how closely she can approximate the 'good mother' image, whatever that may be, within her own culture. For example, daily behaviours can elicit 'shame' for pregnant women, such as not breastfeeding or eating 'take-out' (perceived as unhealthy) too often during pregnancy.

Preserving dignity and privacy in labour is also a universal aspect of women's needs for self-esteem.

In many parts of the world, exposing women's intimate bodily parts is shameful and experienced as embarrassing. Yet, in hospital, this concern is discarded under the license of medical care. Exposing women in labour and birth and ignoring needs for privacy are commonplace in many countries, where delivery rooms and postpartum wards often have glass windows and doors so that staff may easily observe women from adjacent passages. Some justify this exposure by claiming that 'modern' women are more open about nudity so that the impact of exposure on a woman's self-esteem during birth is minimal. There is, however, a vast difference between what women choose to say and do regarding nudity as opposed to what is done to them by others.[9]

Caregivers also need to recognize that birth may not always go the way a woman had hoped and that feelings of disappointment regarding their experiences may well occur. Acknowledging these and assisting the woman to find an explanation for what happened, after birth, may be important and necessary to help her regain her self-esteem. It is never easy to accept that one's body did not perform as well as one would have liked, especially if this is the first time that it has 'let one down'. Understanding that not everything about birth (or the baby and caregiver) is under the woman's control may go a long way towards helping the woman accept what has happened during her pregnancy and birth.

Achieving self-actualization though childbirth is a complex concept. Giving birth is for many, if not most, women a high point in their lives. Many would wish to achieve feelings of fulfilment, pride, inner strength and self-validation through the experience. For some, these feelings emerge; for others, birth can be a disappointment and be psychologically painful. Self-actualization, however, is a uniquely individual experience of self-fulfilment and is not amenable to generalizations that are applicable to all women. Nevertheless, it remains an important need that is acknowledged in the West by the number of societies, organizations and websites that are aimed at helping women achieve feelings of accomplishment through birth.[10] These include the International Childbirth Education Association and Lamaze International in the United States, the National Childbirth Trust in the United Kingdom, the Association for Childbirth and Parenting of Southern Africa and the European-based International Society for Psychosomatic Obstetrics and Gynaecology, among others. Such associations provide recognition for and assistance with the achievement of self-actualization through birth.

Challenges to Working with Childbearing in Different Cultures

Cross-cultural challenges regarding perinatal care occur both when caring for women from different countries who live in our own country and when working in countries other than our own. Both of these will be discussed.

Accommodating Different Cultural Needs within Our Own Society

There are many pitfalls to be avoided when attending to women from different cultural groups than the dominant culture in our own countries. Language differences combined with status inequalities may make it difficult for foreigners' healthcare needs to be met or, indeed, understood in their adopted country.[11] Assistance with translation, at least, is essential. Although this is a necessary first step, the intimate nature of maternity care provides a particular challenge for translators. Expecting children in the family to translate – as they are often the first to acquire a new language – is inappropriate.[12] The partner – who in many cultures plays no part during pregnancy and/or birth – may also be unacceptable. Making sure that the client's physical symptoms are discussed (which itself may be an unacceptable diagnostic procedure, such as in some traditional African cultures[13]) or that the elements of the treatment procedures are understood is challenging but is only the minimum level of communication needed. Greater understanding of the woman's culturally determined needs – perhaps along the lines that Maslow outlined – should also be discussed. Community members can facilitate translation and communication, and written information sheets can sometimes be helpful.

Sensitivity and tolerance are needed when considering traditional practices (such as wearing protective amulets during birthing or traditional methods of disposal of the placenta), and such practices should be encouraged unless they are evaluated as harmful, such as Female Genital Mutilation (FGM).[14] Condemning or disallowing such practices because they are different is inappropriate, for although they may not contribute to biological health (in the caregiver's eyes), they might be essential for psychological well-being. They should be evaluated as biologically beneficial, neither beneficial nor harmful, or harmful. Only the latter forms of traditional care (e.g. giving newborns honey or rubbing ash, dung or oil on the severed umbilical stump) need to be discouraged. Overcoming distrust in different cultural practices is difficult. While many are willing to tolerate these practices, understanding them may not occur, and silent disapproval may well be expressed non-verbally and be abundantly clear.

> In African women, it is customary to tie a piece of string, cut from the same ball, around the abdomen of all family members when one of them leaves home, providing spiritual continuity when separated. In pregnancy, ignorant of its psychological role, Western doctors may remove the string in labour as it is 'dirty', causing immense distress at a particularly vulnerable time.
>
> This is not unique to traditional African women. In the Western world, an item of jewellery or other personal trinket – in my case, a necklace holding a set of charms given to me by each member of my family when I first began to travel extensively – may be carried as a symbol of connectedness with loved ones, and the wearer may be reluctant to remove this in times of stress – or childbearing. Similarly, religious symbols – such as a crucifix – may take on protective meaning for some women and will be relinquished with reluctance, leaving the woman feeling somewhat insecure.

Even when cultural practices are regarded as harmful, caregivers still need to be sensitive when caring for women for whom the practices have meaning. For example, women from countries where FGM is normal practice may be convinced that caesarean section means death. In many of their countries of origin, admission to hospital only occurs after prolonged labour and frequently results in death. Particularly supportive care needs to be provided rather than brusquely discounting fears or simply ignoring the issue altogether though ignorance.

Providing for the spiritual needs of clients, concurrently with physiological needs, is both possible and beneficial.[15] In South Africa, physicians were advised to encourage traditionally oriented clients who feared surgery to seek the blessing of their *sangoma* ('traditional healer') before entering hospital. Conviction that surgery kills does little to support recovery. Praying for one's own or another's recovery is also a global practice.

Healthcare services that cater to multi-cultural clientele need to develop innovative approaches to incorporate these needs into their healthcare services.[16] Encouraging healthcare facilities to offer clients contact with others of a similar cultural background and similar healthcare needs may provide a stronger voice for the expression of these needs to the healthcare authorities. Establishing contact with local community groups and liaison through cultural representatives are other possibilities to explore to provide mutually beneficial, two-way information exchanges. Alternative and/or complementary treatment paradigms should be considered in addition to the Western pharmacopoeia. Finally, it is essential to monitor how well the health needs of clients are being met. This monitoring may involve formal research using techniques such as focus group discussions or survey type assessments and should be an integral and continuous part of the healthcare services offered.[17]

International Perinatal Health Consulting: Working in Other Countries

Numerous difficulties are involved in working with childbirth across cultures.[18] One of these is the obvious and often difficult-to-avoid problem of seeing things through the eyes of one's own culture and judging all others as inferior instead of different.

A second difficulty emerges when trying to assess – usually through research – which approach is clinically 'better'.[19] Western evaluations call for 'scientific facts' when trying to determine which birth practices are most beneficial. Yet data regarding the outcome of birthing procedures in different countries are, unfortunately, not often available and, when they are, may not always be reliable. Records may be hand written and filed, and data aggregation is done manually, slowly and sometimes inaccurately. Less 'hard science' evidence of birth outcomes, such as assessments of patient satisfaction, are not routinely collected in most parts of the world due partly to the challenges of doing so but more often because women's opinions are valued less than clinical indicators. In addition, many of the so-called safe birth practices of Western medicine (e.g. routine, continuous, fetal heart monitoring, induction, epidurals, routine multiple ultrasound scanning, caesarean sections and the lithotomy position for birth) have come under fire from evidence-based studies. What was regarded as good practice is now being discarded as harmful in the light of evidence-based research. What practices should then be used to assess appropriate birth procedures?

Working in the international cross-cultural milieu has raised a number of academic and ethical challenges for me. Questions such as what right do we have to suggest that our or an alternate healthcare system is superior to one already in place in a country in which we consult? How can we assess that what we offer is appropriate for our host country? Could we actually do harm by transforming one system of care into another? How do we avoid the ethical issue of coercion when offering suggestions for alternate systems of care to a country when this advice is offered in the name of international agencies such as the World Health Organization (WHO) or the United Nations Children's Fund (UNICEF) or when it is associated with benefits such as educational opportunities? There are no easy answers to these questions other than to remain sensitive to the implications of our work at all times.

A third difficulty arises in that sophisticated technology may be used inappropriately.[20] Is a 'half-baked' application of Western technology at times more harmful than the traditional way? For example, in parts of Eastern Europe, routine prenatal ultrasound is now available. Research evidence suggests that, on a routine basis, multiple screening is probably not beneficial for mother or baby or cost-effective and that if used at all, one or two routine scans is all that could reasonably be routinely justified. Indicated scanning is, of course, not questioned by this research. In Eastern Europe, however, multiple screening is usually introduced as soon as equipment becomes available, with screening even being done at every prenatal visit. Combined with insufficiently skilled technicians and poor-quality equipment, this misapplication may lead to unnecessary or harmful interventions. Even in Canada, with its high regard for evidence-based clinical care and at a time when only one routine ultrasound was recommended in clinical care, women surveyed by the Maternity Experiences Survey reported an average of three scans during pregnancy.[21]

In our efforts to reform other countries' health practices, we may not readily recognize what aspects of their systems are good and may be even better than our own. For example, some former Soviet practices such as the immensely supportive systematic postpartum follow-up of infants (called 'patronage') was most beneficial not only for its clinical usefulness but also for the psychological support it gave parents.[22] The Western birth environment often leaves this aspect of maternal-child care less well attended, and the Eastern European model could be of value for other countries. Yet this system was dismantled in the rapid overhaul of Soviet healthcare system – with Western assistance – in the 1990s. Simultaneously, specialist paediatricians were forced to retrain as family doctors – a 'missing' category of healthcare provider under the Soviet Union – resulting in intense dissatisfaction among these now 'demoted' caregivers. Local dissatisfaction with this change was not heeded. The 'gung-ho' imposition of our 'superior' models of care on this culture was, at times, breathtaking and potentially harmful.

Local voices must be heard and attended to when making recommendations for changing birth practices. How often is lip service paid to this? How easy is it to influence countries in the name of science and with the authority attributed to the 'foreign expert', especially if wearing a WHO or other United Nations agency hat? How often, too, are practices changed only because locals wish to gain prestige (and income) through collaboration with international consultants?

During my numerous visits to various countries, I often observed how tempting it was for locals to introduce changes that were advocated because their collaboration with 'international experts' enhanced their prestige or their pockets. Sometimes this was harmful, such as distributing free formula samples to new mothers on behalf of international formula industries in return for personal gains. While appearing to be a magnanimous gesture, this action virtually ensured that mothers would fail to breastfeed successfully if they used the product.

Which practices are regarded as harmful, harmless or beneficial also have to be judged against the alternatives that are available in any community.[23] For example, in countries where tight swaddling of babies from head to toe was practiced, we advocated abandoning such swaddling and providing skin-to-skin contact to promote breastfeeding. Although our advice was followed and the tight swaddling was removed, it was replaced by thick towelling bandages around the infant's neck to support the newborn's head, as a 'floppy' baby's head (never seen when babies' heads were tightly swaddled) was regarded as pathological. In addition, our advice created a need for infant clothing – not available in these countries – as they had hitherto not been necessary. Finding the right balance between encouraging practices that are potentially harmless or beneficial and discouraging those that are truly dangerous can be challenging![24]

Cross-cultural misunderstandings also present challenges.[25] Translators vary in quality and do not always understand your perspective. For example, when I was working with a colleague in St Petersburg, we entered a WHO-Euro promoted teenage healthcare centre. We were met with a print of the famous Leonardo da Vinci *Madonna and Child*, the original of which has pride of place in the city's Hermitage Museum. My colleague, the late Marsden Wagner (then regional advisor for maternal and child health in the WHO's Regional Office for Europe) was proudly shown this picture and told that it had been introduced in response to his suggestion, made months earlier, to liven up the walls: to make the place more attractive to teenagers by decorating it with pictures of 'Madonna.' Cross-cultural misunderstandings do occur but are not always as harmless or humorous as this.

We have much to learn about how best to work when striving to improve birth globally.[26] The challenge is to find out how to satisfy the childbirth needs of women and their families within the women's own cultural groups. Simply applying what 'works' in one's own family and culture may be inappropriate and unacceptable in another, such as, for example, when we eradicated swaddling practices. Misuse of technologies also may occur. For example, abuse of prenatal ultrasound with consequent termination of female fetuses in countries such as China and India is increasingly prevalent. The resulting gender imbalance is already leading to crimes of kidnapping, child brides and the sale of increasingly scarce women.[27]

Some well-intentioned international consultants donated 'snugglies' (soft padded surrounds for naked NICU babies) to replace the practice of swaddling those babies in incubators in Eastern Europe. We arrived some time later and were proudly shown the tightly swaddled babies lying peacefully in the centre of the 'snugglies' in the incubators, but far from their padded, comforting edges.

Part of successful inter-cultural integration lies in the need to specify similarities, rather than concentrate on differences, between groups.[28] Although emphasizing differences in childbearing practices in different cultures may be academically interesting, of far more importance, from a healthcare perspective, is the need to determine the similarities within cultures, such as the shared needs of all women who give birth.

Some principles of international health consulting may serve to inform better family-centred caregivers who work with women from differing cultural backgrounds within their own society or who encounter women from different backgrounds when working in other countries.[29] These include

- Recognizing whose needs are being met by practices proposed – those of the woman and her family or those of the caregiver;
- Providing a collaborative approach to care that involves the woman and her family in decision-making about her care;
- Being flexible about clinical care guidelines so as to offer individualized care that suits the woman's particular cultural background but still complies with evidence-based recommendations;
- Acknowledging that some of the women's or their families' wishes may, at times, offer better options than those of the caregiver;
- Remaining sensitive to cultural differences;
- Providing respectful care;
- Ensuring that caregiving advice is sustainable by the woman and her family (and not, for example, too costly for her economic situation or too contradictory to her cultural practices);
- Following up on caregiving advice to assess compliance/agreement;
- Offering a holistic approach to care and not simply biologically based advice;
- Removing social barriers to collaboration such as following acceptable dress codes;
- Fostering a trusting and honest caregiving relationship; and remaining committed to the care of the woman and her family within their cultural framework.[30]

These characteristics of care are essential not only for inter-cultural care but also for care provided for all women and their families.

> Following acceptable dress codes in order to be acceptable to women of differing cultural practices from one's own is often necessary, even if challenging. While working in Tajikistan in an Islamic fundamentalist community, it was essential for me to wear long-sleeved clothing, full-length dresses and head coverings at all times. The women on our team also had to be sure that they never moved out of our Médecins Sans Frontières 'safe house', where we lived during our mission, without a male escort, for fear of being stoned by clearly evident elders who were watching our street and house. Whether one agrees with these restrictions or not is irrelevant if one wants to be effective in providing healthcare advice.

The need for respect, dignity, self-esteem and emotional support during pregnancy and particularly during childbirth is universal. How these needs are met during childbearing can vary from culture to culture and is linked to such issues as privacy, decision-making responsibility and continuity of care. Discerning what healthcare services and practices could enhance each woman's reaction to birth within the confines of a 'safe' birth and her culturally determined expectations is the challenge faced by today's caregivers.

Key Points

- There is no universal 'best' approach to perinatal care.
- It is possible to highlight *universal needs of women* in childbirth rather than *universal means of satisfying them* using Maslow's model of a need hierarchy.
- Cross-cultural challenges regarding perinatal care occur both when caring for women from different countries who live in our own country and when working in countries other than our own.
- Some principles of international health consulting may serve to inform better family-centred caregivers serving differing cultural groups.

Part IV

Meeting Professional Standards

12 Abuse in Obstetric and Gynaecological Care

Principle:
- Care is always non-abusive.

Overview

In recent decades, we have recognized the reality of violence and abuse in our world to the extent that measures of violence (towards children, women and men) have been incorporated into United Nations agencies' healthcare indicators.[1] The incidence of violence against women and children far exceeds our previous expectations and provides a shocking reminder of the progress that we have yet to make in providing a respectful and healthy social environment. This concern is global. This abuse also occurs in perinatal and gynaecological care.

Outline

Sexual, Physical and Emotional Abuse of Women and Obstetric Care
Obstetric Care Procedures May Be Abusive
Gynaecological Procedures May Be Abusive
Emotional Abuse of Women by Caregivers
Abusive Clinical Treatment without Women's Knowledge
Politics and Pregnancy Care
Abusing Social Determinants of Health
Factors Contributing to Abuse

The US Agency for International Development Translating Research into Action (USAID-TRAction) Project conducted by Harvard University School of Public Health identifies seven categories of disrespect and abuse that may and do occur in the perinatal period in a number of countries worldwide. These include physical abuse, non-consensual care, non-confidential care, non-dignified care, discrimination based on specific patient attributes, abandonment of care and detention in facilities.[2] Physical, sexual and emotional abuse may all occur. More recently, a mixed-methods systematic review has led to the establishment of seven categories of abusive or disrespectful care of women during childbirth. These include physical abuse, sexual abuse, verbal abuse, stigma and discrimination, failure to meet professional standards of care, poor rapport between women and providers and health system conditions and constraints.[3]

Sexual, Physical and Emotional Abuse of Women and Obstetric Care

According to a 2013 United Nations global review of available data, 35% of women worldwide have experienced either physical and/or sexual violence. In some countries, this figure rises to 70%.[4] The implications of previous experience of violence, whether sexual, physical or emotional, for obstetric and gynaecological care are more significant than for other areas of healthcare.[5] Sexual violence has obvious ramifications given that the same bodily parts are involved. Memories of physical violence may be aroused through the intimacy of gynaecological or obstetric examinations and procedures, and for this reason, we should heed any male or female caregiver preference. Knowledge of the women's past experience should temper how we touch women, what preparation we give them for obstetric examinations, what supports they might need to cope with such contacts and what advice we give. A caregiver's ability to sensitively probe for such past traumas and to provide appropriate support for women with these experiences may be enhanced by the use of such instruments as the 'Antenatal Psycho-Social Health Assessment Tool' (ALPHA),[6] which explores psychological and social issues that give rise to stress in pregnancy as well as their associated negative obstetric outcomes.

Admitting to and discussing sexual, physical or emotional abuse are difficult for any woman despite many societies' (but not all) increasing recognition and condemnation of such acts.[7] In cultures where such actions are regarded by society as a normal or expected part of life, women have even less chance of being heard sympathetically. Some countries, such as India, are currently struggling to deal with such views. In either setting, we need to protect the confidentiality of such information, once revealed. This results in difficulties regarding the sharing of information with additional caregivers who need to be aware of the woman's past experiences and the importance of not simply recording this information on charts where it is available for indiscriminate inspection. It is necessary to discuss this concern with women and to agree on what information we can share, with whom, and whether verbally or through written documentation. Many cultures and countries are reluctant to address the embarrassing issue of family violence and abuse directly. Few have implemented effective training programmes for medical and allied healthcare workers to assist them to deal with the abusive experiences of their clients, such as that described by the Public Health Agency of Canada.[8] Even fewer have considered that their own practices may add to that abuse. It is past time to do so.

Obstetric Care Procedures May Be Abusive

Although abusive social situations are increasingly recognized and exposed, there are also situations that women regard as abusive but which are, or were at the time of their experience, considered necessary or beneficial by caregivers.[9] We can classify some aspects of standard obstetric care as practiced in some technologically advanced societies and in parts of the developing world as violence against women. Those procedures are, and have been, usually performed with the best interests of the woman in mind and supported by the available scientific evidence of the time. Regardless of the best intentions of the caregivers, they are abusive. These practices include routine episiotomy, repair of minor perineal lacerations, lack of appropriate anaesthesia or analgesia for such perineal procedures, exploration of the uterus or exteriorization and visualization of the cervix following vaginal delivery, swabbing of the vagina with antiseptic after birth, anal exploration after delivery, and less painful procedures such as routine perineal and pubic shaving and enemas during labour. Even the embarrassing lithotomy position with its emotional and physical associations of helplessness and loss of control for the woman, as well as its clinically blatant exposure of psychologically and socially private body parts, may be regarded as abusive by women. Today, not being allowed to have a companion during labour and birth may be regarded as abusive. In South Africa, in 2007, 84.5% of women were not allowed to have companions in childbirth.[10] In Brazil, in 2008, 41.8% of women were not allowed to have a companion for labour and 98.6% for delivery.[11] Whereas these were accepted and beneficially regarded obstetric routines some time ago, they are no longer supported by evidence.[12] In many developed societies, these practices fortunately have been discontinued, although not completely and not everywhere.[13]

> I have frequently observed outdated and abusive obstetric care practices. Women sometimes emerge from their birth experiences wishing to 'never have another child again' or to 'never go through such an experience again'. Many times they appear physically battered after birth, with extremely painful perineal areas resulting from deep and extensive episiotomies which preclude sitting for some days or even weeks, combined with perineal bruising from excessive manual stretching of the perineum during the second stage of labour, and with extensive bruising of their arms from intravenous lines. Pale and sore, they lie unmoving for hours after birth. I have, however, never met a perinatal healthcare provider who wished to harm his or her patients. Such abusive care, at least in the dozens of countries I have worked in, was based on the best available knowledge of caregivers at that time. Inadequate or out-of-date knowledge; a lack of concern for the perspectives or rights of women; a lack of respect for their dignity, privacy and confidentiality; and inadequate financial resources were characteristics that I associated with abusive care whenever I observed it.

Widespread lack of informed consent for common procedures occurring at the time of birth (non-consensual care), such as for episiotomies, hysterectomies, blood transfusions, sterilization, augmentation of labour and even caesarean sections, have also been reported in many childbirth settings, with some women reporting lack of patient-doctor confidentiality.[14] Many women report painful and frequent vaginal examinations in labour, sometimes conducted in non-private settings, and withholding of pain relief.[15] Others have reported being neglected or ignored in labour (and even at delivery), having long wait times, being 'punished' for not booking prior to delivery, having 'rushed' care and feeling that they were 'bothering' or 'putting the caregiver out'. Women often report inadequate explanations about potential complications or impending delivery and that these explanations were often rushed if provided at all.[16]

Worse still is the blatant physical abuse and non-dignified care of women during labour and birth in a number of countries through, for example, hitting or slapping with an open hand or instrument; pinching, particularly on the thighs; kicking, shouting at, or scolding the mother; exerting excessive pressure on her abdomen to get the baby out; performing episiotomies or other procedures, sometimes for financial gain; repairing episiotomies without pain relief; or even tying the woman down during labour or using mouth gags.[17]

In Southern Sudan, I was present with a woman entering the second stage of labour in a local rural clinic being attended by a Sudanese, Western-trained healthcare provider/midwife. The recumbent woman struggled to lift herself into a seated position only to be pushed down onto the delivery bed and told to lie flat. This series of movements was repeated a few times, with the caregiver forcibly pushing the woman down each time. Ignorant of the benefits of an upright position for birth and disdainful of traditional upright delivery positions, this aggressive and inappropriate care was clearly the result of poor training combined with a lack of respect for the birthing woman's needs.

Verbal abuse of women in childbirth is also reported. This includes the use of harsh or rude language, judgemental statements, threats of poor outcomes or withholding treatment if women were noncompliant, most commonly from midwives and nurses and less often from doctors. Women from lower socio-economic groups, migrants, those from ethnic minorities, adolescents and older mothers of high parity report discriminatory care.[18] The words most commonly used by women to describe the verbal abuse they experience include 'rude, harsh language, sarcasm, swear, snap at, mock, threaten, scold, scream/yell/shout/raise voice, degrade, belittle, dehumanize, intimidate, ridicule, name-calling, humiliate and insult', reflecting the wide array of disrespectful treatment provided for these women.[19]

Sexual abuse during labour has also emerged from Kenya, where a male healthcare provider examined a woman in labour forcefully while touching his own genitals, roughly pulling her legs apart and repeatedly shoving his fingers into her vagina.[20] In Nigeria, sexual abuse of women by a healthcare worker is reported by 2% of women.[21]

A further abusive practice involves the payment of bribes to doctors, nurses, midwives, receptionists and guards. These bribes take the form of money, food or drinks, jewellery or other gifts and are expected in many countries around the world. Women believe that such payments ensured better care, more timely care or the provision of medications.

In my international perinatal care work, I have frequently encountered the expectation for women to pay bribes for 'better care'. In many cases these payments ensured the availability of pain-relieving medications for labour and birth and even for the repair of episiotomies or perineal tears, the use of private rooms, access to water births and care from more senior members of the healthcare facility. In some cases, such payments ensured cleaning of the women's rooms. 'Private' hospitals have emerged that offer such services – often basic clinical care practices – for (large) fees, thus, in a sense, formalizing the informal bribery system. While 'luxury' care (e.g. more comfortable rooms, better food or a choice of meals and private TVs) can perhaps be viewed as justifying private payment systems, the provision of standard evidence-based care that is essential good clinical practice should never warrant special bribes, as frequently occurs.

Recognition of such abuse is growing, albeit slowly. Venezuela, for example, in 2007 published a new 'Organic Law on the Right of Women to Be Free from Violence' that addresses violence in the obstetric care setting.[22] The law defines obstetric violence as 'the appropriation of the body and reproductive processes of women by health personnel, which is expressed as dehumanized treatment, an abuse of medication, and to convert the natural processes into pathological ones, bringing with it loss of autonomy and the ability to decide freely about their bodies and sexuality, negatively impacting the quality of life of women'.[23] According to this act, obstetric violence includes

- Untimely and ineffective attention to obstetric emergencies;
- Forcing the woman to give birth in a supine position, with legs raised, when the necessary means to perform a vertical delivery are available;
- Impeding the early attachment of the newborn with his or her mother without medical cause, thus preventing early attachment and the possibility of holding, nursing or breastfeeding immediately after birth;
- Altering the natural process of low-risk delivery by using acceleration techniques without obtaining voluntary, expressed and informed consent of the woman.
- Performing delivery via caesarean section when natural childbirth is possible without obtaining voluntary, expressed, and informed consent from the woman.

Gynaecological Procedures May Be Abusive

Also of importance worldwide is that most of the women who experience abusive birth procedures are still in their reproductive years and continue to require obstetric care for future pregnancies, as well as gynaecological care between pregnancies and after their childbearing years.[24] In particular, gynaecological procedures (which are not accompanied by the positive experience of a baby emerging from all the 'unpleasant' medical procedures) may evoke traumatic memories of medical encounters during earlier births. The gynaecologist needs to remain alert and sensitive to such background experiences. While these issues are not explored in depth here, they are touched on to acknowledge their importance in this context.

It would be valuable to explore alternate methods of conducting vaginal procedures, thereby reducing the psychological stress of pelvic examinations and avoiding the emotional trauma that can be evoked through memories of personal or healthcare-related abuse experienced by some women.[25] Whereas obstetric care is moving towards a more sensitive approach to care, gynaecological procedures have generally escaped criticism. In preference to intimate examinations, non-invasive techniques of diagnosis should be explored and developed. Alternatives to the lithotomy position for vaginal examination are desirable. We sorely need exploration of what would make women's experiences of vaginal procedures more palatable. For instance, simple changes such as conducting routine examinations while standing at the woman's side with her legs bent and feet resting on the bed rather than with the caregiver seated directly opposite her splayed legs in a lithotomy position may be far less embarrassing and exposing and much more acceptable.[26]

In South Africa, while I was working at Chris Hani (formerly Baragwanath) Hospital in Soweto, I shared obstetrics education for fourth- and sixth-year medical students at the University of the Witwatersrand with an obstetrician, Dr James McIntyre. We routinely expected our students to role-play the part of a pregnant woman or a woman in labour, requiring them to assume a lithotomy position with their legs in stirrups – while remaining fully dressed. A second student acted the doctor's role.

> Student reflections on their emotions during this role-play revealed embarrassment, powerlessness, vulnerability and fear – a worthwhile exposure for them that led to far greater sensitivity regarding women's experiences during care.[27]

Emotional Abuse of Women by Caregivers

Whereas clinical procedures may inflict painful experiences on women during pregnancy and birth, other actions may be psychologically abusive. Lack of respect for a woman's dignity, privacy and confidentiality may result in emotional abuse and non-dignified care and is a commonly reported theme from many women around the world.[28] Non-confidential care related to sensitive patient information such as human immunodeficiency virus/acquired immunodeficiency virus syndrome (HIV/AIDS) status, age, marital status or medical history increases the women's likelihood of discriminatory care and may deter her from using healthcare facility care in the future.[29] Failure of a physician to provide a follow-up visit for a woman following assisting with her delivery (leaving this to midwives or nurses) may engender a feeling of her unimportance (together with a lack of respect for her doctor!). Avoiding women or minimizing contact with them following adverse pregnancy outcomes (again leaving this to midwives or nurses) is simply unacceptable – and at times – cowardly. Reports from South Africa, Ghana, Sierra Leone, Kenya, Africa, Brazil and India indicate that some caregivers abandon women, leaving them to labour and give birth alone.[30]

Abusive Clinical Treatment without Women's Knowledge

Unwelcome to acknowledge, as it may seem almost unbelievable, is the increasing recognition that doctors sometimes 'behave badly' in operating theatres.[31] Comments passed and actions taken when a woman is anaesthetized may be 'inappropriate and disrespectful of patients, harmful to students, and derogatory towards colleagues'. In 2015, the *Annals of Internal Medicine* published an anonymous account of such behaviours, including the attending physician's comment, while swabbing a woman's labia and inner thighs prior to a vaginal hysterectomy, that 'I bet she's enjoying this.'[32] Other inappropriate and derogatory, sometimes racist comments may be made and are often not countered by embarrassed – and often junior – colleagues. Singh and Posner also reported hearing openly homophobic, anti-Semitic and sexually charged comments in the operating theatres with little done to stop them.[33] As they advised, 'If you wouldn't say it with the patient awake and your mother in the room, don't say it.'[34] As they noted, the patient should be cared for with the utmost respect whether awake or asleep. There is, for example, no place to undertake pelvic examinations in the operating theatre for the purpose of instruction without the patient's prior knowledge and consent. It is up to caregivers themselves to assume responsibility for ending such bad and abusive behaviours.

Politics and Pregnancy Care

Political systems play a significant role in determining whether childbirth is supportive or abusive of mothers and their families. There are myriad examples of how political systems have abused childbearing women, including among Black women in South Africa under Apartheid, women giving birth in the former Soviet Union under Communist rule, women growing up in societies that practice Female Genital Mutilation (FGM), often believed to be religiously required, and women in genocidal situations including Cambodia, Rwanda and other current African conflict zones where rape is increasingly used as a weapon of war with its traumatic consequences for childbearing and rearing.[35] Horrific medical experimentation on reproduction, childbearing and sexuality was a distinct policy under Nazi rule in its efforts to either eliminate the Jewish people and others deemed to be 'undesirable' or to promote reproduction among so-called Aryans that met Nazi-approved racial standards.[36] Sexuality, pregnancy, childbearing and newborn care were systematically abused during the Holocaust as well.[37] Less violent but also emotionally and physically abusive experiences face women in China living under a predominantly one-child-only political policy, although this is now changing.

Abusing Social Determinants of Health

For some decades now, we have been aware of the social determinants of health as contributors to perinatal outcomes. Poverty, however it is defined, is a major predictor of health outcomes. So too are related factors such as education, income, race and disability. Although these are important and essential societal-level factors, they are sometimes used to avoid individual responsibility in advocating for strengthening perinatal practices. It is far too easy for caregivers to relegate less than optimal outcomes among poorer women to their disadvantaged social situation instead of considering whether their care for these women has also been discriminatory and partially responsible for their health.

Although Western societies do not express this so openly, a similar prejudiced view emerges more subtly in practice. In Canada, for example, where perinatal care is among the best in the world and where equity in access to healthcare services is a matter of national pride, a recent cross-country survey reported that women with higher education and socio-economic levels were least likely to have shaves, enemas or pushing on their abdomens during delivery or to lie in a supine position for birth – in other words, practices that are not evidence-based.[38] This is an extremely concerning finding. Benchmark standards in these situations should be zero and, even if practiced, should not be discriminatory based on socio-economic factors.

In Mexico, too, planned caesarean sections are positively associated with years of schooling and a higher socio-economic status.[39] In some reports, women who have been unable to pay for their care have either had their newborns detained by the facility after birth or have themselves been detained until payment was made, weeks or even months later.[40] Discriminatory care based on social and personal characteristics of women such as economic status, age, education, HIV/AIDS status, race, obesity, immigrant status and traditional practices is deplorable.

Although an extremely sensitive issue, the question must be asked whether remuneration packages influence the use of technology and present a barrier to equitable family-centred care. No attempt is being made to level this accusation at any one or any group of practitioners through this book, although there is clear evidence to indicate that where fee-for-service remuneration packages are in place for caregivers, the rates of technological interventions increase. For example, surveyed obstetricians in South Africa acknowledged that some caesarean sections were performed for financial incentives.[41] In countries where both fee-for-service and salaried medical service structures co-exist, the technological intervention rate can be almost twice as high in fee-for-service systems. This occurs most frequently when there is private health insurance available to higher socio-economic groups compared with salaried-care services that often care for families at lower socio-economic levels.[42] It is obvious that where we financially reward caregivers for interventions, they, not surprisingly, intervene more.

We do not often examine social determinants of health as mediators of abusive obstetric practices, perhaps because it is unbelievable to think that such prejudices find outlet in practice or because they are too embarrassing to expose. Increasing attention to these concerns should be a central issue in current and future family-centred care.

Factors Contributing to Abuse

Abuse is inappropriate whether it is psycho-social, sexual, physical, emotional, financial or medical. Factors contributing to such abuse include the normalization of disrespect and abuse during labour as part of standard care, lack of community engagement and oversight, financial barriers, lack of women's empowerment or autonomy, lack of national laws and policies regarding human rights and ethics and lack of respect for some types of care providers.[43]

> In war-torn Southern Sudan, I asked a number of traditional birth attendants with whom I was working, if they could have any wish they wanted, what things they would most want to obtain, that would enable them to provide better care for women in childbirth? They agreed that the most important item was a uniform that others would recognise as a sign of their status so that they would be treated with respect. They also asked for rubber boots for wading through the mud caused by heavy summer rains to reach outlying women in labour and that would keep their uniforms clean and their appearance dignified. They clearly perceived their lack of status as an obstacle to their providing care for mothers. Years of international pressure to give birth in formal healthcare facilities rather than with the aid of traditional birth attendants has led locals to lose respect for traditional birth attendant women, who are frequently the only available healthcare provider in this huge, largely rural country.

Perinatal healthcare providers need to consider whether they are contributing to abuse or can play a role in ameliorating its impact. Strengthening healthcare provider training to facilitate care that is more respectful, shows increased awareness of psychological and social issues in childbearing, champions a rights-based approach to care and provides legal and accountability interventions is needed to reduce abuse during obstetric and gynaecological care.[44] The World Health Organization (WHO), in association with other United Nations aid agencies, has recently issued a statement endorsing the importance of preventing the mistreatment of women during childbirth and at the same time promoting their respectful care.[45] It is hoped that in their proposed future developments of standards and indicators of respectful care and interventions to reduce mistreatment, the needs of the family are considered and not only those of mothers.

Key Points

- The incidence of violence against women and children provides a shocking reminder of the progress that we have yet to make in providing a respectful and healthy social environment. This concern is global.
- Physical, psycho-social, sexual, financial, emotional and medical abuse all may occur during perinatal care.
- Some situations are regarded as abusive by women but are, or were at the time of their experience, considered necessary or beneficial by caregivers. In many developed societies, these practices have been discontinued, although not completely and not everywhere.
- Women who experience abusive birth procedures continue to require obstetric care for future pregnancies as well as gynaecological care between pregnancies and after their childbearing years. Their trust in caregivers may be lost.
- Lack of respect for a woman's dignity, privacy and confidentiality may result in emotional abuse: non-dignified care is reported commonly around the world.
- Comments passed and actions taken in the operating theatre when a woman is anaesthetized may be inappropriate and disrespectful of patients, harmful to students and derogatory towards colleagues.
- Political systems play a significant role in determining whether childbirth is supportive or abusive of mothers and their families.
- Discriminatory care based on social and personal characteristics of women occurs.
- Caregiver remuneration packages may influence the use of technology and present a barrier to equitable family-centred care.
- In some countries, 'under the table' payments lead to discriminatory care.
- Abuse is inappropriate whether it is psychological, social, sexual, emotional, physical, financial or medical.

Chapter 13

Monitoring, Evaluation and Research

Principle:
• Feedback from families is encouraged and facilitated and then is monitored and rigorously evaluated by caregivers and the healthcare facility.

Overview

An efficient system of national and regional perinatal data collection that is reliable, timely and standardized is necessary for effective monitoring and evaluation of perinatal care and the development of national guidelines for care. The challenges faced when collecting both clinical and psycho-social perinatal data globally, and nationally, are addressed. The use of such data for both health promotion and research is examined.

Outline

Perinatal Data Collection
Clinical and Psycho-Social Indicators
Local Data Collection
Health Promotion versus Health Research
Cultural Difficulties in Implementing Health Research
Conflicting Goals of Health Research and Health Promotion

The World Health Organization's (WHO's) European Regional Office maintains an ongoing database (Health for All Database[1]) that co-ordinates key indicators of health, including perinatal health, across all its member states. Although this is exceptionally valuable and provides a means of global inter-country comparison, as well as within-country progress over time, the vast health framework that is covered limits the number of indicators that can be followed, as well as the depth of inquiry that can be made into perinatal issues. Individual countries also retain ongoing data-collection systems that include perinatal indicators such as the Public Health Agency for Canada's Perinatal Surveillance System[2], the American Pregnancy Risk Assessment Monitoring System (PRAMS)[3] and the American Listening to Mothers[4] survey. Many, if not most, of these programmes need to expand their perinatal health surveillance coverage to give a broader understanding of family-centred perinatal care issues.

Perinatal Data Collection

A major challenge to national perinatal database collection is obtaining data in a timely fashion. Frequently data collected at the hospital level has to be collated and forwarded to regional authorities before being sent to national data-collection centres. The integration of these multiple sources of data is then required, together with validation that data submitted are accurate. This is often a lengthy process, resulting in data that is several years old being the most up-to-date available. Real-time data collection is still not the norm, although with an increasing application of web-based technology, assessment and integration of current perinatal events should become more accessible in the future. The Ontario, Canada, Better Outcomes Registry and Network (BORN) is a rapidly expanding perinatal monitoring system designed with this goal in mind.[5] In addition, databases vary from one centre or region to another, making integration of disparate measures difficult or impossible. The need for a nationally accepted perinatal data-collection method is obvious, even though reaching agreement across a country (and across the globe) as to just what indicators should be included and when they should be recorded is challenging.

Even when this is collected, the use and dissemination of national perinatal data are hindered by concerns for privacy of the information. The result may be that local planning services do not obtain the necessary information they need on which to base predictions of services needed, particularly when these refer to remote areas or infrequently occurring health events as such events must often be amalgamated with other information in the database to protect privacy. Rare events, that may require suppression, may be the most severe or life threatening and could be the most important to have available for evaluation and future preventive planning.

Data collection is open to corruption or manipulation. When conducting hospital assessments in some countries, I frequently asked to examine the monthly records of maternity hospital wards or other hospital records, particularly when I detected possible inconsistencies. In many places, records were hand written and frequencies amalgamated without any arithmetical aids such as calculators or computers. I frequently uncovered errors in these calculations when I checked them. I soon realized that such miscalculations may not have been always accidental. Hospital budgets were allocated to care for a fixed number of specific incidences. For example, 'pathological wards' were expected to have a certain number of women (or neonates) in them each month. If the records indicated that fewer pathologies had occurred than were anticipated, funding for these (often more lucrative wards) was cut. The result of this may have been a 'fudging' of numbers so that reports conformed to the expected standards set by the health authorities – hence the correct entry of cases into records but the incorrect totalling of some pathological incidences when these records were amalgamated. While I cannot prove that this did occur, certainly the temptation was there to encourage such misrepresentations. An alternative practice was to allocate 'physiological' ('normal') mothers and babies to pathological wards to ensure that the numbers looked 'appropriate'.

Clinical and Psycho-Social Indicators

The lesson that has been learned from analysis of the importance of social support in labour and birth lends urgent support to the need to develop psycho-social perinatal indicators. Outcomes of studies regarding labour support acknowledge the emotional, cognitive, social and cultural needs of parents as well as their biological/medical requirements. Perinatal data collection has, however, traditionally focussed on clinical events or practices. Psycho-social and cultural issues are not usually included in large-scale perinatal databases either routinely or even at all. However, data-monitoring approaches can, and should, contribute to family-centred care.

Some countries have occasionally conducted national surveys of women's experiences of their perinatal care through federal government agencies, for example, the Maternity Experiences Survey in Canada,[6] the US surveys of women's birth experiences encompassing about 78% of all births in the United States, the Pregnancy Risk Assessment Monitoring System (PRAMS)[7] and a number of surveys conducted in the United Kingdom.[8] Other countries have, at times, supported regional or local surveys of women's (and sometimes men's) experiences of their perinatal care.[9] Assessing women's (and sometimes men's[10]) satisfaction with their care is commonly a central focus of such surveys, although multiple issues, including clinical events, are usually explored.

> A follow-up survey, currently in progress, of published academic papers in response to the Canadian Maternity Experiences Survey of women's experiences and perceptions of their care, as well as application of the findings to healthcare policy developments, reveals that, to date, 57 peer-reviewed publications have been based on this survey and three Canadian healthcare policies have incorporated its findings. Clearly, such surveys are valuable sources of information for clinical and psycho-social perinatal care analysis.

Comparing perinatal practices across countries poses a number of challenges. Primary among these is that questionnaires used in each country/survey are different and not often comparable. Even when similar issues are explored, questions regarding them vary, as do methods of response analysis. In addition, the items not reported in these comparisons may be even more valuable to address than those that are included. For example, some interventions such as pushing on the top of the abdomen to help push the baby down in labour were only included in the Canadian and US surveys, where reported rates were, surprisingly, as high as 15 and 17%, respectively. No surveys included questions regarding routine cervical examination after birth or even exteriorizing the cervix for this purpose, as was widespread traditional practice some time ago and may or may not be continuing in some places. Nor were questions regarding routine sweeping of the membranes before or during labour or routine artificial rupture of the membranes commonly included in all surveys. Women's reactions to such practices were, consequently, also not examined. There is clearly a need for the development of a uniform international perinatal assessment process that includes a careful analysis of the family-centredness of this care from the perspective of women and their families.

The nature of issues that are addressed when comparing perinatal indicators across countries is a further concern. It is likely that agreement could be reached regarding traditionally measured indicators of clinical care. However, should we not be developing indicators of successful birthing beyond the biological level to include social, psychological and cultural implications? Can we adequately determine when technology is truly beneficial – in a family-centred and holistic sense - and when it leads to more harm than good when we do not often assess its psycho-social impact? Evaluating psycho-social and cultural issues in perinatal care is difficult, but this does not justify their omission. Given that many issues, particularly psycho-social issues, often cannot be addressed through randomized, controlled trials, how valuable is our current emphasis on such trials as the primary basis for our practice? What is the real, holistic evidence for the use of technology in maternal and child healthcare? We need to consider, and value, alternate research paradigms to randomized, controlled trials if we are to measure the complexity of psycho-social outcomes, particularly when randomization to psychologically differing groups is unethical. We also need to incorporate research findings into a model that emphasizes an individualized approach to care. This is difficult to do when the application of quantitative research findings in care relies on an average group response to an intervention.

> It is also not always possible to test potential clinical care practices through randomized, controlled trials, sometimes for psychological reasons. For example, current attempts to study the value of inositol in addition to folic acid on reducing neural tube defects in women who have already experienced this adverse outcome in a previous pregnancy are almost impossible to undertake. Women are, understandably, unwilling to be randomized to a placebo group when inositol appears to be potentially protective and harmless based on animal research and some human case studies.[11] Obtaining adequate/randomized, controlled trial evidence of its value or potential harm may never be possible.

Agreement regarding which psycho-social issues to explore in perinatal surveys is difficult to reach. In addition, the range of items that can be included, the variety of ways such questions can be asked and the lack of unanimity as to just which of these are crucial indicators of psycho-social perinatal health make it extremely difficult to reach agreement on a universal set of indicators.

It is not only the mother's experiences that are of importance in family-centred data monitoring but also those of her chosen family support persons. Just as some countries have begun to examine women's perceptions of their care, a few are becoming concerned about partners' views as well.[12] In a family-centred approach, the experiences of extended family members, who are an integral part of many families' experiences at this time, will also be considered.

The benefits that can be gained from conducting national and international comparisons of perinatal practices are immense. On the one hand, such surveys provide a global standard against which any country, city or even maternity service can compare itself so that it can identify areas in need of improvement as well as areas of strength. On the other hand, such comparisons reveal intriguing differences across regions, such as the higher rates of partner support in labour in North America and the United Kingdom compared to lower rates in many other countries or the higher proportion of Baby Friendly Hospitals (BFHs) in European centres compared to those in North America.[13] Comparisons also may facilitate monitoring changes in rates over time if surveys are repeated.

Local Data Collection

In addition to national or regional perinatal data collection, it is important for maternity hospitals to conduct local surveys of women's and their partners' experiences of their perinatal care in order to monitor and evaluate their own particular policies and practices. Findings are useful for hospital self-improvement. Assessing women's or families' satisfaction and the family-centredness of care offered – through follow-up evaluations of their hospital experiences – should be as much a part of such surveys as the medical procedures routinely documented by hospitals, such as how many caesarean sections were done, and the occurrence of adverse pregnancy outcomes. Ideally, all these variables will be considered in evaluating hospitals' and caregivers' effectiveness. To facilitate such assessment, a bank of possible questions and issues that assess family-centred practice, family-centredness of healthcare facilities (either locally or nationally) and women's perceptions of the family-centredness of their care is provided in Appendix 1. This list can provide a starting point for caregivers, facilities and countries to develop a customized assessment tool for themselves and for the women for whom they care.

Health Promotion versus Health Research

The conflict between health promotion and research has been prominent in my work, particularly in Eastern Europe. While research has remained a primary interest, the ethical question of whether it is appropriate to indulge in academic research when countries are struggling with basic educational and technical needs is paramount. United Nations agencies support health-promotional programmes and are not often directly concerned with research unless this is clearly beneficial for the host country. When resources are scare, bringing existing knowledge to countries that desperately need it is far more important than answering new questions. Once basic priority issues (e.g. reducing maternal and infant mortality) are managed reasonably well, there can be time for more academic research pursuits. Notwithstanding these accepted priorities, combining the two approaches of health promotion and research has remained a challenge for me throughout my years of work.

Data collection globally is not only for the purposes of monitoring and evaluation but is also essential for research. Contrary to common belief, research into health issues – whether international or local – does not necessarily result in or imply health promotion. Such research may also be unethical. In the international arena, the ideological value of 'contributing to the improvement of global health' does not always justify exploiting the resources of developing countries by means of research without the host countries/organisations receiving any benefit.

In theory, local researchers can gain from participating in international research trials by obtaining knowledge of hitherto unknown research methodologies, employment income and (possibly) some academic credit. However, they seldom gain sufficient understanding of the research methods followed to enable them to replicate or generalize the methods, report or publish the research findings locally or offer any direct benefit to study participants. The study findings may also lack any relevance to the countries participating in the research or may fail to be implemented locally to benefit the population. It is possible, too, that some research could put local collaborators at risk, particularly if governments are not sympathetic to the research outcomes or proposed changes.

International perinatal research often fails to address health concerns that are a priority for developing countries. Multicenter studies that include developing countries should address both their needs and those of the developed world. For example, the Term Breech Trial,[14] one of the largest multinational randomized, controlled trials to be undertaken in recent years in perinatal care, addressed the issue of the optimal method of delivering babies presenting in a breech position at term. In some of the countries participating in this trial, where maternal and neonatal mortality rates are at extremely high levels due to a multitude of unrelated challenges, this issue was likely not a priority, although still relevant for them. The controversial conclusions of this trial, which have contributed significantly to increased caesarean section rates worldwide, raise concerns about the applicability of the findings and the resulting promotion of caesarean sections in developing countries.

> In rural African communities, a woman having a caesarean section may find the experience so unpleasant and unwanted that she might avoid seeking medical care for her next pregnancy, choosing instead to give birth at home with support from local, untrained traditional birth attendants, thereby increasing her chances of potential mortality or morbidity. In some cases, even if she were willing to seek medical care, her lack of access to healthcare facilities (common in the vast tracts of rural African lands) would increase her risk. Increasing the rate of caesarean section for all but the most essential indications in such environments therefore can have life-threatening consequences.

In considering whether or not to participate in such trials, countries need to fully explore the consequences of potential findings on their own healthcare settings. Ethics committees that review such trials and researchers developing such studies need to be aware of and consider these implications. While the research itself may be admirable and well conducted, the implications of its findings for the development of local guidelines for practice that address the needs of local families need to be carefully considered within each cultural context.

Cultural Differences in Implementing International Research

Donor and local health systems frequently differ in their systems of change and reform.[15] While democratic decision-making processes may be the standard of the donor country or consultants, the hosts may be more familiar with autocratic decision-making. Integrating such different models can be a challenge. International consultants should consider both the ethical and psychological effects of trying to change these differing approaches. For example, healthcare providers accustomed to autocratic approaches may find Western ethical research requirements foreign at best, if not needlessly constraining. Requirements such as those for obtaining informed consent, providing the freedom to refuse participation without fear of reprisal and for fully informing participants of the requirements of participation may be viewed as unnecessary in some host countries. They may even be perceived as challenging to the authority of healthcare providers or signalling their apparent weakness. Family-centred care in such an authoritarian setting is unlikely to be well established. Research protocols need to incorporate a value of family-centred care and involvement in both understanding and consenting to the research process, as well as to the clinical intervention being offered.

The globally significant Promotion of Breastfeeding Intervention Trial (PROBIT) in Belarus was confronted with the challenge of conducting research respectfully, with due consideration of women's and hospitals' rights to refuse to participate. Local researchers were accustomed to 'ordering' patients to do whatever they wished. In this case, as the study had the backing of the Ministry of Health, non-compliance with it was frowned upon. The research team, however, emphasized that women had the right to refuse to participate in the study without penalty, and devoted a great deal of time to this issue in the training of our research collaborators. We made it clear that we did not expect any centres potentially eligible for inclusion in the trial to comply with it against their wishes, and one or two did withdraw before randomization, as they were not willing to be potentially allocated to the control arm of the study. Bridging this cultural difference was challenging.

Conflicting Goals of Research and Health Promotion

Combining research and health promotion can be difficult.[16] It may easily be possible to test the effects of an intervention in a randomized, controlled trial where one arm of the trial contains the 'new' intervention and the other does not. Research grants will usually support the application of the 'new' approach to the experimental group. If this treatment proves beneficial, there is, however, no provision in the usual research grant to provide the intervention for the control group as well. Nor is there funding available to ameliorate the effects of an unsuccessful or even harmful intervention.[17] From a health-promotional and ethical point of view, this is unacceptable, as both groups should benefit from the research findings. From a family-centred viewpoint, this is potentially harmful for those participating in the study. Reversing any negative effects of research interventions in the experimental group at the conclusion of the study, as well as applying the findings to the control group, if found to be beneficial, should be built into all research grants. At present, this does not occur. Some re-thinking of the ethical consequences of grant funding policy is needed. Study populations – meaning women and their families in perinatal care – continue to be viewed simply as guinea pigs and are expected to be willing to contribute to lofty ideological goals such as the 'betterment of care in future'[18] – or to somewhat less ideological goals of advancing the individual researchers' career aspirations.

It is rare, but not impossible, to conduct major international health research studies differently by (unusually) incorporating the potential outcomes of the studies into their intervention programmes. For example, PROBIT[19] did consider the ethical implications of manipulating populations for the purposes of gaining research findings. This study of over 17,000 Belarusian mother–baby pairs revealed clear infant health benefits to being born in a hospital that followed the requirements of the BFHI. We did not ask the granting agencies that supported the trial for funding to provide the intervention to the control group in the event of a positive impact of the intervention (or withdrawal of the intervention from the experimental group should the intervention have been shown to be harmful). A request of this nature would have been regarded as 'beyond the scope of the proposed research' and may have resulted in the entire study being refused funding. I, however, was not comfortable proceeding without implementing the appropriate intervention as a consequence of the findings. My team members and I chose, instead, to obtain further funding for follow-up interventions. As a result, we provided training for hospitals that had agreed not to implement the BFHI during the trial (the control-group hospitals) after the conclusion of the study, supported by additional funding from the WHO Regional Office for Europe.[20]

We accept that a trial should be stopped if an interim analysis reveals clear negative consequences if it were to be continued. Yet a positive interim analysis does not result in a decision to apply the findings to all.[21] One could also argue that completed research without implementation of its findings is of little value. A significant body of work has been published with the altruistic hope that others will read it and apply it in practice. Sadly, we have learned that dissemination and application of research findings are a neglected area as well as a generally unsuccessful or, at least, lengthy one. If research grants required implementation of positive research outcomes – thus blending research and health promotion – this would be far more effective. At present, women provide the data collected in much perinatal research, researchers publish these data and enhance their careers, professional bodies disseminate guidelines based on the research findings to their members and few professionals, if anyone, assess whether these findings have been implemented to the benefit of the mothers who provided the data in the first place – or at least their counterparts. This is hardly a woman- or family-centred approach.

International research and international health-promotion programmes raise thorny issues. Conflicts between the goals and methods of research, health promotion and family-centred care remain despite attempts to improve international research standards.[22]

Key Points

- An efficient system of national and regional perinatal data collection that is reliable, timely and standardized is necessary for effective monitoring and evaluation of perinatal care and the development of national guidelines.
- Perinatal data collection has traditionally focussed on clinical events or practices. Psycho-social and cultural issues are not usually included, although they should be.
- Conducting national surveys of women's experiences of their perinatal care is essential.
- There is a need for a uniform international perinatal assessment process that includes a careful analysis of the family-centredness of care.
- Evaluating psycho-social and cultural issues in perinatal care is difficult, but that does not justify their omission.
- It is not only the mother's experiences that are of importance in family-centred data monitoring but also those of her chosen family support persons.
- Maternity hospitals should conduct local surveys of women's and their partners' experiences of their perinatal care in order to monitor and evaluate their own particular policies and practices.
- Research into health issues – whether international or local – does not necessarily result in, or imply, health promotion. Combining research and health promotion can be difficult.

Goals, Ethics and Rights in Family-Centred Perinatal Care

14

Principles:

- Care addresses the needs of women, their newborn(s) and their chosen family supports during pregnancy, birth and postpartum.
- Care respects the reproductive and sexual rights of women and their families.

Overview

Perinatal care services can be greatly improved. Our emphasis on technological development in recent decades has benefitted many but has been accompanied by a loss of concern and respect for women's emotional and intellectual needs. We need to give birthing and babies back to families. This book addresses many of these issues. The characteristics of a family-centred maternity facility are listed in this chapter together with reference to the chapters in which they are discussed, providing a goal for strengthening care. The development of reproductive ethics and rights through United Nations declarations is discussed. Recent developments of rights relating to mothers during childbearing and those of newborns are examined. Moreover, the rights and ethics-based issues reviewed in this book are also listed together with reference to the chapters in which they are discussed.

Outline

Characteristics of a Family-Centred Maternity Facility
Ethics and Rights in Reproductive Healthcare
The Rights of Mothers and Families during Pregnancy and Childbirth
The Rights of the Child
The Rights of Newborns
Rights and Ethics-Based Issues Addressed in This Book

Characteristics of a Family-Centred Maternity Facility

Women having vaginal or caesarean births will generally

- Be cared for with an individualized family-centred approach (Chapters 1, 2, 8 and 14).
- Be provided with up-to-date, evidence-based care (Chapter 6).
- Receive psycho-socially sensitive care (Chapter 7).
- Have care that is culturally appropriate (Chapters 10 and 11).

- Have care that is respectful of the woman's, and her family's, dignity, confidentiality and privacy (Chapter 7).
- Be cared for in a facility that conforms to the World Health Organization/United Nations Children's Fund (WHO/UNICEF) Baby Friendly Hospital Initiative (BFHI) (Chapters 4 and 5).
- Have access to multiple caregivers capable of caring for both medical and psycho-social needs (Chapters 9, 15 and 16).
- Be able to discuss their birth experiences with their birth caregivers and be entitled to full, honest and transparent information about all aspects of their care (Chapter 7).
- Be offered an apology if avoidable negative outcomes occur (Chapter 7).
- Have non-abusive care (Chapter 12).
- Have access to publicly available, aggregated and understandable information regarding the facility's maternity care practices and outcomes (Chapter 16).

Women having vaginal or caesarean births will prenatally

- Have the option to attend prenatal classes, together with their chosen companion, designed to assist families with the physical, psychological and social changes occurring during pregnancy, birth and the first months of parenthood (Chapters 4, 5 and 8).
- Always have access to their maternity records – whether in hard copy or through electronic access – no matter where they are (Chapter 3).
- Take an active role in decisions about their or their baby's care, together with their chosen support companion(s), based on comprehensive evidence-based information, without coercion (Chapter 8).

Women having vaginal or caesarean births will in labour and birth

- Be attended at labour and birth by the companion(s) of their choice such as their partner, doula, family member or friend (Chapter 3).
- Avoid a supine position and the use of stirrups in labour and birth except when instrumental or surgical delivery is performed (Chapter 6).
- Be cared for using only essential, evidence-based interventions without discrimination (Chapter 6).
- Be offered a variety of non-pharmacological pain management methods as alternatives to pharmacological options. Caesarean section will preferably be conducted with regional rather than general anaesthetic (Chapter 6).
- Hold their newborn skin-to-skin from the moment of birth onwards (unless medically unreasonable to do so) and breastfeed when the baby shows signs of readiness for a feed – usually within the first hour or so after birth (Chapters 3, 4 and 5). Be supported to feed the baby with breastmilk substitutes if the mother has chosen this option.
- Give birth in an atmosphere that is caring and gentle and remains so after birth (Chapter 3).

Women having vaginal or caesarean births will after birth

- Room-in for 24 hours a day after birth with their newborn and a family member/companion (Chapters 4 and 5).
- Take an active role in caring for their newborns (Chapters 4, 5 and 8).

- Room-in with their baby and a family member/companion in the neonatal intensive care unit (NICU) if the baby needs NICU care and share extensively in the baby's care, including breastmilk feeding or breastfeeding (Chapter 5).
- Be referred to available community parenting support services and activities on discharge. Ensure that appropriate systems are in place to transfer families in need of further medical care back to the healthcare services/team (Chapters 4 and 5).
- Be provided with a means of offering feedback to the facility on their maternity care experiences, which are then rigorously monitored, evaluated and incorporated into future care by the facility (Chapter 13).

Ethics and Rights in Reproductive Healthcare

Reproductive rights have become an increasingly important focus in recent decades. In 2014, the Centre for Health and Gender Equity (CHANGE) declared April 11 as the International Day for Maternal Health and Rights.[1] This movement aims to encourage rights-based, respectful care of women during pregnancy and childbirth. This day promotes the importance of dignity, respect and skilled care for women during pregnancy and birth and acknowledges the growing evidence about the disrespect and abuse that women can face in countries at all levels of development. The importance of such rights applies equally to the child and the family. Since the 1990s, the United Nations health agencies have spearheaded reproductive rights in obstetric and neonatal care as universal developments.[2] Some countries have led the field in moving towards appropriate care of women and their families, as well as in relation to reproductive health. Most of the member countries of the United Nations support, at least in theory, these principles, although it may still take some time to implement these mandates in practice and through national legislation.

A series of global consensus conferences has led to UN declarations of action agendas for socially equitable and sustainable development in the twenty-first century.[3] These conferences, including the Fourth World Conference on Women (Beijing 1995), the World Summit for Social Development (Copenhagen 1995), the International Conference on Population and Development (Cairo 1994) and the World Conference on Human Rights (Vienna 1993), resulted in a progressive agenda for development. Arising from these conferences have been the Convention on the Rights of the Child, the Convention on the Elimination of All Forms of Discrimination against Women and the Declaration on the Elimination of Violence against Women. In essence, these declarations reflect a policy of people-centred development based on the following key principles[4]:

- All individuals should be able to enjoy all human rights and fundamental freedoms. Achieving social equality and justice is a priority objective of the global community, in particular, for girls and women and indigenous and other vulnerable groups.
- Empowering people and eradicating poverty, especially through access to information, resources and democratic institutions, are the key to unleashing human potential and securing peace and development for all.
- Women's rights are human rights. National development cannot be achieved without the full and equal participation of women in public and private decision-making and their access to equal opportunities in all aspects of social and economic activity.
- Men's shared responsibilities and participation in all aspects of family and household roles, including child rearing and child support, sexual and reproductive behaviour and family planning practice, must be encouraged to enable men and women to develop partnerships based on equality and mutual respect.

- Health and education for all are core factors of development that must be dealt with as a part of inter-related social, economic and poverty eradication efforts.

These principles form the basis of numerous international initiatives designed to safeguard sexual and reproductive rights, to ensure conformity to ethical and human rights and standards and to monitor these through research and development.

The initial priority of many of these agendas was the development of rights regarding reproduction, specifically focussing on the right to bear only as many children as wanted and when wanted. In consequence, many of these recommendations, such as the 1968 Tehran Human Rights Conference, the 1994 International Conference on Population and Development held in Cairo, the 1995 Fourth World Conference on Women held in Beijing and the 2008 Sexual Rights Declaration of the International Planned Parenthood Federation, focus primarily on family planning and freedom of choice. While the newly endorsed United Nations Sustainable Development Goals do include some reproductive and sexual health targets, these cover family planning, adolescent fertility and sexual education (Targets 3.7 and 5.6).[5] Issues such as safe abortion, non-discrimination based on sexual orientation or gender identity, sexual satisfaction, gender-based violence and the importance of high-quality, confidential and timely sexual and reproductive services are inadequately endorsed by these goals due to opposition from some member states and their conservative allies to abortion, adolescent sexual and reproductive health services and sexual rights. In consequence, *The Lancet*, together with the Guttmacher Institute, has established a commission aiming to develop broad-ranging, evidence-based priorities for sexual and reproductive health and rights for the coming decades.[6]

> Early on in my career I questioned the value of the numerous documents outlining rights, charters, declarations, guidelines and recommendations that were scattered throughout the literature. I rapidly learned that these documents provide some of the strongest arguments that can be used to influence changes in practices. They are usually developed by groups of experts following considerable thought, debate and research. Despite their validity, their value is sometimes underrated, particularly in countries where professionals regard their way as 'the best', even if this way is in contradiction to such (usually) globally applicable recommendations.
>
> Because the United Nations health organizations focus their attention more on developing nations – where there is greatest need for assistance – than on the technologically sophisticated world – which should have the resources to help themselves – their charters and recommendations are often discounted by these more developed nations as not applicable to them. This can clearly lead to better healthcare systems being introduced in developing countries than exist in wealthier nations. The earlier and more extensive implementation of the Baby Friendly Hospital Initiative (BFHI) in developing countries compared to more affluent parts of the world is a case in point – much to the potential detriment of babies born in the latter countries.

The Rights of Mothers and Families during Pregnancy and Childbirth

More recently, initiatives have developed that are expanding the concern for reproductive health rights to include that of the mother during pregnancy and childbirth. The White

Ribbon Alliance for Safe Motherhood, with support from United States Aid (USAID), is leading the campaign to promote respectful maternity care. The White Ribbon Alliance has developed The Respectful Maternity Care Charter: The Universal Rights of Child-bearing Women (2011).[7] It identifies that in addition to bringing vital, potentially life-saving health services, women's experiences with maternity caregivers have the potential to empower and comfort or to inflict lasting damage and emotional trauma. Women's memories of their childbearing experiences stay with them for a lifetime. The White Ribbon Alliance is attempting to build national, regional and global awareness which envisions a world in which a woman's right to 'respectful maternity care' is embedded at all levels of all maternal health systems around the globe and that these rights are reflected in a sense of entitlement among women. The charter addresses the issue of disrespect and abuse among women seeking maternity care. It asserts that all childbearing women need and deserve respectful care and protection. This includes care to protect the mother–baby pair as well as marginalized or vulnerable women (e.g. adolescents, ethnic minorities and women living with physical or mental disabilities or with human immunodeficiency virus (HIV) infection).

Other national organizations have emphasized the rights of women during childbearing, for example, Childbirth Connection in the United States in 2012 proposed The Rights of Childbearing Women.[8] The rights listed reflect practices that occur during pregnancy, birth and the postpartum period. Childbirth Connection asserts that we must ensure that all childbearing women have access to information and care based on the best scientific evidence now available and have opportunities to exercise their right to make healthcare decisions. Access to legal or other recourse to address their grievances is needed by women whose rights are violated.

The Breastfeeding Mothers' Bill of Rights, promoted by the Department of Health, State of New York (2010)[9] and the US Center for Reproductive Rights Declarations[10] (1992–2013) are two further examples of locally developed rights-based documents that support women during this period. The Canadian Society for Obstetricians and Gynaecologists has also developed a charter of sexual and reproductive rights and health that focuses on sexual issues and includes mention of reproductive health issues.[11]

The preceding rights-based reproductive health programmes have been predominantly directed towards women in keeping with the 'woman-centred' approach to care that has superseded previous 'physician-centred' or 'baby-centred' attitudes. There is still a dearth of attention being paid to a rights-based approach to 'family-centred' perinatal care.

The Rights of the Child

The United Nations Convention on the Rights of the Child (UNCRC, 1989)[12] extended reproductive rights concerns towards the child. Some organizations within member countries, such as the Canadian Institute of Child Health, have adapted this declaration to address national circumstances, as in the Rights of the Child in the Healthcare System.[13] This document presents a revised set of children's rights in relation to the healthcare system and describes the relevant article(s) from the UNCRC. The document identifies 11 specific rights:

- I have the right to live and to have my pain and suffering treated, even if I am unable to communicate my need. I have this right regardless of my age, gender or income.
- I have the right to be viewed first as a child, then as a patient.

- I have the right to be treated as an individual with my own abilities, culture and language.
- I have the right to be afraid and to cry when I feel hurt.
- I have the right to be safe in an environment that is unfamiliar to me.
- I have the right to ask questions and receive answers that I can understand.
- I have the right to be cared for by people who perceive and meet my needs even though I may be unable to explain what they are.
- I have the right to speak for myself when I am able and to have someone speak on my behalf when I am unable.
- I have the right to have those who are dear to me close when I need them.
- I have the right to play and learn even if I am receiving care.
- I need to have my rights fulfilled.

The Rights of the Newborn

The rights of the child outlined earlier do not specifically address the rights of the newborn and, even more essential, the rights of the sick or preterm baby cared for in an NICU. A current global initiative is addressing this issue with a petition submitted, in 2014, to the UN Child Rights Committee to amend its declaration to incorporate family-centred neonatal intensive care.[14] This petition was signed by 135 newborn healthcare providers from 26 countries. Specifically, it requests that Article 24(e) of the Convention on the Rights of the Child be amended to read

> To ensure that all segments of society, in particular parents and children, are informed, have access to education and are supported in the use of basic knowledge of child health and nutrition, the advantages of breastfeeding, *which includes healthy newborns, and also infants admitted to the intensive care unit where the mother (family) has full access to the baby*, hygiene and environmental sanitation and the prevention of accidents [suggested amendment shown in italics].

To date, we have yet to see any changes made to the UNCRC Rights of the Child to incorporate a focus on newborn care, although other groups are addressing this issue. An Italian group, for example, have developed the 'Parma Charter of the Rights of the Newborn',[15] which incorporates many of the ideals outlined in this book. This charter incorporates the following:

1. Every newborn is entitled to life at the best levels of health.
2. Every live newborn is entitled to appropriate assistance during delivery.
3. Every newborn, be he healthy or ill, is entitled to the best care, social protection and safety available.
4. Every newborn has the right to be born in the most suitable place.
5. The newborn must be guaranteed vicinity to his parents.
6. No medical procedure, including those for research purpose, may be performed on the newborn without the informed consent of his parents or legal guardian.
7. Every newborn is entitled to be adequately fed.
8. In the case of the birth of a severely ill newborn, appropriate treatment must be guaranteed.
9. Every newborn is entitled to be registered after birth, to be given a name and to acquire a nationality.
10. The newborn is a person.

Clause 3 of this charter specifies that 'special attention must be granted to the medical, social and psychological care of the unborn child and the mother, during pregnancy and delivery, on account of the close implications for the newborn's health'. Clause 5 requires that all healthy newborns room-in with their mother. Babies cared for in NICUs must have family-centred care providing support for parents who should be involved as far as possible in caring for the baby and in related decision-making processes. Breastfeeding is to be facilitated and encouraged as the optimal feeding method, as addressed in Clause 7.

Rights and Ethics-Based Issues Addressed in This Book

This book has moved beyond mother- or baby-centred care to emphasize the importance of the family during pregnancy, birth and the first months of parenthood. It has incorporated the rights and ethics-based issues highlighted by UN agencies as well as various national organizations involved in perinatal care. The family-centred perinatal care rights that have been raised in this book are listed below, noting the chapter(s) in the text where they are discussed. They are applicable regardless of type of delivery, either vaginal or caesarean, and to the care of mothers, fathers/partners' and newborns with either optimal or adverse outcomes.

I, my baby and my family have

- The right to family-centred maternal and newborn care (Chapters 1, 2 and 14)
- The right to consideration of pregnancy and birth as normal, healthy events until proved otherwise (Chapters 3 and 4).
- The right to the best available evidence-based care (Chapter 6).
- The right to have interventions used only when essential (Chapter 6).
- The right to care that is sensitive to my psycho-social needs (Chapters 6 and 7).
- The right to companionship during care (Chapters 3 and 7).
- The right to culturally sensitive and informed care (Chapters 10, 11 and 15).
- The right to individualized care (Chapter 8).
- The right to care from interdisciplinary caregivers as needed (Chapters 9, 15 and 16).
- The right to caregivers trained in family-centred care (Chapter 9).
- The right to a holistic approach to care (Chapters 1 and 2).
- The right to appropriate preparation for parenthood (Chapter 8).
- The right to breastfeed with appropriate support (Chapters 4 and 5).
- The right to active involvement in the birth process (Chapters 3 and 7).
- The right to active involvement in the care of our newborn (Chapters 4, 5 and 8).
- The right to informed, rather than coerced, consent (Chapter 8).
- The right to knowledge of potential adverse outcomes arising from care (Chapter 5).
- The right to privacy, dignity and confidentiality (Chapter 7)
- The right to non-abusive care (Chapter 12).
- The right to open and honest communication (Chapter 7).
- The right to safety and to apology (Chapter 7)
- The right to provide feedback on care (Chapter 13).
- The right to have access to information about hospital practices and outcomes (Chapter 16).

In recent decades, considerable advances have been made in strengthening perinatal care by focussing on evidence-based obstetric practices together with a more family-centred approach. Evidence-based knowledge has provided striking and necessary technological improvement in maternal and newborn care, but the application of a family-centred approach, particularly when complications develop for either mother or baby in pregnancy and childbirth, has lagged behind. The goals of family-centred care are based on recognition of human rights in perinatal care. A comprehensive, holistic approach that is truly family-centred is needed if this is to become the normative standard.

Key Points

- Our emphasis on technological development in recent decades has benefitted many but has been accompanied by a loss of concern and respect for women's emotional and intellectual needs. We need to give birthing, and babies, back to families.
- Characteristics of a family-centred maternity care facility are outlined.
- Respect women's and families' rights.
- Respect the rights of the newborn.

Part

V

An Unfinished Agenda

Best Practices from Global Settings

Principles:
- Care is inter-disciplinary requiring co-ordination among caregivers.
- Care is culturally sensitive and informed.

Overview

In the industrialized world, we are inclined to believe that our systems of care are superior to those offered in the developing world. Yet we can learn a great deal from alternate cultural approaches to healthcare, such as the training of perinatal psychologists that has been introduced into Moldova, hospital hotels in some Scandinavian countries and the Humane Perinatal Care Initiative of Estonia (see Chapter 5). Learning from these programmes, as well as exploring national or even local innovations, can lead to a betterment of perinatal care for all concerned. This chapter explores a national programme that shows an effective and psycho-socially integrated implementation of both the World Health Organization/United Nations Children's Fund (WHO/UNICEF) Baby Friendly Hospital Initiative (BFHI)[1] and the WHO Regional Office for Europe's Effective Perinatal Care Programmes[2] within a single country as well as a number of local initiatives from countries around the world that offer alternate, interesting models that strengthen perinatal services.

Outline

A National Programme: Strengthening Perinatal Care in the Republic of Moldova

A Model for Terms of Reference for Psychologists in Perinatal Care Centres

Best practices from Estonia, the United Kingdom, Scandinavia, Canada and South Africa

A National Programme: Strengthening Perinatal Care in the Republic of Moldova

Since the collapse of the former Soviet Union in 1989, the countries of Central and Eastern Europe (CCEE), the Newly Independent States (NIS) and the Central Asian Republics and Kazakhstan (CARK) have undertaken massive reform programmes for all aspects of their functioning. Not least among these is that relating to healthcare. Although all aspects of healthcare have been and still are in the process of reform, maternity and newborn care has received considerable targeted assistance due to the high levels of maternal and infant mortality and morbidity that existed in these countries.

Not all countries have made similar progress in strengthening their perinatal care services. Differing priorities; availability of open-minded, committed or qualified personnel; selective sources of funding for reform; and political will (or lack thereof) result in differing rates of progress in changing the status quo. One country, the Republic of Moldova, however, stands out as particularly impressive in its eager and whole-hearted embracing of modern perinatal care knowledge, attitudes and practices. Its success story is still incomplete, although its key perinatal outcome indicators already show remarkable improvement. For instance, maternal mortality dropped from 44 per 100,000 live births in 1990 to 15 per 100,000 in 2011[3] using WHO-recommended indicator definitions. Perinatal mortality dropped from 15.3 per 1,000 births in 1990 to 12.5 per 1,000 in 2011 and early neonatal mortality from 8.8 per 1,000 births in 1990 to 5.4 per 1,000 births in 2011. These figures indicate a significant improvement.

Changes introduced in the country cover a wide range of simultaneous reform measures within the framework of perinatal care. In 1997, supported by UNICEF and in part by other donor agencies, a National Programme to Improve Perinatal Health was initiated in Moldova, following a great deal of international aid agency activity in the country commencing in the early 1990s.

The first programme to be introduced in the country following the breakup of the Soviet Union was the WHO/UNICEF BFHI. It was welcomed locally as it offered to reinforce a long-held cultural value (breastfeeding) that was hitherto, despite local encouragement, largely unsuccessful due to inappropriate healthcare systems that were in place. As in many countries of the world where the use of breastmilk substitutes has been encouraged, knowledge of the principles and practices of effective breastfeeding technique, as embodied in the Ten Steps to Successful Breastfeeding,[4] was largely unknown in 1992 when the CCEE/NIS/CARK BFHI initiative was launched in St Petersburg, Russian Federation. Moldovan representatives at this conference returned home to encourage local authorities to follow this initiative. Training on the BFHI began shortly after, with the assistance of the WHO and UNICEF. In 1996, I assessed the first three hospitals in Moldova for accreditation as Baby Friendly Hospitals and a year or two later, a further two. The programme has continued with ongoing training of new healthcare centres, evaluation of new hospitals and re-evaluation of existing accredited centres.

The positive effects of the BFHI, as well as the exposure it brought to developments in perinatal care, led to further reform movements. From 1997 onwards, the national programme to improve perinatal health was implemented, taking a number of steps, including

- *Training* of national facilitators in the WHO-Euro 'Essential Antenatal, Perinatal and Postpartum Care Course', the 'Essential Newborn Care and Breastfeeding Course' and the WHO Making Pregnancy Safer Programme.
- Developing evidence-based *national guidelines for perinatal care* to replace the older 'edicts' set by Moscow[5] and two sets of guidelines: the National Perinatal Care Guideline A, *The Foundational Principles of Organization and Delivery of Perinatal Care,* and Guideline B, *Regionalized Perinatal Care: Levels and Contents.*
- The WHO-Euro courses raised awareness of the need for a more humane, family-centred approach to healthcare. This, in turn, resulted in two developments. The first was the implementation of a *Survey of Women's Perceptions of their Perinatal Care* based on my earlier work in St Petersburg, Russian Federation, and other countries.[6] This initial survey was later used to assess the impact of the initial introduction of evidence-based practices in some regions of the country, and the results were published in 2002.[7]

- The second consequence of the WHO-Euro courses was growing awareness of the *importance of multi-disciplinary approaches to perinatal care*. The importance of the midwife in care, as well as of family doctors in addition to obstetricians and neonatologists, became a national concern. Family doctors were developed as primary caregivers, and the UNICEF 2004 Plan of Action specifically targeted the strengthening of the midwife's role in perinatal care.

- Moldova has taken reform even further than most. In 2003, the country sought international guidance again to highlight the role of the *psychologist in perinatal care*, and I trained national trainers in psycho-social aspects of pregnancy, birth and postpartum care. This training led to the establishment of *terms of reference for psychologists in perinatal healthcare* services by local health authorities. The UNICEF 2004 Plan of Action for Moldova, in consequence, targeted the establishment of psychologists in most perinatal care centres throughout the country. These psychologists were to assist with standard needs such as coping with pregnancy loss, difficult birth experiences and postpartum depression. They were also to assist with two problems of considerable concern in Moldova (and other Eastern European countries): trafficking of women and abandonment of babies.

- In 1998, as a further development focussed on psycho-social issues in perinatal care, Moldova requested that I offer specialized training for those responsible for *preparation of families for pregnancy, birth and parenthood,* a recommendation of their National Guidelines for Perinatal Care.

- A three-level system of *regionalized perinatal care* was put into place. The system comprises the following levels: level I (district level), level II (*judets* or county level) and level III (the republican level) reflecting increasing levels of specialization.

- *Perinatal care records* were refined, and a *Guide for Would-Be Mothers* was developed and distributed among pregnant women. Nine sets of posters on various perinatal care subjects were publicly distributed. To raise public understanding and support for the benefits of new perinatal care approaches, 35 radio programmes called 'I Want to Become a Mother' and 25 TV programmes entitled, *Perinatal Care Guide for Parents,* were aired on local TV/radio stations.

- Two grants from the government of Japan helped to equip the National Maternal and Child Health Center and 11 second-level perinatal care facilities, as well as train their staff in the use and maintenance of *new equipment.*

- In an effort to set up a sustainable system to *monitor and evaluate perinatal care,* the Centres for Disease Control and Prevention (CDC) in Atlanta offered three workshops to train health workers from various Moldovan counties in quality management in perinatal care. Old statistical reporting forms were brought in line with the perinatal care technologies promoted under the programme. Process, impact and outcome indicators for monitoring and evaluating ante-, intra- and postpartum care were developed.

- *Immunization programmes* were strengthened. This included ensuring an uninterrupted supply of vaccines, syringes and safety boxes for the National Immunization Programme; improving quality and safety of immunization services; strengthening the managerial skills of the workers; fortifying vaccine-preventable surveillance systems and promoting public trust in vaccines.

- The *Nutrition* component of the Maternal Child Health Project aimed at eliminating iodine deficiency disorders and reducing anaemia prevalence among pregnant women and children. Core strategies included promotion of universal salt iodization and flour fortification with iron. These are being complemented by iron and folic acid supplements for pregnant women and children under age five.

- Implementation of the *Integrated Management of Childhood Illness* (IMCI) Programme encompassed interventions in the healthcare system, in the community, and at home aiming at reducing childhood deaths, illnesses and disability and improving children's growth and development. IMCI strategy improves health workers' skills as well as family and community practices related to child health and nutrition and strengthens the healthcare system for effective management of childhood illnesses.

The training that took place was rapid and extensive. By 2002, a quarter of all obstetricians and family doctors had undertaken training on perinatal care and almost half of all midwives and other medical assistants. Moldova has incorporated a strong emphasis on psychological and social considerations into its evidence-based and de-medicalized approach to perinatal care This is incorporated into their *Terms of Reference for Perinatal Psychologists Working in All Perinatal Care Services* that were established in 2003 through a consensus reaching process within the National Perinatal Association of Moldova. The Ministry of Health committed to establishing formal positions for psychologists in all perinatal healthcare centres. Their terms of reference provide a valuable model to follow.

Terms of Reference for Psychologists in Perinatal Care Centres

In general,

- All healthcare providers should respect the privacy, dignity and confidentiality of women in perinatal care.
- All healthcare providers should avoid emotional or physical violence or abuse when caring for women.
- Psychologists will support women and their partners, as well as healthcare providers.
- Psychologists will work with families when necessary or when requested to do so by the family.
- Healthcare providers should refer women for psychological assistance when this is perceived to be needed.
- The psychologist should be regarded as an integral member of a multidisciplinary perinatal team and should attend and contribute to clinical case review meetings within perinatal departments.
- The psychologist should work together with social workers and other specialists in collaborating with local authorities such as welfare agencies.
- Psychologists should assist with conflict between healthcare providers and patients.

In prenatal services, psychologists should

- Contribute to antenatal preparation for women and their families regarding pregnancy, birth and the postpartum period, together with other members of the healthcare team.
- Provide counselling for women who experience spontaneous or medical abortions.
- Provide counselling in the case of antenatal fetal death or loss of a close family member or similar tragedy in the perinatal period.
- Provide counselling for women in difficult situations, such as single mothers, teenage mothers, trafficked women, women pregnant after rape, women experiencing domestic

violence, women in incomplete families (such as when the partner is away from home) or women at risk of abandonment of their babies.

- Provide counselling for women and their partners if they are human immunodeficiency virus (HIV) positive.
- Provide counselling for women with unwanted pregnancy.

In intra-partum services,

- Psychologists should endeavour to ensure the presence of a companion at birth for all women and particularly for women in difficult situations such as teenagers, single mothers or other vulnerable women.

In postpartum services, psychologists should

- Assist women and their families in the event of neonatal death or newborn abnormalities.
- Assist the mothers and families of babies in the neonatal intensive care unit (NICU).
- Conduct discussion groups with new mothers in postpartum units to discuss issues of psycho-social concern for new mothers, such as the birth experience, difficulties with breastfeeding or baby care, integrating the new baby into the family, and marital concerns.
- Provide counselling for women with unwanted babies (including women with denial of pregnancy or birth and those intending to give the baby up for adoption).
- Assist women who have psychological concerns about breastfeeding.
- Assist women with postpartum depression.

Educational needs to achieve the preceding include the following:

- Healthcare workers need knowledge and skills in counselling.
- Psychologists should be trained about perinatal care.
- Training is needed for those providing antenatal preparation for women and their families.
- Healthcare workers should be educated about the role of the psychologist in perinatal care.

Moldova is also incorporating ideas from other countries (such as Sweden and Estonia) and is providing postpartum units that accommodate both parents together with their healthy or preterm/sick newborn baby, in the same room, during the postpartum period.

Outcomes

Systematic evaluation of the perinatal care programme allows Moldova to identify and assess gaps in knowledge and skills of health workers, as well as to pinpoint failures in the care delivered to pregnant women, women in labour, postpartum women and newborns on an annual basis. As a matter of routine, these findings are carefully examined, and less successful, more change-resistant areas where rigorous efforts are needed to achieve a breakthrough are easily exposed. This evaluation helps to set the priorities for the programme for the forthcoming year.

Obstacles to Programme Implementation

A number of factors hinder the implementation of changes in perinatal care in Moldova – as in many countries. Financial limitations restrict the provision of adequate facilities for care, supplies, equipment and training, but these are less challenging than other problems. More difficult to resolve are the remnants of traditional thinking about perinatal care that may persist, particularly among the more senior caregivers. Although new information and approaches to perinatal care are disseminated widely and are incorporated into the revised national guidelines, it is hard for older practitioners to accept that healthcare systems in place for most of their lives are no longer regarded as appropriate. Such changes appear to negate the value of their lifetime contributions to the care of women during pregnancy and birth. It is necessary to emphasize that they, as caregivers, have always done what is best for women based on their available knowledge, although the knowledge which they were provided was lacking, not their professional integrity.

The lessons to learn from Moldova are legion. With its challenging social, political, economic and infrastructure difficulties, it has achieved a great deal with very little. UNICEF, in particular, has played a major role in assisting with perinatal healthcare reform in Moldova. The success of the programme, however, is due to the remarkable perinatal healthcare workers in Moldova, who, through personal commitment and enthusiasm for improving their services, have undertaken tasks far beyond their normal call of duty, often with little financial compensation for their additional efforts. A number of singular individuals who led this programme for many years, including Dr Octavian Bivol of UNICEF and Professor Petru Stratulat of the Ministry of Health in Moldova, can take pride in their accomplishments.

Local Programmes

Innovative local programmes and approaches to strengthening family-centred perinatal care in some countries are described. They are not exhaustive, nor are they representative of models that could be emulated; they are simply examples of intriguing ideas that show promise. There are many others.

Scandinavia: Family Maternity Hotels

In some Scandinavian countries, 'family maternity hotels' have been developed adjacent to maternity hospitals and connected to them by (often underground) passages. They are 'five star' hotels that offer every modern convenience traditionally associated with top-class hotels – in addition to offering health clinics on each floor with midwifery attendance every day to provide postpartum care for both mothers and newborns. The hotels allow families to stay together from the first day after their baby is born and to receive any needed clinical care together in the privacy and comfort of a 'hotel'. This is a fascinating idea that provides a family-centred alternative to postpartum wards in hospitals.

Estonia: Postpartum Family Rooms

Estonia offers another alternative in the form of 'family rooms' in maternity hospitals. Although an increasing number of hospitals are allowing partners to remain with the mother after childbirth, they make little, if any, provision for their comfort or care during this time. Some hospitals in Estonia have taken advantage of their lowered birth rate in recent decades to provide family rooms supplied with two beds, allowing for both the mother and her partner to stay together with their newborn (family rooming-in) for the duration of their postpartum care. Partners are free to come and go as they wish but are also welcome to stay throughout the woman's hospitalization. This model is certainly a valuable one to foster.

> When visiting a postpartum family room in Estonia, I asked to take a photograph of the room to use as a teaching tool for sharing this model of care elsewhere. The father in the room quickly jumped up, lifted his baby from its bassinet and held the baby for the photo while seated next to the mother on the bed. His pride and excitement at being part of the postpartum experience were tangible.

United Kingdom: Effective Knowledge Translation

Reading every paper that is published in one's field can be an overwhelming task. Having the information summarized for you or integrated into a readily accessible resource is a boon for many caregivers. The Midwifery Information and Resource Service (MIDIRS) is one such resource that provides a valuable model to follow. Whereas the Internet certainly makes publications more accessible, services that provide an integration of sound knowledge are a model for the future. Not only does MIDIRS provide summary documents that integrate findings of multiple articles relating to a similar issue for healthcare providers, it also provides evidence-based fact sheets for mothers and families regarding multiple aspects of evidence-based and family-centred perinatal care.

Canada: Antenatal Assessment of Psycho-Social Risk

Growing awareness of the potential to predict women most at risk for adverse psycho-social outcomes after birth led to the development of a prenatal assessment scale that has been shown to assist in identifying women at potential risk of psychological complications of pregnancy and birth.[8] This useful scale (the Antenatal Psycho-Social Health Assessment Scale or ALPHA Scale[9]), together with the evidence available for each of the potential outcomes, has been actively implemented in practice in parts of Canada and was included in the WHO-Euro training programmes designed to strengthen maternity care in the European region.

South Africa: Combined Psycho-Social and Obstetric Teaching

In 1990, Dr James McIntyre at Baragwanath Hospital and I introduced innovative combined psycho-social and obstetric teaching for fourth- and sixth-year medical students during obstetric blocks. Sharing and exchanging the teaching baton with equal facility, we exposed students to both the psycho-social and medical issues of obstetric care through jointly offered rounds. For example, if diagnosis of an intra-uterine death was being studied, we considered clinical symptoms and diagnostic procedures and then challenged students to consider what they would have said to the mother during this process. Students' common reactions were to say, most inappropriately, 'Call the nurse to discuss this with the mother!' We emphasized how important it was to care for the woman's emotional concerns and needs for information simultaneously with clinical care and gave consideration as to just how to manage difficult situations such as this. Students' reactions to this approach to teaching were evaluated and were extremely positive.[10]

> The South African climate of high-achievement motivation combined with a strong endorsement for innovation and excellence lay behind the willingness of academic professionals to undertake such a non-conventional teaching approach. A lack of bureaucratic hindrances also allowed this programme to be implemented and assessed in a timely manner much to the satisfaction of the students and to the benefit of women and their families.

In addition, allied healthcare professionals were provided courses on perinatal health psychology: these courses were part of the standard curricula for students of social work, nursing, physiotherapy, occupational therapy and psychology.

South Africa: Multi-Disciplinary Professional Perinatal Associations.

In the 1980s, South Africa's multi-disciplinary and multi-culturally focussed developments led, not surprisingly, to the formation of a multi-disciplinary and multi-cultural *Association for Childbirth and Parenthood* that gained the approval of the *African National Congress*. The association was at the vanguard of anti-Apartheid changes that were emerging throughout the county. It blazed innovative paths as it collapsed the common 'disciplinary silo' approach to maternity care education – an approach that is still the norm in many countries around the world. Rather than focussing on issues of importance to any single professional group, this organization addressed issues of concern to parents and caregivers and facilitated discussions about them across disciplines in order to develop solutions. WHO-Euro's willingness to accept this model of inter-disciplinary education in their Essential Perinatal Care Courses is indicative of its longer-term impact.

All too often technologically developed countries regard their approaches to care as superior and – somewhat paternalistically – worthy of sharing with less developed societies. Global and national examples of better ways to educate and care for women in a holistic and family-centred framework are, however, evident in many places. The greatest obstacle to benefitting from them is our reluctance to consider that other countries or cultures may have better ideas than our own. Studies comparing inter-country perinatal healthcare practices are useful tools for evaluating how well our own systems compare with those of other countries.[11] A far more welcoming and open-minded approach is needed, not just to listen to the ideas of others but to actively seek them out and adopt them when appropriate.

Key Points

- We can learn a great deal from alternate cultures' approaches to healthcare.
- A national perinatal strengthening programme implemented in Moldova shows an effective and psycho-socially integrated implementation of family-centred and evidence-based care.
- A number of local initiatives across the globe can provide exciting models to consider, including Scandinavian maternity hotels, postpartum family rooms in Estonia, effective knowledge translation in the United Kingdom, Canadian assessments of psycho-social risk and South African combined obstetrics and psycho-social education, as well as multidisciplinary perinatal professional associations.

Chapter 16

The Road Ahead

Principles:
- Aggregated information about family-centred psycho-social and clinical practices and outcomes is made publicly available and accessible regardless of socio-economic or educational background.
- Care is inter-disciplinary, requiring co-ordination among caregivers.

Overview

Providing a holistic approach to care is not a new idea. It is embodied in the World Health Organization's (WHO's) definition of health, included in the WHO Constitution of 1948. Despite considerable improvements in perinatal care, we have not managed to do justice to this component of our caregiving service, and rectifying this remains a challenge for the coming decades. A series of issues must still be addressed. Although solutions to these problems are not always easy to achieve, as a start, we need to think about them before doing more harm than good in the future. Labour is difficult for women: making it easier for women and their families is difficult for caregivers.

Outline

Promoting Family-Centred Care
Family-Centred Professional Development
Promoting Multi-Cultural Awareness
Implementing Our Knowledge
Funding Family-Centred Research
Conclusion

Promoting Family-Centred Care

Evaluating Caregivers and Care Facilities

Perinatal surveillance systems tend to aggregate data to reflect practices in a country or perhaps a region within the country. Families are not usually able to obtain this information or to evaluate the practices, policies and outcomes that occur in any one healthcare service. Although many countries offer mothers/families a choice of healthcare service or provider, there is no objective means available to them on which to base this choice. When choosing a caregiver or a place in which to give birth or seek healthcare, hearsay and convenience are simply not sufficiently valid considerations. Maintaining secrecy about the practice outcomes of individual healthcare providers or facilities is usually rationalized on the grounds of protecting privacy. There is, however, a vast difference between privacy and secrecy. Although we must respect privacy, secrecy should be unthinkable and may be unethical. From the mother's/family's perspectives, it is precisely this need for privacy – or perhaps secrecy – regarding psycho-social and clinical perinatal practices and, especially, outcomes that is a concern. If there is nothing to hide, then why hide it? When purchasing any major product or service, we almost routinely seek out valuations of its efficacy: How well does this work? How often does it break down? Have previous clients been satisfied with their results? We try to answer these basic questions, yet answers to these questions are not available for perinatal care facilities or for individual caregivers within them. Providing a transparent national (or regional) 'psycho-social and clinical perinatal practices and outcomes database' for families as well as for caregivers and facilities is long overdue not only for perinatal care but indeed for all healthcare services. Such a database should be freely accessible to potential mothers/families and written in jargon-free language that is accessible to all individuals regardless of their educational or socio-economic background. Published responses to many, if not most, of the questions suggested in the Appendix, by individual caregivers and by maternity care facilities, as well as by mothers who have been cared for in these facilities or by these caregivers, would go far towards providing such a local, regional or national database.

Midwifery Care

Are we addressing the issue of what constitutes skilled attendance at delivery in developing and developed countries adequately? The findings of meta-analyses of randomized trials support the growth of midwifery.[1] Women's higher satisfaction with midwifery care compared to that offered by obstetricians, family doctors or nurses also strongly endorses an increased role for midwives.[2] Taking place on almost a worldwide level and growing in momentum, midwifery does offer an optimal alternative to highly specialized Western, medically based obstetrics and will help to de-medicalize birth and to provide a more family-centred and holistic approach to perinatal care.[3] Midwives – if well trained and competent – are able to meet the needs of scientific medicine for effective care of the normal pregnancy and are able to satisfy the psychological, social and cultural expectations of women and their families at this time.

In developing countries, methods of co-operation between traditional birth attendants and professional caregivers to ensure appropriate use of technology for safe birth require sensitive consideration. Traditionally, we have emphasized physician-based care in both the developed and developing worlds. The time is ripe to encourage alternate or expanded caregiver models, such as care from independent midwives or shared care from skilled traditional birth attendants together with trained caregivers in developing countries.[4]

In 2001, I was asked by the United Nations Children's Fund (UNICEF) agency in what was then Southern Sudan to develop an evidence-based psycho-socially sensitive and culturally respectful training course for illiterate traditional birth attendants. The importance of upgrading the knowledge and skills of traditional birth attendants had been recognized as an important need, in addition to providing better-trained healthcare providers in formal hospital or clinic settings. This is particularly important as there is a shortage of midwives and most perienatal care services, and healthcare facilities, are distant from women who primarily give birth at home. I developed a pictorial course using virtually no wording.

The UNICEF agency's progress report for Southern Sudan in 2005 revealed that historically, 60 to 80% of deliveries in the region were home births. It is gratifying to note that the same report notes that pregnancy outcomes have been improved in the region as trained traditional birth attendants have been increasingly attending births.[5]

The skills of traditional birth attendants need to be upgraded to incorporate them into the healthcare system. Such training has proved to be successful.[6] Sharing decision-making between traditional birth attendants and programme co-ordinators ensures the selection of the most appropriate candidates for obstetric/midwifery training. Providing non-verbal but evidence-based and psycho-socially sensitive training manuals for use with illiterate traditional midwives, such as the manual I developed for use in Southern Sudan,[7] may also help to reduce the exceedingly high rates of maternal and infant mortality that occur in such countries. Skilled physicians, who so often remain sceptical of traditional birth attendants, need to accept their value as well as the pictorial manuals that can assist them to upgrade their knowledge and skills. Overcoming prejudices about traditional birth attendants – who are frequently illiterate – is needed if we are to contribute towards improving care for women in remote and inaccessible regions (as is characteristic of many African and Asian countries). Such approaches also offer an opportunity to integrate the traditional family-centred approach of births surrounded by trusted caregivers and family members with some evidence-based clinical care methods.

In countries such as South Africa, Southern Sudan (now South Sudan) and Ethiopia there are clear physical barriers to in-hospital care for all women during childbirth. Vast land expanses, no roads, minimal public transport services, and male-dominated and poor communities make access to hospitals impossible for most women in rural regions. Providing clean water, education regarding hygiene and local – preferably with some training – support people is probably the best that will be available for many years to come. Motorcycles with sidecars or motorcycles or bicycles adapted to carry a passenger behind them that could navigate narrow walkways might be the best option to introduce as a means of transport from rural villages to available health centres when essential. At present, women are transported by being carried on a makeshift stretcher or, more commonly, being dragged through the bush on such a stretcher behind a horse or cow – if the husband is prepared to pay for this transport. Water wells, wheels and wiser women are probably far better interventions to seek than high-technology obstetric care training in urban centres, if we are to reduce the disastrously high maternal mortality rates in such countries.

Family-Centred Professional Development

Interdisciplinary Perinatal Care Education

At undergraduate level, all medical students receive the same education. In later years, even closely related areas – such as obstetrics/gynaecology and paediatrics – diversify to focus on their own areas. Education of midwives, nurses, psychologists and other healthcare providers also follows distinctive programmes, and there is little overlap of teaching or learning opportunities for these various branches of healthcare-related students. It is not surprising, then, that clinical care has become separated along disciplinary lines and that professional interchange is limited. Family-centred care challenges this traditional breakdown of professional silos. Care of families during the perinatal period requires interprofessional contact, communication, co-ordination and collaboration. This should start during undergraduate training and continue into later years of specialization. Complete integration is unrealistic, however, because today's knowledge base is so broad. Instead, we need frequent opportunities for shared learning and exchange through, for example, integrated lectures or courses, where appropriate, and multi-disciplinary meetings conferences and professional organizations. Fortunately, an awareness of such needs is growing, albeit slowly.

Creating Inter-Professional Bodies

In addition to our established, uni-disciplinary professional bodies, we need integrated professional organizations that bring together all professionals caring for families during their transition to parenthood. We need to include the family perspective in these interactions as well. Rather than only concentrating on a single professional perspective, we need to be problem focussed so that we can consider the perspectives of each type of professional involved in the care of any one problem, as well as the views of recipients of care, side by side. It is likely that such integrated approaches to care will reveal innovative and sensitive solutions to issues that any one, single approach would not have considered. Diversified thinking will be far more effective than a uni-disciplinary or parallel multi-disciplinary approach. The multi-disciplinary and multi-cultural Association for Childbirth and Parenthood of Southern Africa model described in Chapter 15 is well worth further consideration and development for global application.

Qualifying Perinatal Psychologists

How well developed are divisions of health psychology, and particularly perinatal health psychology, in North America, Australia, or indeed any country? Psychological associations cater for the more severe forms of mental ill-health and usually emphasize clinical psychology. We train few professionals to care for the normal emotional and intellectual challenges faced by people experiencing common medical interactions. The field of perinatal care is no exception. We desperately need schools of psychology to strengthen their education of both psychology students and those from other healthcare disciplines regarding psycho-social issues in health, particularly perinatal health. Whereas social and legal issues are well cared for by social workers, the psychological and interpersonal concerns of women and caregivers that arise during the transition to parenthood are currently underserved.

Promoting Multi-Cultural Awareness

We clearly need to develop greater understanding of cultural differences in beliefs, attitudes towards and practices regarding health and healthcare across cultures. This applies to differing cultural groups within our own societies as well as when working in countries other than our own. A recent survey of obstetrics and gynaecology departments across Canada revealed that only a third of departments (36%) include a global women's health component, and few of the programme directors or senior residents within these programmes thought that their existing programmes offered sufficient education in these issues. Yet 90% of programme directors reported that prospective residents inquired about global health opportunities. Young graduates would obviously like to learn more about multi-cultural women's health concerns, but their needs are not being met.[8]

Implementing Our Knowledge

We need to reassess the systems in place that are not succeeding in the implementation of research findings. Waiting for others to read publications of our findings and then to consider implementing them in practice leads to remarkably lengthy delays in knowledge dissemination and application.

> The levonorgestrel-releasing intra-uterine device for contraception (with a valuable side effect of minimizing menorrhagia) was developed and licensed in Finland in 1990 and acknowledged and included in the United Kingdom's Royal College of Obstetricians and Gynaecologists clinical guidelines for many years before it was introduced into the United States and Canada in about 2001–2. To this day, it is used far less often in this part of the world than in Scandinavian and European countries. In fact, North Americans use intra-uterine devices for contraception less often than in all global areas other than sub-Saharan Africa. Despite this, the intra-uterine device is now the leading global reversible method of contraception.[9]
>
> Menorrhagia is the presenting symptom among most women who undergo hysterectomy. Instead of recommending the levonorgestrel-releasing intra-uterine device, hysterectomies continue to be one of the most commonly performed surgeries in North America.[10] In Canada, for example, hysterectomies were among the top five reasons for in-hospital surgeries in 2012–13.[11] Reasons for this are speculative but could include long-standing fears regarding the safety of intra-uterine devices, slow dissemination of information about their usefulness, over-reliance on a medicalized approach rather than a woman-centred treatment or, perhaps, the relative financial gain to be obtained from hysterectomy surgery.

Professional bodies usually assume responsibility for disseminating evidence-based information in the form of guidelines. National or regional perinatal surveillance systems collect information regarding practices, but we hold no one accountable when evidence-based findings and guidelines are not implemented (unless a problem reaches disastrous consequences that invoke legal action). At the very least, the individual practitioner should be responsible for ensuring that his or her knowledge and practice remain up-to-date. Likewise, each departmental head within a healthcare facility should be responsible and accountable for the practices in place in that department or facility. It is time for us to designate personnel who are responsible for disseminating current research findings within healthcare facilities, implementing them and taking action to ensure that we follow these findings when deviations from these standards occur.

Funding Family-Centred Research

Research funding agencies are contributing to our current emphasis on biological outcomes rather than psycho-social concerns. Many commonly believe that perinatal health research proposals have greater difficulty gaining funding support if they do not include clear-cut objective markers as primary outcomes. Although it is possible to develop psycho-social outcome measures that are objective, it is more difficult to do so and easier to use readily available clear-cut customary measures of biological functioning. The result is a plethora of studies with mortality or clearly measureable morbidity as the primary outcome and a scarcity of studies explaining less definitive concepts such as personal well-being. And yes, this should also include well-designed qualitative studies.

> We need to acknowledge that human beings are complex; that health is a balance between physiological, psychological, social and spiritual levels of functioning; and that care for the whole person requires attention from specialists in each of these areas working in co-ordination. At the risk of sounding science fictional, *Star Trek* provides a possible model to follow by combining the care offered by a medical doctor with that of a ship's counsellor. Traditional societies seek balance between the elements of their world. Our Western pharmacopeia could, perhaps, benefit by learning from this model.

Social scientists are also partly to blame for this gap in research. We need well-developed and well-defined outcome measures that are convincing enough to warrant significant research funding. The questions suggested for inclusion in a measure of family-centredness of perinatal care in the Appendix might provide a starting point for developing appropriate insights into at least this aspect of perinatal care. In addition, we need to consider whether research programmes should include support for the implementation of research findings – or at least the amelioration of any harmful outcomes – and not only for conducting a study.

Conclusion

Many of the issues raised in this book, including those just highlighted, are controversial. Addressing them will be difficult and perhaps even disturbing. Traditionalists who wish to 'protect their turf' will be unwilling to change. Although caution, care and sensitivity will be required before acting on any of them, failure to consider the issues that this book raises and to institute programmes that might resolve the problems inherent in them might constitute major errors of omission. It is my hope that this book will serve to stimulate further action on some of these difficult challenges.

Key Points
- Providing transparent psycho-social and clinical perinatal practices and outcomes reports for families as well as for caregivers is long overdue.
- Midwives – if well trained and competent – are able to care for normal pregnancy and may best satisfy the psychological, social and cultural expectations of women and their families.

- In developing countries, co-operation between traditional birth attendants and professional caregivers requires sensitive consideration.
- Care of families during the perinatal period requires inter-professional contact, communication, co-ordination and collaboration. This model should be initiated during undergraduate training and continue into later years of specialization
- In addition to creating professional bodies that focus on individual disciplines, we need integrated professional organizations that bring together all professionals caring for families during their transition to parenthood. We also need to include the family perspective.
- Schools of psychology need to strengthen their education of both psychology students and those from other healthcare disciplines regarding psycho-social issues in health, particularly perinatal health. Whereas social and legal issues are well cared for by social workers, psychological and counselling issues require knowledge that is more specialized.
- We need to develop greater understanding of cultural differences in beliefs, attitudes and practices regarding health and healthcare across cultures. This applies to differing cultural groups within our own societies as well as when working in countries other than our own.
- We need to designate personnel who are responsible for disseminating current research findings within healthcare facilities, implementing them and taking action to ensure that these findings are followed.
- Research funding agencies are contributing to our current emphasis on biological outcomes rather than psycho-social concerns.
- Research funding programmes should include support for the implementation of research findings – or at least the amelioration of any harmful outcomes – and not only for conducting a study.

Appendix: Family-Centred Care Monitoring Questions

Three sets of monitoring questions follow. The first list is intended for use by individual caregivers of any professional group, with the second being directed at the institutional level. The third list provides a sample of questions that mothers could be asked to address. These are not formalized, 'ready-to-use' questionnaires but provide a 'question bank' or an 'issue bank' that can serve as a source of potential questions to ask caregivers or healthcare facilities regarding the family-centredness of their care. The healthcare service or caregivers for which it is intended would need to adapt these questions to suit their circumstances. Response categories (e.g. never, sometimes, often), layout and spacing have not therefore been attempted here to leave these options to be customized by the user. These questions are not exhaustive or all-inclusive. They can be expanded on if a topic is of particular concern, deleted if not applicable and be supplemented by additional issues of interest. A number of surveys of women's perceptions of their maternity care have been developed and used in large-scale surveys, and it would be advisable for any facility planning to implement such surveys to explore these in more depth.[1] The questions included here for completion by women/families focus specifically on issues that reflect the family-centredness of their care rather than on the full array of their perinatal care experiences.

Individual Caregiver Questions

Are You Offering Family-Centred Prenatal Care?

- What proportion of women carries their own case records or has a means to access their electronic records?
- What proportion of prenatal care visits is attended by both the mother and her partner or chosen companion?
- What proportion of primiparas in your care attends prenatal preparation classes?
- What proportion of classes is attended by both the mother and a chosen companion/partner?
- How often do you weigh women attending you for prenatal care?
- How often do you advise obese women to lose a considerable amount of weight while they are trying to get pregnant and/or during pregnancy?
- How many ultrasounds do you routinely do during a pregnancy?
- How often do you counsel women on the possible consequences of adverse outcomes of prenatal screening tests and their likely courses of action in response?
- How often do you discuss families' expectations regarding their care during labour and birth?
- Do you provide evidence-based information to families on which they can base their expectations and decisions regarding their perinatal care?

Are You Offering Family-Centred Care during Labour and Birth?

- What proportion of mothers giving birth under your care have

  - planned Caesarean sections?
  - Caesarean sections following attempted vaginal births?
  - vaginal births?

- What proportion of mothers giving birth under your care by vaginal, caesarean section following attempted vaginal birth or planned caesarean sections have

  - induction?
  - augmentation of labour?
  - pubic shaving?
  - perineal shaving?
  - enemas?
  - labour monitored using a partograph?
  - unrestricted ambulation throughout labour?
  - pharmacological pain relief?
  - non-pharmacological pain management such as baths, relaxation techniques, TENS, massage, position changes and ambulation?
  - epidural or spinal analgesia?
  - supine position for birth with the use of stirrups?
  - supine position for birth without stirrups?
  - an upright or side-lying birth position?
  - a partner and/or companion at birth?
  - a doula at birth?

- episiotomy?
- pushing on the abdomen to help get the baby down?
- forceps or vacuum deliveries?
- tears?
- stitches?
- exteriorization of the cervix to check for tears?
- delivery of the newborn directly onto the mother's abdomen?
- skin-to-skin care immediately after birth?
- skin-to-skin care for the first hour or more after birth?
- separation of mother and baby during the first hour after birth?
- breastfeeding within the first hour or so after birth, when the baby shows signs of readiness for a feed?
- minimal or no interruptions for clinical care procedures, for at least the first hour after birth?

- What proportion of women giving birth under your care has a companion of choice with them

  - in labour?
  - at birth?

- Who makes decisions about implementing each of the preceding practices?
- How much say did the mother/family have in each of these decisions?

Are You Offering Family-Centred Breastfeeding Support after Birth?
- Have you received more than 1 or 2 hours of formal education regarding breastfeeding?
- Have you attended an 18- to 20-hour (or similar) breastfeeding training programme based on the BFHI?
- What proportion of newborns you assist to deliver is put to the breast too quickly, within minutes of birth?
- How long after birth do newborns spontaneously show an interest in breastfeeding if no interventions in this process are instituted?
- What proportion of mothers do you show how to 'hand express' milk?
- What proportion of mothers in your care do you advise to give their newborns liquids other than breastmilk?
- What proportion of mothers do you encourage to breastfeed according to

  - a regular schedule?
  - a baby-led, cue-, or demand-based programme?

- Do you encourage mothers to give their newborns pacifiers/dummies?
- How often are you offered gifts or promotions from formula-producing companies in return for using or promoting their breastmilk substitutes?
- How often do you accept these gifts?

Are You Offering Family-Centred Care in NICUs?
- What proportion of mothers in your care who give birth to babies that require NICU care gets to hold their babies before the baby is transferred to intensive care?

- What proportion of mothers with babies in NICU room-in with their newborns? Do you encourage this on a full-time (24/7) basis?
- Have you ever felt the need to discuss the stresses of your work with someone who is familiar with these challenges?

  . Were you able to?

- How competent do you feel you are to care for women or families who have experienced major perinatal losses such as termination of pregnancy, birth of a baby with congenital anomalies, stillbirth or neonatal loss?

  . Were you ever given training on this issue?
  . Should you have?

- Do you routinely contact mothers who have had serious pregnancy complications (such as stillbirth, termination of pregnancy for fetal anomalies or birth of a baby with anomalies) in the post-birth/termination period, to provide support and information for them?

Are You Providing Psycho-Socially Sensitive Family-Centred Care?
- Do you ever ask how the woman and her partner/support companion feels about their labour and birth experience?
- Do you offer an opportunity for them to discuss their feelings with you and for you to provide any information or explanation they might need?
- Do you allow a companion to accompany a woman when she is having an obstetrical or gynaecological procedure performed?
- Have you ever offered this option to any woman?
- Do you routinely provide non-problematic results to women or only test findings that require further medical attention?

  . What proportion do you personally speak to by telephone?
  . What proportion is called and asked to make an appointment for them to see you to learn of their test results?

Do You Routinely Monitor the Family-Centredness of Your Care?
- Have you ever taken any courses on medical humanities or psycho-social concerns in the perinatal period?
- How often do you meet with mothers or families after a difficult birth experience (e.g. a miscarriage, still birth or unwanted caesarean section) simply to discuss what happened and why?

  . How comfortable would you be to enter into this type of discussion?

- Are you able to refer women or their family members to a perinatal psychologist (or similar qualified professional) for counselling regarding any aspect of their perinatal experience if needed?
- How often do women request consideration of their spiritual needs during the perinatal period?

  . Are you able to grant these requests?

- How often do women under your care seek a 'second opinion'?
- Have often do you ask women in your care such questions as

  . How happy are you to give birth in hospital/at home?
  . Are you afraid of hospitals? Doctors? Birth?
  . Would you like to talk to anyone about this?
  . What can I do to make you feel more comfortable about your forthcoming birth? Is there anything you would like to do – or like me to do or not to do – that would make you feel happier about the prospect of birth?
  . Who would you like to have with you in labour and at birth?

- How often do you visit a woman you have assisted during the birth of her baby on the day after birth?
- Do you use the ALPHA scale (or similar) to assist in determining psycho-social risk factors in your patients?
- Have you ever had any training on how to indicate to women that you are open to discussion about sexually related abuse without causing them emotional distress by the way you ask about this?
- How do you share such information with colleagues who may need to know about the woman's history of abuse?
- What position do you adopt for routine vaginal examinations of women:

  . Do you stand at her side?
  . Do you station yourself at the foot of the bed?

- Is information about your perinatal practices and outcomes publicly available?

Are You Providing Family-Centred Multi-Disciplinary Care?

- Do you participate in or contribute to any perinatal association's activities that are not your primary professional focus?
- How often do you contribute to or participate in perinatal activities organized by women's groups?
- What proportion of your training was devoted to normal pregnancy and birth?
- What percentage to complications of pregnancy and birth?
- Were you ever given training in perinatal care by members of other professions than your own, such as by midwives, neonatologists, family doctors, obstetricians or perinatal psychologists?
- Do you share teaching programmes offered to healthcare students with professionals from other disciplines?
- Is there a multi-disciplinary healthcare association in your country that is dedicated to inter-disciplinary perinatal care rather than to issues of importance to one primary discipline such as obstetrics?

Are You Providing Family-Centred and Culturally Sensitive Care?

- What proportion of women in your care come from cultural backgrounds different from your own?
- How often do you explore their cultural needs with regard to pregnancy, birth and postpartum?

- Do you routinely perform caesarean sections for women who have previously had Female Genital Mutilation?
- Are you familiar with the laws in your country regarding repair of the perineum of such women following a vaginal birth?
- Should caregivers be prosecuted for re-infibulating a woman after a vaginal birth?
- Do you confirm with women that the advice you are giving them is feasible or possible within their social and cultural contexts?
- Do you check with women of different cultural backgrounds regarding their needs for privacy, particularly during clinical examination and at birth?
- Have you ever considered a woman's differing cultural practice to be preferable to your own?

Satisfaction with Care

- Do you routinely ask families how satisfied they are with
  - their care during pregnancy?
  - their care during labour and birth?
  - their care in the postpartum period?

Institutional Questions

Are You Offering Family-Centred Prenatal Care?
- Does your healthcare facility offer prenatal care classes? Do mothers/families pay a fee to attend them?
- How many ultrasounds are done in your facility during routine prenatal care, and when?
- Does your institution provide evidence-based information to families on which they can base their expectations and decisions regarding their perinatal care?

Are You Offering Family-Centred Care during Labour and Birth?
- What proportion of mothers giving birth in your healthcare facility has
  - caesarean sections?
  - vaginal births?

- What proportion of mothers giving birth in your healthcare facility by vaginal, caesarean section following attempted vaginal birth or planned caesarean section have
  - induction?
  - augmentation of labour?
  - pubic shaving?
  - perineal shaving?
  - enemas?
  - labour monitored using a partograph?
  - unrestricted ambulation throughout labour?
  - pharmacological pain relief?
  - non-pharmacological pain management such as baths, relaxation techniques, TENS, massage, position changes or ambulation?
  - epidural or spinal analgesia?
  - supine position for birth with the use of stirrups?
  - supine position for birth without stirrups?
  - an upright or side-lying birth position?
  - a partner and/or companion at birth?
  - a doula at birth?
  - episiotomy?
  - pushing on the abdomen to help get the baby down?
  - forceps or vacuum deliveries?
  - tears?
  - stitches?
  - exteriorization of the cervix to check for tears?
  - delivery of the newborn directly onto the mother's abdomen?
  - skin-to-skin care immediately after birth?
  - skin-to-skin care for the first hour or more after birth?
  - separation of mother and baby during the first hour after birth?

.   breastfeeding within the first hour or so after birth, when the baby shows signs of readiness for a feed?

.   minimal or no interruptions for clinical care procedures for at least the first hour after birth?

- Are there differences in the rates of use of the preceding interventions between obstetricians, family doctors and midwives in your facility? If so, are these clinically justifiable?

- What proportion of women giving birth in your facility has a companion of their choice with them

    .   in labour?
    .   at birth?

- To what extent do families make decision about each of these practices? Do you attempt to monitor this?

Are You Offering Family-Centred Care after Birth?

- Do you expect caregivers in your facility to ask how families felt about their labour and birth experience? Do they discuss family members' feelings and provide information or explanations that families might need?

- What proportion of partners room-in with the new mother in the postpartum ward for the full duration of her stay? What facilities are provided for them:

    .   a comfortable chair?
    .   a bed?
    .   meals?

- What proportion of your staff (obstetricians, neonatologists, family doctors, midwives and nurses) is trained on at least an 18- to 20-hour course on the BFHI?

- What proportion of your clients is exclusively breastfeeding their babies on discharge?

- Does your facility have a written breastfeeding supportive policy that is based on the WHO/UNICEF BFHI?

- If you are an educational facility, what proportion of students receives 18 to 20 hours of education on breastfeeding?

    .   Medical students?
    .   Allied medical profession students?

- Do you provide preparation for breastfeeding for pregnant women and their families?

- What proportion of mothers in your facility practices rooming-in 24 hours a day

    .   following vaginal birth?
    .   following caesarean section?
    .   when their babies are in an NICU?

- Are mothers referred to breastfeeding support resources in your area after discharge?

- Does your facility accept gifts from formula-producing companies in return for using or promoting their breastmilk substitutes?

- Is your healthcare facility accredited as a Baby-Friendly Hospital/Institute?

Are You Offering Family-Centred Care in NICUs

- What proportion of mothers (or families) of babies in NICU can stay with their infants for 24/7 in your facility?
- What proportion of babies in NICUs has

  - single-room family care?
  - multi-bed ward care?

- Do mothers actively share care for their preterm or sick newborns in NICUs with healthcare providers? What proportion of the baby's/babies' care do mothers provide?
- What proportion of NICU babies in your facility is exclusively breastfed on discharge?
- Do you have perinatal psychologists in your facility?

  - What proportion is full-time staff?
  - What proportion is part-time staff?
  - What proportion is occasional consultants?

- Does your facility routinely follow up 'graduates' of NICU care to monitor their progress and development?
- Do you continue to offer medical, psychological and social support and assistance with the care of these babies if this is needed?
- Do you routinely contact mothers who have had serious pregnancy complications (such as stillbirth, termination of pregnancy for fetal anomalies or birth of a baby with anomalies) in the post-birth/termination period, to provide support and information for them?

Are You Providing Psycho-Socially Sensitive Family-Centred Care?

- Do students in your facility have to take courses in psychological, social or cultural aspects of medical/perinatal care?

  - If so, are they appropriately family-centred?

- Does your institute (if it is a teaching institute) provide training for perinatal psychologists?
- Does the university nearest to you offer training in perinatal health psychology?
- In your facility, to what extent are families involved in decisions about

  - their care?
  - the health services offered?
  - education programmes for your students?

- To what extent do you think that women in your facility make decisions about their care

  - based on truly informed consent?
  - based on informed coercion?

- Could maternity hotels serve as a model to follow in your facility?

Are You Providing Family-Centred Inter-Disciplinary Care?

- Does your healthcare facility encourage inter-disciplinary collaboration and co-ordination
  - with regard to patient care? How?
  - with regard to student education? How?
  - with regard to professional development? How?

Are You Providing Family-Centred and Culturally Sensitive Care?

- What cultural groups are cared for in your facility?
- Do you have sufficient resources in your facility to overcome the challenges of language and cultural differences in your practice?

Do You Routinely Monitor the Family-Centredness of Your Care Facility?

- Does your facility collect perinatal healthcare data?

  - Does this include psycho-social indicators?
  - Are these data collected in real time?

- Does your facility assess women's reactions to their perinatal care?
- Does it seek the reactions of other family members such as those of the partner?
- Is your facility able to compare your own perinatal database findings with those of other hospitals/regions/national databases?
- Does your facility assess women's and their families' experiences of

  - normal perinatal experiences?
  - complications of pregnancy, birth or the newborn?

- Does your facility seek information from women of differing cultural backgrounds regarding their satisfaction with their perinatal care?
- Is information about your perinatal practices and outcomes published in a form that is readily available to the public?

Satisfaction with Care

- Does your facility routinely ask families how satisfied they are with
  - their care during pregnancy?
  - their care during labour and birth?
  - their care in the postpartum period?

Women's Questions

Did You Have Family-Centred Prenatal Care?

- Did you carry you own healthcare records in some form (e.g. paper or electronic access to records) while you were pregnant?
- Did you attend prenatal care classes?
  - . What proportion of prenatal care visits did your chosen support person/partner attend?
- How often were you weighed during your pregnancy care visits?
  - . At the first visit only?
  - . At almost every visit?
- How many ultrasounds did you have, and when, in your pregnancy?
- Did you have any prenatal screening tests (e.g. to check for a Down syndrome baby)?
  - . Did your caregiver discuss what you might do if the test results showed that there might be a problem with your baby?
  - . Did your caregiver call you personally to give you the results of your tests, did a nurse call you, or were you asked to come into the office to get the results?
- Did your caregiver ever provide an opportunity for you to talk about possible abuse in your life?
- Did your caregiver discuss possible methods of delivery with you such as the possibility of having a caesarean section?
- Did your caregiver discuss any of the following regarding birth with you prior to the onset of your labour?
  - . Who you would like to have with you in labour and at the birth?
  - . Whether you were afraid of birth or of doctors or hospitals?
  - . What your caregiver could do to make you more comfortable about these concerns?
  - . How you wanted to manage your pain in labour?
  - . Whether you wanted to be in an upright position for birth?
  - . Whether you wanted to have your feet in stirrups?
  - . Whether you wanted an enema?
  - . Whether you wanted to have your public or perineal hair shaved?
  - . Whether you wanted your baby delivered directly onto your abdomen at the time of birth?
  - . Who you would like to cut the cord?
  - . Whether you wanted to hold your baby skin-to-skin immediately after birth?
  - . Whether you wanted to breastfeed shortly after your baby was born?
- How much say do you feel you had in deciding on any of these practices?
- Were you ever given evidence-based information on which to base your expectations and decisions regarding your care during pregnancy, birth and the postpartum period?

Did You Have Family-Centred Care during Labour and Birth?

- Did you have

    . a spontaneous-onset vaginal birth?
    . an emergency caesarean section (following a planned vaginal birth)?
    . a planned caesarean section (decided on before labour started)?

- Did you have

    . an induced labour (labour was started by the caregiver with medications)?
    . augmentation of labour (labour was speeded up after it started with medications)?
    . your pubic hair shaved?
    . your perineal hair shaved?
    . an enema?
    . the ability to walk around in labour as you pleased?
    . pain relief by means of drugs/medications?
    . non-pharmacological pain management such as baths, relaxation techniques, TENS, massage, position changes and ambulation?
    . an epidural or spinal analgesia?
    . your baby while in a supine (flat-lying) position for birth with your legs in stirrups?
    . your baby while in a supine (flat-lying) position for birth without stirrups?
    . an upright or side-lying birth position?
    . your partner and/or a companion of your choice at the birth?
    . a doula at the birth?
    . an episiotomy (or cut to your perineum to make it easier for the baby to come out)?
    . pushing on your abdomen to help get the baby down?
    . a forceps or vacuum delivery?
    . tears to your perineum?
    . stitches in your perineum?
    . exteriorization of the cervix (pulling it down after delivery) to check for tears?
    . delivery of the newborn directly onto your abdomen?
    . skin-to-skin care immediately after birth?
    . skin-to-skin care for the first hour or more after birth?
    . your baby with you continuously during the first hour after birth?
    . the opportunity to breastfeed your baby within the first hour or so after birth, when the baby showed signs of readiness for a feed?
    . minimal or no interruptions for clinical care procedures for at least the first hour after birth?

- Do you feel that you were treated with respect during your pregnancy, labour and birth?
- Were your caregivers concerned with maintaining your dignity during pregnancy, labour and birth?
- Did you think your caregivers were competent to care for you during pregnancy, labour and birth?

- Did you have a good relationship/good interactions with your caregivers during your labour and birth?
- Did your caregivers respect your cultural practices/needs during pregnancy, labour and birth?
- Were your privacy and confidentiality respected during pregnancy, labour and birth?
- Were your partner's/chosen support person's needs cared for during labour and birth?
- Was your companion ever asked to leave the room just when you felt you wanted him or her with you most?
- Did the doctor/caregiver who helped you deliver your baby come to see you in the postpartum wards/at home in the days after giving birth?
- Did you have the same caregiver during pregnancy, labour and birth?
  - If not, would this have been your preference?
  - If yes, was this what you wanted?

Did You Have Family-Centred Support after the Birth?

- Did any of your caregivers ever ask how you felt about your labour and birth experience? Did they discuss your feelings with you and provide any information or explanation that you might have needed regarding them? Was your partner/support companion asked these types of questions?
- If you gave birth in a hospital, was your partner/chosen support person able to stay with you 24/7 after the birth?

  If yes, what was provided for your companion?

  - A bed?
  - A comfortable chair?
  - Meals?

- Did you try to breastfeed your baby?

  If yes, then

  - For how long did you breastfeed your baby (number of days, weeks, months, still breastfeeding)?

- Did anyone teach you about breastfeeding and how to hold or position your baby on the breast *before* the baby was born?
- Did anyone teach you about breastfeeding and how to hold or position your baby on the breast *after* the baby was born?
- How soon after birth did you first breastfeed your baby?
- Did your baby stay with you in the same postpartum room from the time of delivery onwards?
- For how long did you breastfeed exclusively (gave your baby no other foods or liquids other than breastmilk)?
- When did you add other liquids to your baby's diet?
- When did you add solid food to your baby's diet?
- Did you breastfeed 'on demand' (on baby's cue) or according to a schedule?
- Did you give your baby a pacifier/dummy? If so, when was this introduced?

- Were you given free formula samples?
  - Were these given in the hospital?
  - By your caregiver?
  - In the mail or though other sources?
- Were you contacted by a formula-producing company with free offers for baby goods, even if these did not include baby formula, baby bottles/teats?
- How supportive of breastfeeding was/were
  - your partner?
  - your mother?
  - other family members?
  - your caregivers?

- How helpful with regard to breastfeeding was/were
  - your partner?
  - your mother?
  - other family members?
  - your caregivers?

- Was breastfeeding difficult for you?
- Did you have problems getting help with breastfeeding?
- Did you decide to give up breastfeeding because of these problems?
- Were you made to feel guilty for not being able to continue with breastfeeding?
- If you have another baby, do you think you will try to breastfeed that baby?

If you did not breastfeed,
- Did you receive assistance with formula-feeding your baby?
- Were you made to feel guilty about not breastfeeding?
- If you have another baby, will you try to breastfeed that baby?

If Your Baby Was Admitted to an NICU
- Did you hold your baby before he or she was taken to the NICU, even if only for a moment or two?
- Was your baby's condition explained to you fully as soon as it was possible to do so?
- Did the caregiver who looked after you during birth personally explain the problems that your baby faced?
- Were you able to stay with your baby in the NICU?
  - All day and night (24/7) from birth until the baby was discharged?
  - Some hours of the day until the baby was discharged?
  - For a night or two prior to discharge?
  - Hardly ever?

- Was it possible for your partner/chosen support person to stay with you and the baby in the NICU 24/7?
  - Would this have been your preference?

- Did the NICU have single-family rooms available for some families?
- Were you made to feel welcome in the NICU? Alternatively, did you feel like a visitor?
- What proportion of the baby's care were you encouraged to undertake yourself?
- Could you easily ask questions or get help when you needed it?

  - With regard to your baby's health?
  - With regard to your own worries and concerns?

- Were your own personal worries and concerns discussed with you in the NICU?
- After your baby was discharged from the NICU, did anyone from the care facility follow up with you about your own or your baby's progress?

If You Experienced a Pregnancy Loss, Had a Baby with a Congenital Anomaly or Had an Otherwise Very Difficult Birth Experience

- Did your caregiver meet with you to explain what had happened?
- Did you feel that you had as much time as you needed with your caregiver to discuss what happened?
- Do you still have unanswered questions?
- Were you ever given the name and contact details of someone with whom you could discuss these difficult experiences?

  - Did you ever contact that person?
  - Would you have preferred the person to call you rather than you calling him or her?

- Did you want to discuss these experiences with a spiritual advisor (e.g. a priest, rabbi or other religious person)?

  - If yes, were you able to do this?
  - Did your health caregivers help you to arrange this?

Satisfaction with Care

- Overall, how satisfied are you with the care you received during pregnancy?
- Overall, how satisfied are you with the care you received during labour and birth?
- Overall, how satisfied are you with your postpartum care?

Notes

Chapter 2

1. E. Zwelling and C. R. Phillips, 'Family-Centered Maternity Care in the New Millennium: Is It Real or Is It Imagined?', *Journal of Perinatal and Neonatal Nursing* 15, no. 3 (2001).

2. Public Health Agency of Canada (PHAC), *Family-Centred Maternity and Newborn Care Guidelines* (PHAC, 2017, in preparation).

3. The Transforming Maternity Care Vision Team, '2020 Vision for a High-Quality, High-Value Maternity Care System', *Women's Health Issues* 20, no. 1 (2010).

4. J. Smith, F. Plaat and N. Fisk, 'The Natural Caesarean: A Woman-Centred Technique', *BJOG: An International Journal of Obstetrics and Gynaecology* 115, nos. 1037–42 (2008).

5. Public Health Agency of Canada. *Family-Centred Maternity and Newborn Care Guidelines* .

6. J. R. Roudebush and others, 'Patient- and Family-Centered Perinatal Care: Partnerships with Childbearing Women and Families', *Journal of Perinatal and Neonatal Nursing* 20, no. 3 (2006).

7. Zwelling and Phillips, 'Family-Centered Maternity Care in the New Millennium'.

8. World Health Organization (WHO), *Preamble to the Constitution of the World Health Organization* (Geneva: WHO, 1946).

9. World Health Organization (WHO), *Having a Baby in Europe* (Copenhagen: WHO, 1985).

10. Roudebush and others, 'Patient- and Family-Centered Perinatal Care'.

Chapter 3

1. WHO, 'Safe Motherhood: Mother-Baby Package – Implementing Safe Motherhood in Countries', World Health Organization, Maternal Health and Safe Motherhood Programme, 2013, available at http://whqlibdoc.who.int/hq/1994/WHO_FHE_MSM_94.11_Rev.1.pdf.

2. B. Chalmers, 'Psychosocial Factors and Obstetric Complications', *Psychology and Medicine* 13, (1983).

3. UK National Collaborating Centre for Women's and Children's Health, 'Antenatal Care: Routine Care for the Healthy Pregnant Woman', 2008, available at www.Nice.Org.Uk/Nicemedia/Live/11947/40145/40145.pdf.

4. *Ibid.*

5. S. M. Phelan and others, 'Impact of Weight Bias and Stigma on Quality of Care and Outcomes for Patients with Obesity', *Obesity Reviews* 16 (2015); R. Puhl and K. D. Brownell, 'Bias, Discrimination, and Obesity', *Obesity Research* 9, no. 12 (2001).

6. WHO, 'Safe Motherhood: Mother-Baby Package – Implementing Safe Motherhood in Countries'.

7. B. Chalmers and R. Porter, 'Assessing Management of Normal Labour: The Bologna Score', *Birth* 28, no. 2 (2001).

8. Society of Obstetricians and Gynaecologists of Canada, 'Joint Policy Statement on Normal Birth', *Journal of Obstetrics and Gynaecology of Canada* 30, no. 12 (2008).

9. Royal College of Obstetricians and Gynaecologists, Royal College of Midwives and National Childbirth Trust, *Making Normal Birth a Reality: Consensus Statement from the Maternity Care Working Party* (London: Maternity Care Working Party, 2007).

10. *Ibid.*

11. B. Chalmers, V. Mangiaterra and R. Porter, 'WHO Principles of Perinatal Care: The Essential Antenatal, Perinatal and Postpartum Care Course', *Birth.* 28 (2001).

12. F. Althabe and J. F. Belizan, 'Caesarean Section: The Paradox', *Lancet* 368 (2006); L Gibbons and others, *The Global Numbers and Costs of Additionally Needed and Unnecessary Caesarean Sections Performed Per Year: Overuse as a Barrier to Universal Coverage*, 2010; WHO, 'Appropriate Technology for Birth', *Lancet* 8452 (1985).

13. E. Declercq and B. Chalmers, 'Mothers' Reports of Their Maternity Experiences in the USA and Canada', *Journal of Reproductive and Infant Psychology* 26, no. 4 (2008).

14. B Chalmers, 'Childbirth across Cultures: Research and Practice', *Birth* 39, no. 4 (2012).

15. J. S. Mercer and others, 'Evidence-Based Practices for the Fetal to Newborn Transition', *Journal of Midwifery & Women's Health* 52, no. 3 (2007).

16. H. Goer and A. Romano, *Optimal Care in Childbirth: The Case for a Physiologic Approach* (Seattle, WA: Classic Day Publishing, 2012); A. M. Romano and J. A. Lothian., 'Promoting, Protecting and Supporting Normal Birth: A Look at the Evidence', *Journal of Obstetrics, Gynecology and Neonatal Nursing* 37 (2008).

17. M. L. DeRegil and others, 'Effects and Safety of Periconceptional Folate Supplementation for Preventing Birth Defects', *Cochrane Database of Systematic Reviews* 10 (2010).

18. S. S. Adams, M. Eberhard-Gran and A. Eskild, 'Fear of Childbirth and Duration of Labour: A Study of 2,206 Women with Intended Vaginal Delivery', *BJOG* 119:1238–46 (2012).

19. J. Rush, 'A Randomized Controlled Trial of the Effects of the Bath in Labour', PhD dissertation, University of Toronto, 1999.

20. P. Simkin, 'Non-Pharmacological Methods of Pain Relief during Labour', in *Effectiveness and Satisfaction in Pregnancy and Childbirth*, ed. M. Enkin I. Chalmers and M. Keirse. (Oxford Medical Publications, 1989).

21. E. D. Hodnett and others, 'Continuous Support for Women during Childbirth', *Cochrane Database of Systematic Reviews* 10: CD003766 (2012).

22. B. Chalmers and others, 'Breastfeeding Rates and Hospital Breastfeeding Practices in Canada: A National Survey of Women', *Birth.* 36, no. 2 (2009).

23. B. Chalmers, 'Breastfeeding Unfriendly in Canada?', *Canadian Medical Association Journal* 185, no. 5 (2013).

24. V. Berghella and others, 'Preconception Care', *Obstetrical & Gynecological Survey* 65, no. 2 (2010); M. C. Lu, 'Recommendations for Preconception Care', *American Family Physician* 76, no. 3 (2007).

25. J. Scott, 'Folic Acid Consumption throughout Pregnancy: Differentiation between Trimesters', *Annals of Nutrition & Metabolism* 59, no. 1 (2011).

26. Berghella and others, 'Preconception Care'.

27. S. F. Posner and others, 'Where Are the Data to Drive Policy Changes for Preconception Health and Health Care?', *Women's Health Issues* 18, no. 6 (2008); M. Whitworth and T. Dowswell, 'Routine Pre-Pregnancy Health Promotion for Improving Pregnancy Outcomes', *Cochrane Database of Systematic Reviews* 4 (2009).

28. J. M. Dodd and others, 'Antenatal Interventions for Overweight or Obese Pregnant Women: A Systematic Review of Randomised Trials', *BJOG* 117, no. 11 (2010).

29. K. Melzer and others, 'Effects of Recommended Levels of Physical Activity on Pregnancy Outcomes', *American Journal of Obstetrics and Gynecology* 202, no. 266 (2010).

30. M. I. Cedergren, 'Maternal Morbid Obesity and the Risk of Adverse Pregnancy Outcomes', *Obstetrics and Gynaecology* 103, no. 2 (2004).

31. E. Abalos and others, 'Antenatal Care for Health Pregnant Women: A Mapping of Interventions from Existing Guidelines to Inform the Development of New WHO Guidelines on Antenatal Care', *BJOG* 123 (2015).

32. G. Novick, 'Women's Experience of Prenatal Care: An Integrative Review', *Journal of Midwifery and Women's Health* 54, no. 3 (2009).

33. S. Downe and others, 'What Matters to Women: A Systematic Scoping Review to Identify the Processes and Outcomes of Antenatal Care Provision That Are Important to Healthy Pregnant Women', *BJOG* 123(4) (2015).

34. Pelvic Obstetric and Gynaecological Physiotherapy, 'Pregnancy-Related Pelvic Girdle Pain (PGP): For Health Professionals Formerly Known as Symphysis Pubis Dysfunction (SBD)', available at http://pogp.csp.org.uk/

publications/pregnancy-related-pelvic-girdle-pain-pgp-health-professionals (accessed 24 April 2015); National Health Services, 'Pelvic Pain in Pregnancy', UK Government, available at www.nhs.uk/conditions/pregnancy-and-baby/pages/pelvic-pain-pregnant-spd.aspx (accessed 24 April 2015).

35. M. Hatem and others, 'Midwife-Led versus Other Models of Care for Childbearing Women', *Cochrane Database of Systematic Reviews* 4, CD004667 (2008); Novick, 'Women's Experience of Prenatal Care'.

36. Public Health Agency of Canada, *What Women Say: The Maternity Experiences Survey* (Ottawa, ON: PHAC, 2009).

37. *Ibid.*

38. A. P. Alio and others, 'Feto-Infant Health and Survival: Does Paternal Involvement Matter?', *Maternal Child Health Journal* 14, no. 6 (2010).

39. UK National Institute for Health and Care Excellence, 'Weight Management before, during and after Pregnancy: Quick Reference Guide', 2010, available at www.nice.org.uk/nicemedia/live/13056/49929/49929.pdf.

40. B. Chalmers and others, *Essential Antenatal, Perinatal and Post-Partum Care Course* (Copenhagen: WHO Regional Office for Europe, 1999).

41. C. M. O'Leary and others, 'A Review of Policies on Alcohol Use during Pregnancy in Australia and Other English-Speaking Countries, 2007', *Medical Journal of Australia* 186, no. 9 (2007).

42. M. Enkin and others, *A Guide to Effective Care in Pregnancy and Childbirth*, 3rd edn. (Oxford University Press, 2000).

43. Chalmers and others, *Essential Antenatal, Perinatal and Post-Partum Care Course.*

44. UK National Collaborating Centre for Women's and Children's Health, 'Antenatal Care'.

45. H. C. Brown and H. J. Smith, 'Giving Women Their Own Case Notes to Carry during Pregnancy', *Cochrane Database of Systematic Reviews* 2, CD002856 (2004).

46. M. P. Austin and others, 'The Antenatal Risk Questionnaire (ANRQ): Acceptability and Use for Psychosocial Risk Assessment in the Maternity Setting', *Women Birth* 26, no. 1 (2013); D. Midmer and others, *The Alpha Form: Antenatal Psychosocial Health Assessment Form*, 2nd edn. (University of Toronto, Faculty of Medicine, Department of Family and Community Medicine, 1966).

47. Chalmers, 'Psychosocial Factors and Obstetric Complications'; B. Chalmers, 'Types of Life Events and Factors Influencing Their Seriousness Ratings', *Journal of Social Psychology* 121 (1983); W. P. Witt and others, 'Measuring Stress before and during Pregnancy: A Review of Population-Based Studies of Obstetric Outcomes', *Maternal-Child Health Journal* 18, no. 1 (2014).

48. P. Cavalli and A. J. Copp, 'Inositol and Fresistant Neural Tube Defects', *Journal of Medical Genetics* 39, no. e5 (2002); P. Cavalli and others, 'Effects of Inositol Supplementation in a Cohort of Mothers at Risk of Producing a NTD Pregnancy', *Birth Defects Research A: Clinical and Molecular Teratology* 91, no. 11 (2011).

49. S. Harvey and others, 'A Randomized Controlled Trial of Nurse-Midwifery Care', *Birth* 23 (1996); Hatem and others, 'Midwife-Led versus Other Models of Care for Childbearing Women'; W. Hueston and M. Rudy, 'A Comparison of Labour and Delivery Management between Nurse-Midwives and Family Physicians', *Journal of Family Practice* 37, no. (1993); D. Oakley and others, 'Comparisons of Certified Nurse-Midwives and Obstetricians', *Journal of Nurse-Midwifery* 40 (1995).

50. Hodnett and others, 'Continuous Support for Women during Childbirth'; J. Hofmeyr and others, 'Companionship to Modify the Clinical Birth Environment: Effects on Progress and Perceptions of Labour and Breastfeeding', *BJOG* 98 (1991); M. Klaus and others, 'Effects of Social Support during Parturition on Maternal and Infant Morbidity', *British Medical Journal* 293 (1986).

51. S. R. Magee and others, 'Promotion of Family-Centered Birth with Gentle Cesarean Delivery,' *Journal of the American Board of Family Medicine* 27, no. 5 (2014); M. S. McClellan and W. A. Cabianca, 'Effects of Early Mother-Infant Contact Following Cesarean Birth', *Obstetrics and Gynecology* 56 (1980); J. Smith, F. Plaat and N. Fisk, 'The Natural Caesarean: A Woman-Centred Technique', BJOG 115, no. 1037–42 (2008).

52. I. Chalmers, M. Enkin and M. Keirse, *Effective Care in Pregnancy and Childbirth* (Oxford University Press, 1989).

53. J. Winberg, 'Mother and Newborn Baby: Mutual Regulation of Physiology and Behavior – A Selective Review', *Developmental Psychobiology* 47 (2005).

54. E. R. Moore and others, 'Early Skin-to-Skin Contact for Mothers and Their Healthy Newborn Infants', *Cochrane Database of Systematic Reviews* 5 (2012).

55. D. Affonso and others, 'Reconciliation and Healing for Mothers through Skin-to-Skin Contact Provided in an American Tertiary Level Intensive Care Nursery', *Neonatal Network* 12 (1993); G. C. Anderson, 'Current Knowledge about Skin-to-Skin (Kangaroo) Care for Preterm Infants', *Journal of Perinatology* 11 (1991); S. M. Ludington, 'Energy Conservation during Skin-to-Skin Contact between Premature Infants and Their Mothers', *Heart and Lung* 19 (1990).

56. WHO/UNICEF, *Protecting, Promoting and Supporting Breastfeeding: The Special Role of Maternity Services* (Geneva: WHO and UNICEF, 1989).

57. M. S. Fabic and Y. Choi, 'Assessing the Quality of Data Regarding Use of the Lactational Amenorrhea Method', *Studies in Family Planning* 44, no. 2 (2013).

58. P. Simkin and others, 'Roundtable Discussion on the Language of Birth', *Birth* 39, no. 2 (2012).

59. B. Chalmers, 'Shame on Us!', *Birth* 38, no. 4 (2011).

60. M. Stewart, 'Talking to, and about, Women in Labour: In Roundtable Discussion on the Language of Birth', *Birth* 39, no. 2 (2011).

61. B. Shearer, 'Failure to Progress or Failure to Wait? In Roundtable Discussion on the Language of Birth', *Birth* 39, no. 2 (2011).

62. M. Keirse, 'Just ROAR: Rely on Acronym Rhetoric – Roundtable Discussion on: The Language of Birth', *Birth* 39, no. 2 (2012).

63. B. Chalmers, 'Terminology Used in Early Pregnancy Loss', *BJOG* 99 (1992).

64. *Ibid.*

Chapter 4

1. Y. R. Hong and J. S. Park, 'Impact of Attachment, Temperament and Parenting on Human Development', *Korean Journal of Pediatrics* 55, no. 12 (2012); K. Ma, 'Attachment Theory in Adult Psychiatry, Part 1: Conceptualisations, Measurement and Clinical Research Findings', *Advances in Psychiatric Treatment* 12 (2006); L. A. Sroufe, 'Attachment and Development: A Prospective, Longitudinal Study from Birth to Adulthood', *Attachment and Human Development* 7, nos. 349–67 (2005); S. L. Warren and others, 'Child and Adolescent Anxiety Disorders and Early Attachment', *Journal of the American Academy of Child and Adolescent Psychiatry* 36 (1997); H. I. Yoo and others, 'Parental Attachment and Its Impact on the Development of Psychiatric Manifestations in School-Aged Children', *Psychopathology* 39 (2006).

2. B. Chalmers and others, 'Breastfeeding Rates and Hospital Breastfeeding Practices in Canada: A National Survey of Women', *Birth* 36, no. 2 (2009).

3. Hodnett and others, 'Continuous Support for Women during Childbirth'; Hofmeyr and others, 'Companionship to Modify the Clinical Birth Environment'.

4. B. Chalmers and others, 'Cesarean and Vaginal Birth in Canadian Women: A Comparison of Experiences', *Birth* 37, no. 1 (2010); V. Zanardo and others, 'Elective Cesarean Delivery: Does It Have a Negative Effect on Breastfeeding?', *Birth* 37, no. 4 (2010).

5. World Health Organization (WHO), *Code of Marketing of Breastmilk Substitutes* (Geneva: WHO, 1981); WHO/UNICEF, *Protecting, Promoting and Supporting Breastfeeding*.

6. N. Rollins and others, 'Why Invest, and What Will It Take to Improve Breastfeeding Practices?', *Lancet* 387, no. 10017 (2016); C. Victora and others, 'Breastfeeding in the 21st Century: Epidemiology, Mechanisms and Lifelong Effect', *Lancet* 387, no. 10017 (2016).

7. M. S. Kramer and R. Kakuma, 'Optimal Duration of Exclusive Breastfeeding', *Cochrane Database of Systematic Reviews* 8 (2012).

8. WHO/UNICEF, *Global Strategy for Infant and Young Child Feeding* (Geneva: WHO and UNICEF, 2003).

9. WHO/UNICEF, *Protecting, Promoting and Supporting Breastfeeding*.

10. WHO, *Code of Marketing of Breastmllk Substitutes*.

11. B. Chalmers, 'Implementing the Baby Friendly Hospital Initiative', *Journal of the Society of Obstetricians and Gynaecologists of Canada* 20 (1997).

12. M. Kramer and others, 'Breastfeeding and Child Cognitive Development: New Evidence from a Large Randomized Trial', *Archives of General Psychiatry* 65, no. 5 (2008); M. Kramer and others, 'Promotion of Breastfeeding Intervention Trial (Probit): A Cluster-Randomized Trial in the Republic of Belarus', *Journal of the American Medical Association* 285 (2001).

13. Public Health Agency of Canada, *What Women Say: The Maternity Experiences Survey*.

14. Chalmers and others, 'Breastfeeding Rates and Hospital Breastfeeding Practices in Canada'.

15. Chalmers and others, 'Breastfeeding Rates and Hospital Breastfeeding Practices in Canada'.

16. R. Fox, S. McMullen and M. Newburn, 'UK Women's Experiences of Breastfeeding and Additional Breastfeeding Support: A Qualitative Study of Baby Cafe Services', *BMC Pregnancy & Childbirth* 15 (2015).

17. Chalmers, 'Breastfeeding Unfriendly in Canada?'

18. *Ibid.*

19. B. L. Horta and others, 'Evidence on the Long-Term Effects of Breastfeeding', World Health Organization, 2007; R. A. Lawrence and R. M. Lawrence, *Breastfeeding: A Guide for the Medical Profession*, 7th edn. (New York: Elsevier, Mosby, 2011).

20. Kramer and others, 'Breastfeeding and Child Cognitive Development'; Kramer and others, 'Promotion of Breastfeeding Intervention Trial (Probit)'.

21. Victora and others, 'Breastfeeding in the 21st Century'.

22. Chalmers, 'Implementing the Baby Friendly Hospital Initiative'.

23. B. Chalmers, 'The Baby Friendly Hospital Initiative: Where Next?', *British Journal of Obstetrics and Gynaecology* 111, no. 3 (2004).

Chapter 5

1. B. Chalmers and A. Levin, *Humane Perinatal Care* (Tallinn, Estonia: TEA Publishers, 2001).

2. E. O. Boundy and others, 'Kangaroo Mother Care and Neonatal Outcomes: A Meta-Analysis', *Pediatrics* 137, no. 1 (2016); N. Charpak, Z. Figueroa and J. G. Ruiz, 'Kangaroo Mother Care', *Lancet* 351 (1998); N. Charpak, J. G. Ruiz-Palaez and Y. Rey-Martinez, 'Kangaroo Mother Program: An Alternate Way of Caring for Low Birth Weight Infants? One Year Mortality in a Two Cohort Study', *Pediatrics* 94 (1994).

3. D. Murdock, 'Handling during Neonatal Intensive Care', *Archives of Diseases in Children* 59 (1984).

4. J. G. Long, J. F. Lucey and A. G. Philip, 'Noise and Hypoxia in the Intensive Care Nursery', *Pediatrics* 65 (1980).

5. H. Lagerkrantz and others, 'Plasma Catecholamines following Nursing Procedures in a Neonatal Ward', *Early Human Development* 14 (1986).

6. Chalmers and Levin, *Humane Perinatal Care*.

7. Sezgi Goksan and others, 'FMRI Reveals Neural Activity Overlap between Adult and Infant Pain', *eLife* 4, no e06356 (2015).

8. Chalmers and Levin, *Humane Perinatal Care*.

9. H. Als, 'Program Guide: Newborn Individualized Developmental Care and Assessment Program. An Education and Training Program for Health Care Professionals', available at www.nidcap.org (accessed

30 August 2013); H. Als, 'Individualized, Family-Focused Developmental Care for the Very-Low-Birthweight Preterm Infant in the NICU', in *The Psychological Development of Low-Birthweight Children*, ed. M. D. Sigman and S. L. Friedman (Norwood, NJ: Ablex, 1992); H. Als and L. Gilkerson, 'The Role of Relationship-Based Developmentally Supportive Care in Strengthening Outcome of Preterm Infants', *Seminars in Perinatology* 21 (1997); H. Als and others, 'Individualized Perinatal Care for the Very-Low-Birth-Weight Preterm Infant', *Journal of the American Medical Association* 11 (1994); D. M. Buchler and others, 'Effectiveness of Individualized Developmental Care for Low-Risk Preterm Infants: Behavioral and Electrophysiological Evidence', *Pediatrics* 96 (1995).

10. A. J. Symington and J. Pinelli, 'Developmental Care for Promoting Development and Preventing Morbidity in Preterm Infants', *Cochrane Library* (2009); L. Wallin and M. Eriksson, 'Newborn Individual Development Care and Assessment Program (NIDCAP): A Systematic Review of the Literature', *Worldviews on Evidence-Based Nursing* 6, no. 54–69 (2009); B. Westrup and others, 'A Randomized, Controlled Trial to Evaluate the Effects of the Newborn Individualized Developmental Care and Assessment Program in a Swedish Setting', *Pediatrics* 105 (2000).

11. Chalmers and Levin, *Humane Perinatal Care*; A. Levin, 'The Mother-Infant Unit at Tallinn Children's Hospital, Estonia: A Truly Baby Friendly Unit', *Birth* 21, no. 1 (1994); A. Levin, 'Where Are You Going, Neonatal Medicine? Letter to Editor', *Intensive and Critical Care Nursing* 11 (1995); A. Levin, 'Viewpoint: Humane Neonatal Care Initiative', *Acta Paediatrica* 88 (1999).

12. S. Montero and others, 'Experiences with Perinatal Loss from the Health Professionals' Perspective', *Revista Latino-Americana de Enfermagem* 19, no. 6 (2011); D. Nuzum, S. Meaney and K. O'Donoghue, 'The Impact of Stillbirth on Consultant Obstetrician Gynaecologists: A Qualitative Study', *BJOG* 121, no. 8 (2014).

13. Boundy and others, 'Kangaroo Mother Care and Neonatal Outcomes'; Chalmers and Levin, *Humane Perinatal Care*.

14. D. Hall and G. Kirsten, 'Kangaroo Mother Care: A Review', *Transfusion Medicine* 18 (2008); Moore and others, 'Early Skin-to-Skin Contact'; M. J. Renfrew and others, 'Breastfeeding Promotion for Infants in Neonatal Units: A Systematic Review and Economic Analysis', *Health Technology Assessment* 13, no. 40 (2009).

15. Chalmers and Levin, *Humane Perinatal Care*; Levin, 'Where Are You Going, Neonatal Medicine?'

16. K. D. Bolton and others, 'Black Mother's Experiences of a Neonatal Care Unit', *Journal of Reproductive and Infant Psychology* 11 (1993); K. E. Kahn, S. Wayburne and M. Fouch, 'Baragwanath Premature Unit: An Analysis of the Case Records of 1,000 Consecutive Admissions', *South African Medical Journal* 28, no. 22 (1954); J. Kennell and M. Klaus, 'The Perinatal Paradigm: Is It Time for a Change?', *Clinical Perinatology* 15 (1988); N. Tafari and S. M. Ross, 'On the Need for Organized Perinatal Care', *Ethiopian Medical Journal* 11 (1973).

17. J. Kennell, 'The Humane Neonatal Care Initiative', *Acta Paediatrica* 88 (1999).

18. K. O'Brien and others, 'Evaluation of Family Integrated Care (FiCare): A Cluster of Randomized, Controlled Trails in Canada and Australia', in *Proceedings of the Pediatric Academic Society Meeting* (Baltimore, 2016); K. O'Brien and others, 'Evaluation of the Family Integrated Care Model of Neonatal Intensive Care: A Cluster of Randomized, Controlled Trials in Canada and Australia', *BMC Pediatrics* 15 (2015).

19. O'Brien and others, 'Evaluation of Family Integrated Care (FiCare)'.

20. Chalmers and Levin, *Humane Perinatal Care*.

21. S. K. Cone, S. Short and G. Gutcher, 'From "Baby Barn" to the "Single Family Room Designed NICU": A Report of Staff Perceptions One Year Post Occupancy', *Newborn Infant Nursing Review* 10, no. 2 (2010); R. Domanico and others, 'Documenting the NICU Design Dilemma: Comparative Patient Progress in Open-Ward and Single Family Room Units', *Journal of Perinatology* 31, no. 4 (2011); L. M. Smithgall, 'Perceptions of Maternal Stress and Neonatal Patient Outcomes in a Single Private Room versus Open Room Neonatal Intensive Care Unit Environment' (East Tennessee State University, 2010); W. F. Walsh, K. L. McCullough and R. D. White, 'Room for Improvement: Nurses' Perceptions of Providing Care in a Single Room Newborn Intensive Care Setting', *Advances in Neonatal Care* 6, no. 5 (2006); R. D. White, 'Recommended Standards for Newborn ICU Design', 2013, available at www.nature.com/jp/journal/v26/n3s/full/7211587a.html; R. D. White, 'Single-Family Room Design in the Neonatal Intensive Care Unit – Challenges and Opportunities' *Newborn Infant Nursing Review* 10, no. 2 (2010).

22. J Muraskas and K Parsi, 'The Cost of Saving the Tiniest Lives: NICU's versus Prevention,' *Virtual Mentor* 10, no. 10 (2008); Westrup and others.

23. WH Northway, 'Bronchopulmonary Dysplasia: Twenty-Five Years Later,' *Pediatrics* 89, no. (1992); CL Yeo, S Choo, and LY Ho, 'Chronic Lung Disease in Very Low Birthweight Infants: A 5 Year Review,' *Journal of Pediatrics and Child Health* 33, no. (1997).

24. B Byland, T Cervin, and O Finnstrom, 'Morbidity and Neurological Function of Very Low Birthweight Infants from the Newborn Period to 4 Years of Age: A Prospective Study from the South-East Region of Sweden,' *Acta Pediatrica* 87, no. (1998); R W Cooke, 'Factors Affecting Survival and Outcome at 3 Years in Extremely Preterm Infants,' *Archives of Disease in Children* 71, no. (1994); GJ Escobar, B Littenberg, and DB Petitti, 'Outcome among Surviving Very Low Birthweight Infants: A Meta-Analysis,' *Archives of Disease in Children* 66, no. (1991); Muraskas and Parsi.

25. M Hack and others, 'School-Age Outcomes in Children with Birthweights Under 750g,' *New England Journal of Medicine* 331, no. (1994); A Hall and others, 'School Attainment, Cognitive Ability and Motor Function in a Total Scottish Very-Low-Birthweight Population at Eight Years: A Controlled Study', *Develpomental Medicine and Child Neurology* 37, no. 12 (1995); M. Ornstein and others, 'Neonatal Follow-up of Very Low Birthweight/ Extremely Low Birthweight Infants to School Age: A Critical Review', *Acta Paediatrica* 80 (1991); E. J. Sell and others, 'Early Identification of Learning Problems in Neonatal Intensive Care Graduates', *American Journal of Diseases of Childhood* 139 (1985); K. Stjernqvist and W. Svenningsen, 'Ten Year Follow-up of Children Born before 29 Gestational Weeks: Health, Cognitive Development, Behaviour and School Achievement', *Acta Paediatrica* 88 (1999).

26. J. E. Grey and D. A. Goldmann, 'Medication Errors in the Neonatal Intensive Care Unit: Special Patients, Unique Issues', *Archives of Disease of Children and Fetal and Neonatal Education* 89 (2004).

27. *Ibid.*

28. Als and others, 'Individualized Perinatal Care'; P, T. Berker and others, 'Outcomes of Developmentally Supportive Care for Very Low Birthweight Infants', *Nursing Research* 40 (1991); L. D. Brown and J, A. Heerman, 'The Effect of Developmental Care on Preterm Infant Outcome', *Applied Nursing Research* 10 (1997); B. E. Fleischer and others, 'Individualized Care for Very Low Birthweight Premature Infants Improves Medical and Developmental Outcome in the Neonatal Intensive Care Unit', *Clinical Pediatrics* 10 (1995); P. Petryshen and others, 'Comparing Nursing Costs for Preterm Infants Receiving Conventional vs. Developmental Care', *Nursing Economics* 15 (1997); B. Stevens and others, 'Developmental vs. Conventional Care: A Comparison of Clinical Outcomes for Very Low Birthweight Infants', *Canadian Journal of Nursing Research* 28 (1996).

29. Chalmers and Levin, *Humane Perinatal Care.*

30. *Ibid.*

31. *Ibid.*

32. *Ibid.*

33. A. Merewood and others, 'The Effect of Peer Counselors on Breastfeeding Rates in the Neonatal Intensive Care Unit: Results of a Randomized, Controlled Trial', *Archives of Pediatric and Adolescent Medicine* 160, no. 7 (2006).

34. Chalmers and Levin, *Humane Perinatal Care.*

35. New Brunswick Department of Health, 'New Brunswick Trauma Program', available at http://horizonnb.ca/ home/facilities-and-services/provincial-programs/new-brunswick-trauma-program/injury-prevention/ intentional-injury/child-abuse-neglect.aspx (accessed June 24 2015).

36. Chalmers and Levin, *Humane Perinatal Care.*

37. B. Chalmers and D. Meyers, 'Babies with Abnormalities: Reactions of Mothers,' *International Journal of Prenatal and Perinatal Studies* 1 (1990).

38. *Ibid.*

39. Chalmers and Levin, *Humane Perinatal Care.*

40. Public Health Agency of Canada, *What Women Say: The Maternity Experiences Survey.*

41. Chalmers and Levin, *Humane Perinatal Care.*

42. *Ibid.*

43. *Ibid.*

44. V. Flenady and T. Wilson, 'Support for Mothers, Fathers and Families after Perinatal Death', *Cochrane Database of Systematic Reviews* 1 (2008); K. J. Gold, V. K. Dalton and T. L. Schwenk, 'Hospital Care for Parents after Perinatal Death', *Obstetrics & Gynecology Clinics of North America* 109, no. 5 (2007); S. Harvey, C. Snowdon and D. Elbourne, 'Effectiveness of Bereavement Interventions in Neonatal Intensive Care: A Review of the Evidence', *Seminars in Fetal and Neonatal Medicine* 13, no. 5 (2008); A. Henley and J. Schott, 'The Death of a Baby before, during or Shortly after Birth: Good Practice from the Parents' Perspective', *Seminars in Fetal & Neonatal Medicine* 13, no. 5 (2008); K. Kobler and R. Limbo, 'The Tie That Binds: Relationships in Perinatal Bereavement', *American Journal of Maternal/Child Nursing* 35, No. 6 (2010); C. Scheidt and others, 'Mourning after Perinatal Death: Prevalence Symptoms and Treatment: A Review of Literature', *Psychotherapy Psychosomatic Medical Psychology* 57, no. 1 (2007).

45. Chalmers and Levin, *Humane Perinatal Care*.

46. Levin, 'Viewpoint: Humane Neonatal Care Initiative.'

47. Kennell, 'The Humane Neonatal Care Initiative.'

48. M. Klaus and J. Kennell, *Parent-Infant Bonding*, 2nd edn. (St Louis: Mosby, 1982).

49. Kennell, 'The Humane Neonatal Care Initiative.'

50. T. Griffin and M. Abraham, 'Transition to Home from the Newborn Intensive Care Unit: Applying the Principles of Family-Centered Care to the Discharge Process', *Journal of Perinatal & Neonatal Nursing* 20, no. 3 (2006); K. H. Nyqvist, 'Breastfeeding Support in Neonatal Care: An Example of the Integration of International Evidence and Experience', *Newborn Infant Nursing Review* 5, no. 1 (2005).

51. Klaus and Kennell, *Parent-Infant Bonding*.

52. UNICEF UK, 'UNICEF-UK Baby Friendly Initiative: Guidance for Neonatal Units', available at www.unicef.org.uk/Documents/Baby_Friendly/Going%20Baby%20Friendly/neonatal%20guidance%20 2015.pdf (accessed 16 January 2016).

53. Nordic and Quebec Working Group, 'BFHI Initiative in Neonatal Units', in *Conference and Workshop on the Expansion of the Baby Friendly Hospital Initiative* (Uppsala, Sweden, 2011).

54. J. Ogloff and R. Schuller, *Introduction to Psychology and Law: Canadian Perspectives* (University of Toronto Press, 2001).

Chapter 6

1. WHO, 'Appropriate Technology for Birth'.

2. M. Enkin, M. Keirse and I. Chalmers, *A Guide to Effective Care in Pregnancy and Childbirth* (Oxford University Press, 1989); Cochrane Library, 'The Cochrane Database of Systematic Reviews', available at www.cochranelibrary.com/cochrane-database-of-systematic-reviews/index.html (accessed 17 April 2015).

3. WHO, *Having a Baby in Europe*.

4. WHO, 'Appropriate Technology for Birth'.

5. B. Chalmers, 'WHO Appropriate Technology for Birth Revisited', *British Journal of Obstetrics and Gynaecology* 99 (1992); Enkin, Keirse and Chalmers, *A Guide to Effective Care in Pregnancy and Childbirth*.

6. Chalmers, 'WHO Appropriate Technology for Birth Revisited'.

7. UK National Institute for Health and Clinical Excellence, 'NICE Guideline: Routine Care for the Healthy Pregnant Woman '(March 2008).

8. WHO, 'Second Meeting of Focal Points of Reproductive Health/Health of Women and Children in the European Region', 1998; WHO, *Workshop on Perinatal Care Proceedings* (Venice, 1998).

9. B. Chalmers and V. Mangiaterra, 'Appropriate Perinatal Technology: A WHO Perspective', *Journal of the Society of Obstetricians and Gynaecologists of Canada* 23 (2001).

10. WHO, *Workshop on Perinatal Care Proceedings.*

11. Chalmers, Mangiaterra, and Porter, 'WHO Principles of Perinatal Care'; WHO, *Essential Antenatal, Perinatal and Postpartum Care Course* (Copenhagen: WHO Regional Office for Europe, 2002).

12. WHO, *Essential Newborn Care and Breastfeeding* (Copenhagen: WHO Regional Office for Europe, 1997).

13. B. Chalmers and others, 'The Canada/WHO/St Petersburg Maternal-Child Health Program,' *Journal of Society of Obstetricians and Gynaecologists of Canada* 20 (1998).

14. Enkin, Keirse, and Chalmers, *A Guide to Effective Care in Pregnancy and Childbirth.*

15. Public Health Agency of Canada, *Family-Centred Maternity and Newborn Care Guidelines.*

16. Althabe and Belizan, 'Caesarean Section: The Paradox'; Gibbons and others, *The Global Numbers and Costs of Additionally Needed and Unnecessary Caesarean Sections*; WHO, 'Appropriate Technology for Birth '.

17. A. P. Betran and others, 'WHO Statement on Caesarean Section Rates,' *BJOG* 123, no. 5 (2016).

18. M. S. Robson, 'Classification of Caesarean Sections', *Fetal and Maternal Medicine Review* 12 (2001).

19. F. Althabe and others, 'Cesarean Section Rates and Maternal and Neonatal Mortality in Low-, Middle- and High-Income Countries: An Ecological Study', *Birth* 33, no. 4 (2006); J. Villar and others, 'Caesarean Delivery Rates and Pregnancy Outcomes: The 2005 WHO Global Survey on Maternal and Perinatal Health in Latin America', *Lancet* 367, no. 9525 (2006).

20. Villar and others, 'Caesarean Delivery Rates and Pregnancy Outcomes'.

21. Public Health Agency of Canada, *Perinatal Health Indicators for Canada 2011*(Ottawa, ON: PHAC, 2012).

22. M. J. K. Osterman and J. A. Martin, 'Primary Cesarean Delivery Rates, by State: Results from the Revised Birth Certificate, 2006–2012', *National Vital Statistics Report* 63, no. 1 (2014).

23. S. Hellerstein, S. Feldman and T. Duan, 'China's 50% Caesarean Delivery Rate: Is It Too High?', *BJOG* (2014).

24. L. Gibbons and others, *The Global Numbers and Costs of Additionally Needed and Unnecessary Caesarean Sections Performed per Year: Overuse as a Barrier to Universal Coverage* (2010).

25. *Ibid.*

26. A. J. Macfarlane and others, 'Wide Differences in Mode of Delivery within Europe: Risk-Stratified Analyses of Aggregated Routine Data from the Euro-Peristat Study', *BJOG* 123, no. 4 (2016).

27. Chalmers, 'Childbirth across Cultures: Research and Practice'.

28. L. F. Beck and others, *PRAMS 1999 Surveillance Report* (Atlanta, GA: Division of Reproductive Health, National Center for Chronic Disease Prevention and Health Promotion, Centers for Disease Control and Prevention, 2003).

29. E. R. Declercq and others, *Listening to Mothers: Report of the First National US Survey of Women's Childbearing Experiences* (New York: Maternity Center Association, 2002); E. Declercq and others, *Listening to Mothers II: Report of the Second National US Survey of Women's Childbearing Experiences* (New York: Childbirth Connections, 2006).

30. Public Health Agency of Canada, *What Women Say: The Maternity Experiences Survey.*

31. J. Garcia and others, *First Class Delivery: A National Survey of Women's Views of Maternity Care* (London: Audit Commission, 1998); J. Green, V. Coupland and J. Kitzinger, 'Expectations, Experiences and Psychological Outcomes of Childbirth: A Prospective Study of 825 Women,' *Birth* 17 (1990); J. M. Green and others, *Greater Expectations: The Inter-Relationship between Women's Expectations and Experiences of Decision Making, Continuity, Choice and Control in Labour, and Psychological Outcomes: Summary Report* (Leeds: Mother & Infant Research Unit, University of Leeds, 2003); J. M. Green, V. A. Coupland and J. V. Kitzinger, *Great Expectations: A Prospective Study of Women's Expectations and Experiences of Childbirth*, 2nd ed. (Cheshire: UK Books for Midwives Press, 1998); M. Redshaw and others, *Recorded Delivery: A National Survey of Women's Experience of Maternity Care* (Oxford: National Perinatal Epidemiology Unit, University of Oxford, 2007); Scottish Programme for Clinical Effectiveness in Reproductive Health, *Maternity Care Matters: An Audit of Maternity Services in Scotland 1998* (Aberdeen: Douglas Baird Centre for Research on Women's Health, 1999).

32. S. Brown and J. Lumley, 'Satisfaction with Care in Labour and Birth: A Survey of 790 Australian Women', *Birth* 21 (1994).

33. U. Waldenstrom and others, 'A Negative Birth Experience: Relevance and Risk Factors in a National Sample', *Birth* 31 (2004).

34. B. Chalmers and others, 'What Women Say about Antenatal Care in St Petersburg, Russian Federation', *Journal of Psychosomatic Obstetrics and Gynaecology* 20 (1999); B. Chalmers and others, 'Women's Experiences of Birth in St Petersburg, Russian Federation Following a Maternal-Child Health Intervention Program', *Birth* 25 (1998), 107–16; B. Chalmers and others, 'What Women Say about Post-Partum Care and Breastfeeding in St Petersburg, Russian Federation', *Journal of the Society of Obstetricians and Gynaecologists of Canada* 21 (1999); B. Chalmers and others, 'Contraceptive Knowledge, Attitudes and Use among Women Attending Health Clinics in St Petersburg, Russian Federation', *Canadian Journal of Human Sexuality* 7 (1998); E. Heiberg and others, 'Women's Experiences of Giving Birth in Northwest Russia in 2000 and 2002 and in Northern Norway 2000', *Acta Obstetrica et Gynecologica Scandinavica* 86, no. 3 (2007).

35. B. Chalmers and D. Jeckaite, 'Giving Birth in Two Maternity Hospitals in Lithuania', *Birth* 37, no. 2 (2010).

36. P. Stratulat and others, 'Evaluarea Rezultatelor Implementarii Technologiilor Programului National De Ameliorare a Asistentei Medicale Perinatale in Republica Moldova', *Buletin de Perinatologie* 3 (2002).

37. B. Chalmers and D. Qulieva, 'A Report of Women's Birth Experiences in Baku, Azerbaijan', *Journal of Psychosomatic Obstetrics and Gynaecology* 25 (2004).

38. Chalmers, 'Childbirth across Cultures: Research and Practice.'

39. B. Chalmers, 'Over-Reliance on a Medical Approach to Care: Some Thoughts for Consideration', *Journal of the Society of Obstetricians and Gynaecologists of Canada* 21, no. 11 (1999); M. Wagner, *Pursuing the Birth Machine: The Search for Appropriate Birth Technology* (Melbourne, Australia: ACE Graphica, 1994).

40. Declercq and Chalmers, 'Mothers' Reports of Their Maternity Experiences in the USA and Canada'

41. *Ibid.*

42. B. Chalmers and others, 'Rates of Interventions in Labor and Birth across Canada: Findings of the Canadian Maternity Experiences Survey', *Birth* 39, no. 3 (2012).

43. F. Bragg and others, 'Variation in Rates of Caesarean Section among English NHS Trusts after Accounting for Maternal and Clinical Risk: Cross-Sectional Study', *British Medical Journal* 341 (2010).

44. J. Nagpal and others, 'Widespread Non-Adherence to Evidence-Based Maternity Care Guidelines: A Population-Based Cluster Randomised Household Survey', *BJOG* (2014).

45. B. Chalmers, J. McIntyre and D. Meyer, 'South African Obstetricians' Views on Caesarean Section', *South African Medical Journal* 82 (1991).

46. Public Health Agency of Canada, *Family-Centred Maternity and Newborn Care Guidelines.*

47. Public Health Agency of Canada, *What Women Say: The Maternity Experiences Survey.*

48. Chalmers and others, 'Rates of Interventions in Labor and Birth across Canada.'

49. *Ibid.*

50. Phelan and others, 'Impact of Weight Bias and Stigma on Quality of Care'; R. Puhl and K. D. Brownell. 'Bias, Discrimination, and Obesity', *Obesity Research* 9, no. 12 (2001): 788–805.

51. S. B. De Joy and K. Bittner, 'Obesity Stigma as a Determinant of Poor Birth Outcomes in Women with High BMI: A Conceptual Framework', *Maternal-Child Health Journal* 19, nos. 693–9 (2015).

52. Public Health Agency of Canada, *Family-Centred Maternity and Newborn Care Guidelines.*

53. National Institute for Health and Care Excellence.

54. Chalmers, Enkin and Keirse, *Effective Care in Pregnancy and Childbirth.*

55. Chalmers and Mangiaterra, 'Appropriate Perinatal Technology: A WHO Perspective.'

56. NICE National Institute for Health and Care Excellence, 'Intrapartum Care: Care of Healthy Women and Their Babies during Childbirth', available at www.nice.org.uk/guidance/cg190.

Chapter 7

1. 'It Happened to Me: Responses to the Stillbirth Series', *Lancet* 377, no. 9779 (2011).

2. Enkin and others, *A Guide to Effective Care in Pregnancy and Childbirth*.

3. *Ibid*.

4. Hodnett and others, 'Continuous Support for Women during Childbirth'.

5. B. Chalmers and D. Meyer, 'What Men Say about Pregnancy, Birth and Parenthood', *Journal of Psychosomatic Obstetrics and Gynaecology* 17 (1996).

6. Enkin and others, *A Guide to Effective Care in Pregnancy and Childbirth*.

7. Public Health Agency of Canada, *What Women Say: The Maternity Experiences Survey*.

8. Hodnett and others, 'Continuous Support for Women during Childbirth'; M. H. Klaus and J. .H Kennell, 'The Doula: An Essential Ingredient of Childbirth Rediscovered', *Acta Paediatrica* **86**, no. 10 (1997).

9. Chalmers and Levin, *Humane Perinatal Care*.

10. *Ibid*.

11. N. Ko and others, 'Can Patient Navigation Improve Receipt of Recommended Breast Cancer Care? Evidence from the National Patient Navigation Research Program', *Journal of Clinical Oncology* 32, no. 22 (2014).

12. Chalmers and Levin, *Humane Perinatal Care*.

13. *Ibid*.

14. *Ibid*.

15. *Ibid*.

16. H. Clinton and B. Obama, 'Making Patient Safety the Centerpiece of Medical Liability Reform', *New England Journal of Medicine* 354 (2006); S. Kraman and G. Hamm, 'Risk Management: Extreme Honesty May Be the Best Policy', *Annals of Internal Medicine* 131 (1999); Ogloff and Schuller, *Introduction to Psychology and Law*.

17. Canadian Medical Protective Association, 'Apology Legislation in Canada: What It Means for Physicians', Is0889-E, originally published September 2008, revised April 2013, available at www.cmpa-acpm.ca/-/apology-legislation-in-canada-what-it-means-for-physicians (accessed 17 April 2015).

18. Public Health Agency of Canada, *What Women Say: The Maternity Experiences Survey*.

19. B. Chalmers and K. Omer-Hashi, *Female Genital Mutilation and Obstetric Care* (Vancouver, BC: Trafford Publishers, 2003).

20. Chalmers and Levin, *Humane Perinatal Care*.

21. *Ibid*.

22. *Ibid*.

23. Brown and Lumley, 'Satisfaction with Care in Labour and Birth'; A. Calder and P. Purton, *Maternity Care Matters: An Audit of Maternity Services in Scotland 1998. Scottish Programme for Clinical Effectiveness in Reproductive Health* (Aberdeen: Douglas Baird Centre for Research on Women's Health, 1999); Declercq and Chalmers, 'Mothers' Reports of Their Maternity Experiences'; Garcia and others, *First Class Delivery*; Public Health Agency of Canada, *What Women Say: The Maternity Experiences Survey*.

24. Public Health Agency of Canada, *What Women Say: The Maternity Experiences Survey*.

25. Declercq and Chalmers, 'Mothers' Reports of Their Maternity Experiences'.

26. Chalmers, 'Childbirth across Cultures'.

27. M. MacDorman, F. Menacker and E. Declercq, 'Trends and Characteristics of Home and Other Out-of-Hospital Births in the United States 1990–2006', *National Vital Statistics Report* 58, no. 11 (2010).

28. *Ibid.*

29. L. Vogel, '"Do It Yourself" Births Prompt Alarm', *Canadian Medical Association Journal* 183, no. 6 (2011).

30. Chalmers, 'Shame on Us!'.

31. *Ibid.*

32. B. Chalmers and S. Dzakpasu, 'Interventions in Labour and Birth and Satisfaction with Care: The Canadian Maternity Experiences Survey Findings'. *Journal of Reproductive and Infant Psychology* (in press) (2015).

33. Public Health Agency of Canada, *What Women Say: The Maternity Experiences Survey.*

34. H. Keedle and others, 'Women's Reasons for, and Experiences of, Choosing a Homebirth following a Caesarean Section', *BMC Pregnancy and Childbirth* 15, no. 206 (2015).

35. Society of Obstetricians and Gynaecologists of Canada, 'Improving Sexual and Reproductive Health: Integrating Women's Empowerment and Reproductive Rights', available at http://iwhp.sogc.org/uploads/File/ISRH_booklet_web.pdf (accessed July 16, 2011).

36. *Ibid.*

37. E. Declercq and others, 'Is a Rising Cesarean Delivery Rate Inevitable? Trends in Industrialized Countries, 1987 to 2007,' *Birth* 38, no. 2 (2011); M. Keirse, 'Commentary: The Freezing Aftermath of a Hot Randomized, Controlled Trial', *Birth* 38, no. 2 (2011); M. Klein and others, 'Attitudes of the New Generation of Canadian Obstetricians: How Do They Differ from Their Predecessors?', *Birth* 38, no. 2 (2011); A. Kotaska, 'Commentary: Routine Cesarean Section for Breech – The Unmeasured Cost', *Birth* 38, no. 2 (2011); A. Kotaska, 'Guideline-Centered Care: A Two-Edged Sword', *Birth* 38, no. 2 (2011); G. W. Lawson, 'Report of a Breech Cesarean Section Maternal Death', *Birth* 38, no. 2 (2011).

38. A. Banaszek, 'Medical Humanities Becoming Prerequisites in Many Medical Schools', *Canadian Medical Association Journal* 183, no. 8 (2011); Enkin and others, *A Guide to Effective Care in Pregnancy and Childbirth.*

39. Public Health Agency of Canada, *What Women Say: The Maternity Experiences Survey.*

40. D. Bower and others, 'Discussions after Death', *South African Medical Journal* 78 (1990); D. Skibniewski-Woods, 'A Review of Postnatal Debriefing of Mothers Following Traumatic Delivery', *Community Practice* 84, no. 12 (2011).

41. B. E. Chalmers and B. M. Chalmers, 'Post-Partum Depression: A Revised Perspective', *Journal of Psychosomatic Obstetrics and Gynaecology* 5 (1986); C. Pesado and others, 'Postpartum Depression and Culture: MCN', *American Journal of Maternal/Child Nursing* 35, no. 5 (2010).

42. F. J. Paulson, D. Sharnail and M. S. Bazemore, 'Prenatal and Postpartum Depression in Fathers and Its Association with Maternal Depression: A Meta-Analysis', *JAMA* 303, no. 19 (2010).

43. Public Health Agency of Canada, *What Women Say: The Maternity Experiences Survey.*

44. M. St-André, P. N. Reebye and J.-V. Wittenberg, 'Infant Mental Health in Canada: Initiatives from British Columbia, Quebec and Ontario', *Journal of the Canadian Academy of Child and Adolescent Psychiatry* 19, no. 2 (2010).

45. C.-L. Dennis and E. Hodnett, 'Psychosocial and Psychological Interventions for Treating Postpartum Depression', *Cochrane Database of Systematic Reviews* 4 (2009).

46. B. Chalmers and D. Meyers, 'Adjustment to the Early Months of Parenthood', *International Journal of Prenatal and Perinatal Studies* 1. (1990); G. W. S. Kong, T. K. H. Chung and I. H. Lok, 'The Impact of Supportive Counselling on Women's Psychological Wellbeing after Miscarriage: A Randomised, Controlled Trial', *BJOG* 121, no. 10 (2014); Skibniewski-Woods, 'A Review of Postnatal Debriefing of Mothers'.

47. Public Health Agency of Canada, *Family-Centred Maternity and Newborn Care Guidelines.*

48. A. Maslow, *Motivation and Personality* (New York: Harper, 1943).

49. B. Chalmers, 'How Often Must We Ask for Sensitive Care before We Get It?', *Birth* 29, no. 2 (2002).

Chapter 8

1. Chalmers and Levin, *Humane Perinatal Care.*

2. *Ibid.*

3. A. J. Gagnon and J. Sandall, 'Individual or Group Antenatal Education for Childbirth or Parenthood, or Both', Cochrane Pregnancy and Childbirth Group (2007).

4. B. Chalmers and J. McIntyre, 'Do Antenatal Classes Have a Place in Modern Obstetric Care?', *International Journal of Psychosomatic Obstetrics and Gynaecology* 15 (1994).

5. B. Chalmers and G. J. Hofmeyr, 'The Gestation of a Childbirth Education Diploma', *Journal of Psychosomatic Obstetrics and Gynaecology* 10 (1989).

6. *Ibid.*

7. L. Gramling, K. Hickman and S. Bennett, 'What Makes a Good Family-Centered Partnership between Women and Their Practitioners? A Qualitative Study', *Birth* 31, no. 1 (2004).

8. A. M. Romano, 'Creating a Culture of Consumer Engagement in Maternity Care', *Journal of Perinatal Education* 19, no. 2 (2010).

9. UK National Institute for Health and Care Excellence: www.nice.org.uk/guidance/published?type=guidelines (accessed 21 July 2014).

Chapter 9

1. Public Health Agency of Canada, *Family-Centred Maternity and Newborn Care Guidelines.*

2. *Ibid.*

3. Hodnett and others, 'Continuous Support for Women during Childbirth'.

4. S. Lewin and others, 'Lay Health Workers in Primary and Community Health Care for Maternal and Child Health and the Management of Infectious Diseases', *Cochrane Database of Systematic Reviews* 3 (2010).

5. Public Health Agency of Canada, *Family-Centred Maternity and Newborn Care Guidelines.*

6. J. Adams and others, 'Attitudes and Referral Practices of Maternity Care Professionals with Regard to Complementary and Alternative Medicine: An Integrative Review', *Journal of Advanced Nursing* 67, no. 3 (2011).

7. V. C. Nikodem and others, 'Do Cabbage Leaves Prevent Breast Engorgement? A Randomized, Controlled Study', *Birth* 20, no. 2 (1993).

8. Chalmers and Levin, *Humane Perinatal Care.*

9. M. Cheyney, P. Burcher and S. Vedam, 'A Crusade against Home Birth', *Birth* 41, no. 1 (2014).

10. Public Health Agency of Canada, *What Women Say: The Maternity Experiences Survey.*

11. J. Ratti and others, 'Playing Nice: Improving the Professional Climate between Physicians and Midwives in the Calgary Area', *Journal of Obstetrics and Gynaecology Canada* 36, no. 7 (2014).

12. Harvey and others, 'A Randomized Control Trial of Nurse-Midwifery Care'; Hueston and Rudy, 'A Comparison of Labour and Delivery Management between Nurse-Midwives and Family Physicians'.

13. Midwives Alliance North America, 'What Is a Midwife?', available at http://mana.org/about-midwives/what-is-a-midwife (accessed 24 June 2015); Canadian Association of Midwives, 'Midwifery in Canada Is Growing', *The Pinard: Newsletter of the Canadian Association of Midwives* 5, no. 1 (2015).

14. Chalmers and Levin, *Humane Perinatal Care.*

15. *Ibid.*

16. B. Chalmers, 'The Case for Perinatal Psychologists', *Perinatology* 6, no. 6 (2004).

17. Chalmers and Levin, *Humane Perinatal Care*.

18. Chalmers, 'The Case for Perinatal Psychologists'.

19. *Ibid.*

20. B. Chalmers, 'Multicultural, Multidisciplinary, Psycho-Social Obstetric Care', *Journal of Obstetrics and Gynaecology of Canada* 21 (1999); Ratti and others, 'Playing Nice'.

21. Chalmers and Levin, *Humane Perinatal Care*.

22. Chalmers, 'Shame on Us!'.

23. Banaszek, 'Medical Humanities Becoming Prerequisites in Many Medical Schools'.

24. *Ibid.*

25. B. Chalmers and J. McIntyre, 'Integrating Psychology and Obstetrics for Medical Students: Shared Labour Ward Teaching', *Medical Teacher* 15, no. 1 (1993).

26. M. D. Avery, O. Montgomery and E. Brandl-Salutz, 'Essential Components of Successful Collaborative Maternity Care Models: The ACOG-ACNM Project', *Obstetrics & Gynecology Clinics of North America* 39, no. 3 (2012); C. S. Homer and others, 'Developing a Core Competency Model and Educational Framework for Primary Maternity Services: A National Consensus Approach', *Women & Birth: Journal of the Australian College of Midwives* 25, no. 3 (2012); D. Siassakos and others, 'More to Teamwork than Knowledge, Skill and Attitude. EBM Reviews: Cochrane Central Register of Controlled Trials', *BJOG* 117, no. 10 (2010); C. Smith and others, 'Ontario Care Providers' Considerations Regarding Models of Maternity Care', *Journal of Obstetrics & Gynaecology Canada* 31, no. 5 (2009).

27. F. Meffe, C. Claire Moravac and S. Espin, 'An Interprofessional Education Pilot Program in Maternity Care: Findings from an Exploratory Case Study of Undergraduate Students', *Journal of Interprofessional Care* 26, no. 3 (2012); L. Saxell, S. Harris and L. Elarar, 'The Collaboration for Maternal and Newborn Health: Interprofessional Maternity Care Education for Medical, Midwifery, and Nursing Students', *Journal of Midwifery and Women's Health* 54, no. 4 (2009).

28. D. D'Amour and I. Oandasan, 'Inter-professional Education for Patient-Centred Practice: An Evolving Framework', in *Interdisciplinary Education for Collaborative, Patient-Centred Practice: Research & Findings Report*, ed. I. Oandasan and others (Ottawa, ON: Health Canada, 2004); I. Oandasan and S. Reeves, 'Key Elements of Interprofessional Education, Part 2: Factors, Processes and Outcomes', *Journal of Interprofessional Care*, Suppl. 1 (2005); University of Toronto, Centre for Interprofessional Education, at http://ipe.utoronto.ca/overview (accessed 20 April 2015).

29. World Health Organization, 'World Health Organization (WHO) Framework for Action on Interprofessional Education and Collaborative Practice', available at www.who.int/hrh/resources/framework_action/en/ (accessed 20 April 2015).

30. Public Health Agency of Canada, *Canadian Hospitals' Maternity Policies and Practices Survey* (Ottawa, ON: PHAC, 2012).

Chapter 10

1. Chalmers and Levin, *Humane Perinatal Care*.

2. B. Chalmers, 'Globalization and Perinatal Health Care', *BJOG* 111, no. 9 (2004); Chalmers and Levin, *Humane Perinatal Care*.

3. B. Chalmers, *African Birth: Childbirth in Cultural Transition* (Sandton, South Africa: Berev Publications, 1990); Chalmers, 'Globalization and Perinatal Health Care'.

4. B. Chalmers, 'Cultural Issues in Perinatal Care', *Birth* 40, no. 4 (2013).

5. Adams and others, 'Attitudes and Referral Practices of Maternity Care Professionals'; Chalmers, *African Birth: Childbirth in Cultural Transition*; B. Chalmers, 'Western and African Conceptualizations of Birth', *Psychology and Health* 12 (1996); Chalmers, 'Multicultural, Multidisciplinary, Psycho-Social Obstetric Care'; B. Chalmers, 'Maternity Care in the Former Soviet Union', *BJOG* 112 (2005); Chalmers, 'Childbirth across Cultures:

Research and Practice'; Chalmers, 'Cultural Issues in Perinatal Care'; Chalmers and Jeckaite, 'Giving Birth in Two Maternity Hospitals in Lithuania'; Chalmers and Omer-Hashi, *Female Genital Mutilation and Obstetric Care*; Chalmers and Qulieva, 'A Report of Women's Birth Experiences in Baku, Azerbaijan'; Chalmers and others, 'Women's Experiences of Birth in St Petersburg, Russian Federation Following a Maternal-Child Health Intervention Program'; Chalmers and others, 'What Women Say about Post-Partum Care and Breastfeeding in St Petersburg, Russian Federation'; Chalmers and others, 'Contraceptive Knowledge, Attitudes and Use among Women Attending Health Clinics in St Petersburg, Russian Federation'.

6. Chalmers, 'Cultural Issues in Perinatal Care'; Chalmers and Levin, *Humane Perinatal Care*.

7. Public Health Agency of Canada, *Family-Centred Maternity and Newborn Care Guidelines*.

8. J. S. Milloy, *A National Crime: The Canadian Government and the Residential School System, 1979–1986* (Winnipeg, MB: University of Manitoba Press, 1999).

9. Library and Archives Canada, Muscowequan Residential School Box 56, File 28, 30 June 1997.

10. C. Reading and F. Wein, *Health Inequalities and Social Determinants of Aboriginal Peoples' Health* (Prince George, BC: National Collaborating Centre for Aboriginal Health, 2009).

11. V. K. Douglas, 'Childbirth among the Canadian Inuit: A Review of the Clinical and Cultural Literature', *International Journal of Circumpolar Health* 65, no. 2 (2006).

12. *Ibid.*

13. T. O'Driscoll and others, 'Delivering Away from Home: The Perinatal Experiences of First Nations Women in Northwestern Ontario', *Canadian Journal of Rural Medicine* 16, no. 4 (2011); Public Health Agency of Canada, *Family-Centred Maternity and Newborn Care Guidelines*.

14. K. J. Miller and others, 'Rural Maternity Care', *Journal of Obstetrics and Gynaecology of Canada* 34, no. 10 (2012); Public Health Agency of Canada, *Family-Centred Maternity and Newborn Care Guidelines*.

15. Government of Canada, *Report of Royal Commission on Aboriginal Peoples* (2006); Public Health Agency of Canada, *Family-Centred Maternity and Newborn Care Guidelines*.

16. National Aboriginal Health Organization, *Cultural Competency and Safety: A Guide for Health Care Administrators, Providers and Educators* (Ottawa, ON: NAHO, 2008); Public Health Agency of Canada, *Family-Centred Maternity and Newborn Care Guidelines*.

17. Public Health Agency of Canada, *Family-Centred Maternity and Newborn Care Guidelines*.

18. Chalmers and Omer-Hashi, *Female Genital Mutilation and Obstetric Care*.

19. *Ibid*; WHO, *Female Genital Mutilation: A Joint WHO/UNICEF/UNFPA Statement* (Geneva: WHO, 1997).

20. Chalmers and Omer-Hashi, *Female Genital Mutilation and Obstetric Care*; WHO, *Female Genital Mutilation*.

21. E. Gilbert, *Female Genital Mutilation: Information for Australian Health Professionals, Victoria* (Victoria: Royal Australian College of Obstetricians and Gynaecologists, 1997).

22. Chalmers and Omer-Hashi, *Female Genital Mutilation and Obstetric Care*.

23. *Ibid*; WHO, *Female Genital Mutilation*.

24. Chalmers and Omer-Hashi, *Female Genital Mutilation and Obstetric Care*; WHO, *Female Genital Mutilation*.

25. Chalmers and Omer-Hashi, *Female Genital Mutilation and Obstetric Care*.

26. B. Chalmers and K. Omer-Hashi, 'What Somali Women Say about Birth in Canada', *Journal of Reproductive and Infant Psychology* 20 (2002).

27. Chalmers and Omer-Hashi, *Female Genital Mutilation and Obstetric Care*.

28. *Ibid.*

29. Public Health Agency of Canada, *Family-Centred Maternity and Newborn Care Guidelines*.

30. Society of Obstetricians and Gynaecologists of Canada, 'Female Genital Cutting: Clinical Practice Guidelines', *Journal of Obstetrics and Gynecology of Canada* 35, no. 11 (2013).

31. Chalmers, *African Birth: Childbirth in Cultural Transition*.

32. B. Chalmers and others, *Essential Antenatal, Perinatal and Post-Partum Care Training Manual*, ed. B. Chalmers (Copenhagen: WHO Regional Office for Europe, 1999). Chalmers, *African Birth: Childbirth in Cultural Transition*.

33. Chalmers, *African Birth: Childbirth in Cultural Transition*.

34. *Ibid.*

35. *Ibid.*

36. *Ibid.*

37. *Ibid.*

38. *Ibid.*

39. *Ibid.*

40. *Ibid.*

41. *Ibid.*

42. Chalmers, 'Maternity Care in the Former Soviet Union'.

43. *Ibid.*

44. *Ibid.*

45. L. Dennis, 'Characteristics of Pregnant Women as Predictors of Utilization of Prenatal Care Services and Satisfaction with Those Services in St Petersburg Russia' (Bloomington: Indiana University Press, 1995).

46. Chalmers, 'Maternity Care in the Former Soviet Union'.

47. *Ibid.*

48. *Ibid.*

49. *Ibid.*

50. *Ibid.*

51. *Ibid.*

52. *Ibid.*

53. *Ibid.*

54. *Ibid.*

55. *Ibid.*

56. *Ibid.*

57. *Ibid.*

58. *Ibid.*

59. *Ibid.*

Chapter 11

1. Chalmers and Levin, *Humane Perinatal Care*.

2. Chalmers, 'Cultural Issues in Perinatal Care'; Chalmers and Levin, *Humane Perinatal Care*.

3. *Ibid.*

4. Maslow, *Motivation and Personality*.

5. Chalmers, 'Cultural Issues in Perinatal Care'; Chalmers and Levin, *Humane Perinatal Care*.

6. *Ibid.*

7. Hofmeyr and others, 'Companionship to Modify the Clinical Birth Environment'.

8. Chalmers, 'Cultural Issues in Perinatal Care'; Chalmers and Levin, *Humane Perinatal Care*.

9. *Ibid.*

10. *Ibid.*

11. Chalmers, 'Globalization and Perinatal Health Care'.

12. Public Health Agency of Canada, *Family-Centred Maternity and Newborn Care Guidelines*.

13. Chalmers, *African Birth: Childbirth in Cultural Transition*.

14. B. Chalmers, 'Psychosomatic Obstetrics and Gynaecology in the New Millennium: Some Thoughts and Observations', *Journal of Psychosomatic Obstetrics and Gynaecology* 19 (1998).

15. Chalmers, 'Cultural Issues in Perinatal Care'; Chalmers and Levin, *Humane Perinatal Care*.

16. Chalmers, 'Psychosomatic Obstetrics and Gynaecology in the New Millennium: Some Thoughts and Observations.'

17. *Ibid.*

18. Chalmers, 'Cultural Issues in Perinatal Care'; Chalmers and Levin, *Humane Perinatal Care*.

19. *Ibid.*

20. *Ibid.*

21. Public Health Agency of Canada, *What Women Say: The Maternity Experiences Survey*.

22. Chalmers, 'Cultural Issues in Perinatal Care'; Chalmers and Levin, *Humane Perinatal Care*.

23. *Ibid.*

24. *Ibid.*

25. *Ibid.*

26. *Ibid.*

27. K. Sutton and B. Chalmers, 'Contraception and Pregnancy Options', in *Human Sexuality*, ed. C. Pukall (Toronto, ON: Oxford University Press, 2014).

28. Chalmers, 'Cultural Issues in Perinatal Care'; Chalmers and Levin, *Humane Perinatal Care*.

29. B. Chalmers, 'What Do International Health Consultants Need to Know?', *Journal of the Society of Obstetricians and Gynaecologists of Canada* 21 (1999).

30. *Ibid.*

Chapter 12

1. UNICEF, 'The State of the World's Children', available at www.unicef.org/sowc/ (accessed 11 April 2014).

2. D. Bowser and K. Hill, *Exploring Evidence for Disrespect and Abuse in Facility-Based Childbirth: Report of a Landscape Analysis* (Washington, DC: USAID-TRAction Project, Harvard School of Public Health and University Research Co., 2010).

3. M. Bohren and others, 'The Mistreatment of Women during Childbirth in Health Facilities Globally: A Mixed-Methods Systematic Review', *PLOS Medicine* (2015).

4. World Health Organization, *Global and Regional Estimates of Violence against Women: Prevalence and Health Effects of Intimate Partner Violence and Non-Partner Sexual Violence* (Geneva: WHO, 2013).

5. Chalmers, 'Psychosomatic Obstetrics and Gynaecology in the New Millennium'; Chalmers and Levin, *Humane Perinatal Care*.

6. Midmer and others, *The Alpha Form*.

7. Chalmers, 'Psychosomatic Obstetrics and Gynaecology in the New Millennium'; Chalmers and Levin, *Humane Perinatal Care*.

8. C. L. O. Schachter and others, *Handbook on Sensitive Practice for Health Care Practitioners: Lessons from Adult Survivors of Childhood Sexual Abuse*. (Ottawa, ON: Public Health Agency of Canada, 2008).

9. Chalmers, 'Psychosomatic Obstetrics and Gynaecology in the New Millennium'; Chalmers and Levin, *Humane Perinatal Care*.

10. Bohren and others, 'The Mistreatment of Women during Childbirth in Health Facilities Globally'.

11. *Ibid.*

12. Enkin, Keirse and Chalmers, *A Guide to Effective Care in Pregnancy and Childbirth*.

13. Chalmers, 'Psychosomatic Obstetrics and Gynaecology in the New Millennium'; Chalmers and Levin, *Humane Perinatal Care*.

14. Bowser and Hill, *Exploring Evidence for Disrespect and Abuse in Facility-Based Childbirth*.

15. Bohren and others, 'The Mistreatment of Women during Childbirth in Health Facilities Globally'.

16. *Ibid.*

17. *Ibid*; Bowser and Hill, *Exploring Evidence for Disrespect and Abuse in Facility-Based Childbirth*.

18. Bohren and others, 'The Mistreatment of Women during Childbirth in Health Facilities Globally'.

19. *Ibid.*

20. Bowser and Hill, *Exploring Evidence for Disrespect and Abuse in Facility-Based Childbirth*.

21. Bohren and others, 'The Mistreatment of Women during Childbirth in Health Facilities Globally'.

22. J. Arnold, '"Obstetric Violence" Introduced as a New Legal Term in Venezuela', available at www.theunnecesarean.com/blog/2010/11/7/obstetric-violence-introduced-as-a-new-legal-term-in-venezue.html (accessed 27 April 2015); Immigration and Refugee Board of Canada, 'Venezuela: Implementation and Effectiveness of the 2007 Organic Law on the Right of Women to a Life Free of Violence', in *Refworld* (Ottawa, ON: Immigration and Refugee Board of Canada, 2008).

23. Arnold, '"Obstetric Violence" Introduced as a New Legal Term in Venezuela'; Immigration and Refugee Board of Canada, 'Venezuela: Implementation and Effectiveness of the 2007 Organic Law on the Right of Women to a Life Free of Violence'.

24. Chalmers, 'Psychosomatic Obstetrics and Gynaecology in the New Millennium'; Chalmers and Levin, *Humane Perinatal Care*.

25. *Ibid.*

26. *Ibid.*

27. Chalmers and McIntyre, 'Integrating Psychology and Obstetrics for Medical Students'.

28. Bowser and Hill, *Exploring Evidence for Disrespect and Abuse in Facility-Based Childbirth*.

29. *Ibid.*

30. *Ibid.*

31. S. Singh and G. Posner, 'Doctors Behaving Badly and the Tyranny of Peer Pressure', *Journal of Obstetrics and Gynaecology of Canada* 37, no. 12 (2015).

32. Anonymous, 'Our Family Secrets', *Annals of Internal Medicine* 163, no. 4 (2015).

33. Singh and Posner, 'Doctors Behaving Badly and the Tyranny of Peer Pressure'.

34. *Ibid.*, 1114.

35. Chalmers, *African Birth: Childbirth in Cultural Transition*; Chalmers, 'Maternity Care in the Former Soviet Union'; Chalmers and Omer-Hashi, *Female Genital Mutilation and Obstetric Care*.

36. B. Chalmers, *Birth, Sex and Abuse: Women's Voices under Nazi Rule* (London: Grosvenor House, 2015).

37. *Ibid.*

38. Chalmers and others, 'Rates of Interventions in Labor and Birth across Canada'.

39. I. Heredia-Pi and others, 'Obstetric Care and Method of Delivery in Mexico:. Results from the 2012 National Health and Nutrition Survey', *PLoS ONE* 9, no. 8 (2014).

40. Bowser and Hill, *Exploring Evidence for Disrespect and Abuse in Facility-Based Childbirth*.

41. Chalmers, McIntyre and Meyer, 'South African Obstetricians' Views on Caesarean Section'; R. de Regt Haynes and others, 'Relation of Private or Clinic Care to the Caesarean Section Birth Rate', *New England Journal of Medicine* 315 (1986); M. Price and J. Broomberg, 'The Impact of Fee-for-Service Reimbursement System on the Utilization of Health Services, Part III: A Comparison of Caesarean Section Rates in White Nulliparous Women in Private and Public Sectors', *South African Medical Journal* 78 (1990).

42. Price and Broomberg, 'The Impact of Fee-for-Service Reimbursement System on the Utilization of Health Services'.

43. Bowser and Hill, *Exploring Evidence for Disrespect and Abuse in Facility-Based Childbirth*.

44. *Ibid*; L. Freedman and M. Kruk, 'Disrespect and Abuse of Women in Childbirth: Challenging the Global Quality and Accountability Agendas', *Lancet*, early online publication 23 June 2014.

45. J. P. Vogel and others, 'Promoting Respect and Preventing Mistreatment during Childbirth', *BJOG* 123, no. 5 (2016).

Chapter 13

1. WHO, WHO Health for All Database, available at www.euro.who.int/en/data-and-evidence/databases/european-health-for-all-database-hfa-db.

2. Public Health Agency of Canada, *Perinatal Health Indicators for Canada 2011*.

3. Beck and others, *PRAMS 1999 Surveillance Report*.

4. Declercq and others, *Listening to Mothers*; Declercq and others, *Listening to Mothers II*.

5. 'BORN: Better Outcomes Registry and Network', available at www.bornontario.ca/en/about-born/ (accessed 1 July 2015).

6. Public Health Agency of Canada, *What Women Say: The Maternity Experiences Survey*.

7. Beck and others, *PRAMS 1999 Surveillance Report*.

8. Green and others, *Greater Expectations: The Inter- Relationship between Women's Expectations and Experiences of Decision Making, Continuity, Choice and Control in Labour, and Psychological Outcomes. Summary Report*; Green, Coupland, and Kitzinger, *Great Expectations: A Prospective Study of Women's Expectations and Experiences of Childbirth*.

9. Brown and Lumley, 'Satisfaction with Care in Labour and Birth: A Survey of 790 Australian Women'; Calder and Purton, *Maternity Care Matters*; Chalmers, *African Birth: Childbirth in Cultural Transition*; Chalmers and Jeckaite, 'Giving Birth in Two Maternity Hospitals in Lithuania'; Chalmers and others, 'What Women Say About Antenatal Care in St Petersburg, Russian Federation'; Chalmers and Qulieva, 'A Report of Women's Birth Experiences in Baku, Azerbaijan'; Chalmers and others, 'Women's Experiences of Birth in St Petersburg, Russian Federation Following a Maternal-Child Health Intervention Program'; Chalmers and others, 'What Women Say about Post-Partum Care and Breastfeeding in St Petersburg, Russian Federation'; Chalmers and others, 'Contraceptive Knowledge, Attitudes and Use among Women Attending Health Clinics in St Petersburg, Russian Federation'; Declercq and others, *Listening to Mothers*; Declercq and others, *Listening to Mothers II*; Heiberg and others, 'Women's Experiences of Giving Birth in Northwest Russia in 2000 and 2002 and in Northern Norway 2000'; P. Stratulat and others, 'Evaluarea Rezultatelor Implementarii Technologiilor Programului National De Ameliorare a Asistentei Medicale Perinatale in Republica Moldova', Buletin de Perinatologie 3 (2002).

10. Chalmers and Jeckaite, 'Giving Birth in Two Maternity Hospitals in Lithuania'; Chalmers and Meyer, 'What Men Say about Pregnancy, Birth and Parenthood'.

11. Cavalli and Copp, 'Inositol and Folate Resistant Neural Tube Defects'; Cavalli and others, 'Effects of Inositol Supplementation in a Cohort of Mothers at Risk of Producing a NTD Pregnancy'.

12. Chalmers and Meyer, 'What Men Say about Pregnancy, Birth and Parenthood'; Freedman and Kruk, 'Disrespect and Abuse of Women in Childbirth'; J. O'Leary and C. Thorwick, 'Father's Perspectives during Pregnancy, Postperinatal Loss', *Journal of Obstetrics, Gynecology, and Neonatal Nursing* 35, no. 1 (2006).

13. Chalmers, 'Childbirth across Cultures: Research and Practice'.

14. M. E. Hannah and others, 'Planned Caesarean Section versus Planned Vaginal Birth for Breech Presentation at Term: A Randomised Multicentre Trial', *Lancet* 356, nos. 1375–83 (2000).

15. Chalmers, 'What Do International Health Consultants Need to Know?'; B. Chalmers, 'What Should International Health Consultants Know?', *Bulletin of the World Health Organization* 77 (1999); B. Chalmers, 'How Ethical Is International Perinatal Research? Challenges and Misconceptions', *Birth* 34, no. 3 (2007).

16. Chalmers, 'How Ethical Is International Perinatal Research?'.

17. *Ibid.*

18. *Ibid.*

19. Kramer and others, 'Promotion of Breastfeeding Intervention Trial (PROBIT): A Cluster-Randomized Trial in the Republic of Belarus'.

20. Chalmers, 'How Ethical Is International Perinatal Research?'.

21. *Ibid.*

22. S. Benatar, 'Reflections and Recommendations on Research Ethics in Developing Countries', *Social Science and Medicine* 54 (2002); G. Lindegger and L. M. Richter, 'HIV Vaccine Trials: Critical Issues in Informed Consent', *South African Journal of Science* 96 (2000).

Chapter 14

1. Editorial, 'Achieving Respectful Care for Women and Babies', *The Lancet* 385, no. 9976 (2015).

2. United Nations, 'Reproductive Rights', available at www.un.org/en/development/desa/population/theme/rights/index.shtml (accessed 1 June 2014).

3. *Ibid.*

4. Family Care International, *Action for the 21st Century: Reproductive Health and Rights for All* (New York: Family Care International, 1994).

5. United Nations General Assembly, *Draft Outcome Document of the United Nations Summit for the Adoption of the Post-2015 Development Agenda*, A/69/L.85, 2015.

6. A. Starrs, 'A Lancet Commission on Sexual and Reproductive Health and Rights: Going Beyond the Sustainable Development Goals', *The Lancet* 386, no. 9999 (2015): 1112.

7. White Ribbon Alliance, *The Respectful Maternity Care Charter: The Universal Rights of Childbearing Women* (Washington, DC, 2011).

8. Childbirth Connection, *The Rights of Childbearing Women* (New York, 2012).

9. New York State Department of Health, *Breastfeeding Mothers' Bill of Rights* (Albany, NY, 2010).

10. Center for Reproductive Rights, *US Center for Reproductive Rights Declarations* (New York, 1992–2013).

11. Society of Obstetricians and Gynaecologists of Canada, 'International Women's Health: Sexual and Reproductive Rights and Health', available at http://iwhp.sogc.org/index.php?page=sexual-reproductive-rights&hl=en_US (accessed 12 March 2013).

12. United Nations, The United Nations Convention on the Rights of the Child (1989), available at www.Unicef.Ca/En/Policy-Advocacy-for-Children/About-the-Convention-on-the-Rights-of-the-Child.

13. Canadian Institute of Child Health (CICH), *Rights of the Child in the Healthcare System* (Ottawa, ON, 2002).

14. A. Levin and B. Chalmers, 'Strengthening Neonatal Intensive Care', available at www.perinat.ee/materjal/UN_letter_4_20130829.doc (accessed 20 February 2014).

15. G. Bevilacqua and others, 'The Parma Charter of the Rights of the Newborn', available at www.uenps.com/media/Parma%20Charter%20Rights%20of%20the%20newborn.pdf (accessed 13 February 2016).

Chapter 15

1. WHO/UNICEF, *Protecting, Promoting and Supporting Breastfeeding.*

2. WHO, *Essential Antenatal, Perinatal and Postpartum Care Course.*

3. WHO, 'WHO Health for All Database'.

4. WHO/UNICEF, *Protecting, Promoting and Supporting Breastfeeding.*

5. Chalmers, 'Maternity Care in the Former Soviet Union'.

6. Chalmers, 'Childbirth across Cultures: Research and Practice'; Chalmers and others, 'What Women Say about Antenatal Care in St Petersburg, Russian Federation'; Chalmers and others, 'Women's Experiences of Birth in St Petersburg, Russian Federation Following a Maternal-Child Health Intervention Program'; Chalmers and others, 'What Women Say about Post-Partum Care and Breastfeeding in St Petersburg, Russian Federation'.

7. Stratulat and others, 'Evaluarea Rezultatelor Implementarii Technologiilor Programului National De Ameliorare a Asistentei Medicale Perinatale in Republica Moldova'.

8. D. K. Midmer and others, *A Reference Guide for Providers: The Alpha Form – Antenatal Psychosocial Health Assessment Form* (Toronto, ON: Department of Family Medicine, University of Toronto, 1996); L. M. Wilson and others, 'Antenatal Psychosocial Risk Factors Associated with Adverse Postpartum Outcomes', *Canadian Medical Association Journal* 154 (1996).

9. Wilson and others, 'Antenatal Psychosocial Risk Factors Associated with Adverse Postpartum Outcomes'.

10. Chalmers and McIntyre, 'Integrating Psychology and Obstetrics for Medical Students: Shared Labour Ward Teaching'.

11. Chalmers, 'Western and African Conceptualizations of Birth'; Chalmers, 'Childbirth across Cultures: Research and Practice'; Declercq and Chalmers, 'Mothers' Reports of Their Maternity Experiences'.

Chapter 16

1. Chalmers and Levin, *Humane Perinatal Care.*

2. B. Chalmers and others, 'The Maternity Experiences Survey: An Overview of Findings', *Journal of Obstetrics and Gynaecology of Canada* 30 (2008).

3. M. J. Renfrew and others, 'Midwifery and Quality Care: Findings from a New Evidence-Informed Framework for Maternal and Newborn Care', *Lancet* (2014).

4. T. Pyone and others, 'Changing the Role of the Traditional Birth Attendant in Somaliland', *International Journal of Gynaecology and Obstetrics* S0020-7292(14)00292–6 (2014).

5. UNICEF, 'UNICEF Southern Sudan Monthly Report', July 2005, available at http://reliefweb.int/report/sudan/unicef-southern-sudan-monthly-report-jul-2005.

6. Pyone and others, 'Changing the Role of the Traditional Birth Attendant in Somaliland'.

7. B. Chalmers, *Training Manual for Use by Traditional Birth Attendants in Southern Sudan, for UNICEF Operation Lifeline Sudan* (UNICEF Operation Lifeline Sudan, 2001).

8. H. C. Millar and others, 'Global Women's Health Education in Canadian Obstetrics and Gynaecology Programs: A Survey of Program Directors and Senior Residents', *Journal of Obstetrics and Gynaecology of Canada* 37, no. 10 (2015).

9. M. M. Ali and others, *Long-Term Contraceptive Protection, Discontinuation and Switching Behaviour: Intrauterine Device (IUD) Use Dynamics in 14 Developing Countries* (London: WHO and Marie Stopes International, 2011); A. Sonfield, 'Popularity Disparity: Attitudes about the IUD in Europe and the United States', *Guttmacher Policy Review* (Fall 2007).

10. Ali and others, Long-Term Contraceptive Protection, Discontinuation and Switching Behaviour; Sonfield, Popularity Disparity.

11. Canadian Institute for Child Health, *Inpatient Hospitalizations, Surgeries and Childbirth Indicators in 2012–2013* (Ottawa, ON, 2014).

Appendix

1. Beck and others, *PRAMS* 1999 Surveillance Report; Chalmers and others, 'The Maternity Experiences Survey: An Overview of Findings'; Chalmers and others, 'What Women Say about Antenatal Care in St Petersburg, Russian Federation'; Chalmers and Omer-Hashi, *Female Genital Mutilation and Obstetric Care*; Chalmers and others, 'Women's Experiences of Birth in St Petersburg, Russian Federation Following a Maternal-Child Health Intervention Program'; Chalmers and others, 'Contraceptive Knowledge, Attitudes and Use among Women Attending Health Clinics in St Petersburg, Russian Federation'; Declercq and others, *Listening to Mothers*; Declercq and others, *Listening to Mothers II*; Garcia and others, First Class Delivery; Green and others, *Greater Expectations: The Inter-Relationship between Women's Expectations and Experiences of Decision Making, Continuity, Choice and Control in Labour, and Psychological Outcomes*; Green, Coupland, and Kitzinger, *Great Expectations: A Prospective Study of Women's Expectations and Experiences of Childbirth*; Midmer and others, *The Alpha Form: Antenatal Psychosocial Health Assessment Form*; Public Health Agency of Canada, *What Women Say*; Public Health Agency of Canada, *Canadian Hospitals Maternity Policies and Practices Survey*; Redshaw and others, Recorded Delivery: A National Survey of Women's Experience of Maternity Care; Healthcare Improvement Scotland, 'The Scottish Woman-Held Maternity Record' (2013), available at www.healthcareimprovementscotland.org/our_work/reproductive,_maternal_child/woman_held_maternity_record/swhmr_maternity_record.aspx; Scottish Programme for Clinical Effectiveness in Reproductive Health.

Bibliography

Abalos, E, M Chamillard, V Diaz, O Tuncalp and AM Gülmezoglu. 'Antenatal Care for Health Pregnant Women: A Mapping of Interventions from Existing Guidelines to Inform the Development of New WHO Guidelines on Antenatal Care'. *BJOG* 123, no. 4 (2015): 519–28.

Adams, J, CW Lui, D Sibbritt, A Broom, J Wardle and C Homer. 'Attitudes and Referral Practices of Maternity Care Professionals with Regard to Complementary and Alternative Medicine: An Integrative Review'. *Journal of Advanced Nursing* 67, no. 3 (2011): 472–83.

Adams, SS, M Eberhard-Gran and A Eskild. 'Fear of Childbirth and Duration of Labour: A Study of 2206 Women with Intended Vaginal Delivery'. *BJOG* 119, no. 10 (2012): 1238–46.

Affonso, D, E Basque, V Wahlberg and J Brady. 'Reconciliation and Healing for Mothers through Skin-to-Skin Contact Provided in an American Tertiary Level Intensive Care Nursery'. *Neonatal Network* 12 (1993): 25–32.

Ali, MM, RK Sadler, J Cleland, TD Ngo and IH Shah. *Long-Term Contraceptive Protection, Discontinuation and Switching Behaviour: Intrauterine Device (IUD) Use Dynamics in 14 Developing Countries* (London: World Health Organization and Marie Stopes International, 2011).

Alio, AP, HM Salihu, JL Kornosky, AM Richman and PJ Marty. 'Feto-Infant Health and Survival: Does Paternal Involvement Matter?' *Maternal Child Health Journal* 14, no. 6 (2010): 931–7.

Als, H. 'Individualized, Family-Focused Developmental Care for the Very-Low-Birthweight Preterm Infant in the NICU'. In *The Psychological Development of Low-Birthweight Children*, ed. MD Sigman and SL Friedman (Norwood, NJ: Ablex, 1992).

——'Program Guide: Newborn Individualized Developmental Care and Assessment Program: An Education and Training Program for Health Care Professionals', available at www.nidcap.org (accessed 30 August 2013).

Als, H and L Gilkerson. 'The Role of Relationship-Based Developmentally Supportive Care in Strengthening Outcome of Preterm Infants'. *Seminars in Perinatology* 21 (1997): 178–89.

Als, H, G Lawhon, FH Duffy, GB McAnulty, R Gibes-Grossman et al. 'Individualized Perinatal Care for the Very-Low-Birth-Weight Preterm Infant'. *Journal of the American Medical Association* 11 (1994): 853–8.

Althabe, F and JM Belizán. 'Caesarean Section: The Paradox'. *Lancet* 368 (2006): 1472–3.

Althabe, F, C Sosa, JM Belizán, L Gibbons, F Jacquerioz et al. 'Cesarean Section Rates and Maternal and Neonatal Mortality in Low-, Middle- and High-Income Countries: An Ecological Study'. *Birth* 33, no. 4 (2006): 270–7.

Anderson, GC. 'Current Knowledge about Skin-to-Skin (Kangaroo) Care for Preterm Infants'. *Journal of Perinatology* 11 (1991): 216–26.

Anonymous. 'Our Family Secrets'. *Annals of Internal Medicine* 163, no. 4 (2015): 321.

Arnold, J. '"Obstetric Violence" Introduced as a New Legal Term in Venezuela', available at www.theunnecesarean.com/blog/2010/11/7/obstetric-violence-introduced-as-a-new-legal-term-in-venezue.html (accessed 27 April 2015).

Austin, MP, J Colton, S Priest, N Reilly and D Hadzi-Pavlovic. 'The Antenatal Risk Questionnaire (ANRQ): Acceptability and Use for Psychosocial Risk Assessment in the Maternity Setting'. *Women Birth* 26, no. 1 (2013): 17–25.

Avery, MD, O Montgomery and E Brandl-Salutz. 'Essential Components of Successful Collaborative Maternity Care Models: The ACOG-ACNM Project'. *Obstetrics & Gynecology Clinics of North America* 39, no. 3 (2012): 423–34.

Banaszek, A. 'Medical Humanities Becoming Prerequisites in Many Medical Schools'. *Canadian Medical Association Journal* 183, no. 8 (2011): c441–2.

Beck, LF, CH Johnson, B Morrow et al. *PRAMS 1999 Surveillance Report* (Atlanta, GA: Division of Reproductive Health, National Center for Chronic Disease Prevention and Health Promotion, Centers for Disease Control and Prevention, 2003).

Benatar, S. 'Reflections and Recommendations on Research Ethics in Developing Countries'. *Social Science and Medicine* 54 (2002): 1131–41.

Berghella, V, E Buchanan, L Pereira and JK Baxter. 'Preconception Care'. *Obstetrical & Gynecological Survey* 65, no. 2 (2010): 119–31.

Berker, PT, PC Grunwald, J Moorman and S Stuhr. 'Outcomes of Developmentally Supportive Care for Very Low Birthweight Infants'. *Nursing Research* 40 (1991): 150–5.

Betran, AP, MR Torloni, JJ Zhang, AM Gülmezoglu and the WHO Working Group on Caesarean Section. 'WHO Statement on Caesarean Section Rates'. *BJOG* 123, no. 5 (2016): 667–70.

Bevilacqua, G, M Corradi, GP Donzelli, V Fanos, D Gianotti et al. 'The Parma Charter of the Rights of the Newborn', available at www.uenps.com/media/Parma%20Charter%20Rights%20of%20the%20newborn.pdf (accessed 13 February 2016).

Bohren, M, JP Vogel, EC Hunter, O Lutsiv, SK Makh et al. 'The Mistreatment of Women during Childbirth in Health Facilities Globally: A Mixed-Methods Systematic Review'. *PLOS Medicine* 12 (2015): e1001847.

Bolton, KD, B Chalmers, P Cooper and E Wainer. 'Black Mother's Experiences of a Neonatal Care Unit'. *Journal of Reproductive and Infant Psychology* 11 (1993): 229–34.

'BORN: Better Outcomes Registry and Network', available at www.bornontario.ca/en/about-born/ (accessed 1 July 2015).

Boundy, EO, R Dastjerdi, D Spiegelman, WW Fawzi, SA Missmer et al. 'Kangaroo Mother Care and Neonatal Outcomes: A Meta-Analysis'. *Pediatrics* 137, no. 1 (2016): 1–16.

Bower, D, C Van Gelderen, B Chalmers and A Hamilton. 'Discussions after Death'. *South African Medical Journal* 78 (1990): 760.

Bowser, D and K Hill. *Exploring Evidence for Disrespect and Abuse in Facility-Based Childbirth: Report of a Landscape Analysis* (Washington, DC: USAID-TRAction Project, Harvard School of Public Health and University Research Co., 2010).

Bragg, F, DA Cromwell, LC Edozien, I Gurol-Urganci, TA Mahmood et al. 'Variation in Rates of Caesarean Section among English NHS Trusts after Accounting for Maternal and Clinical Risk: Cross-Sectional Study'. *British Medical Journal* 341 (2010): c5065.

Brown, HC and HJ Smith. 'Giving Women Their Own Case Notes to Carry during Pregnancy'. *Cochrane Database of Systematic Reviews* 2, CD002856 (2004).

Brown, LD and JA Heerman. 'The Effect of Developmental Care on Preterm Infant Outcome'. *Applied Nursing Research* 10 (1997): 190–7.

Brown, S and J Lumley. 'Satisfaction with Care in Labour and Birth: A Survey of 790 Australian Women'. *Birth* 21 (1994): 4–13.

Buchler, DM, H Als, FM Duffy, GB McAnulty and J Leiderman. 'Effectiveness of Individualized Developmental Care for Low-Risk Preterm Infants: Behavioral and Electrophysiological Evidence'. *Pediatrics* 96 (1995): 923–32.

Byland, B, T Cervin and O Finnstrom. 'Morbidity and Neurological Function of Very Low Birthweight Infants from the Newborn Period to 4 Years of Age: A Prospective Study from the South-East Region of Sweden'. *Acta Pediatrica* 87 (1998): 758–63.

Calder, A and P Purton. *Maternity Care Matters: An Audit of Maternity Services in Scotland 1998. Scottish Program for Clinical Effectiveness in Reproductive Health* (Aberdeen: Douglas Baird Centre for Research on Women's Health, 1999).

Canadian Association of Midwives. 'Midwifery in Canada Is Growing'. *The Pinard: Newsletter of the Canadian Association of Midwives* 5, no. 1 (2015): 5–6.

Canadian Institute for Child Health. *Inpatient Hospitalizations, Surgeries and Childbirth Indicators in 2012-2013.* (Ottawa, ON: CICH, 2014).

Canadian Medical Protective Association. 'Apology Legislation in Canada: What It Means for Physicians', IS0889-E, September 2008 (revised April 2013), available at www.cmpa-acpm.ca/-/apology-legislation-in-canada-what-it-means-for-physicians (accessed 17 April 2015).

Cavalli, P and AJ Copp. 'Inositol and Folate Resistant Neural Tube Defects'. *Journal of Medical Genetics* 39, no. e5 (2002).

Cavalli, P, G Tonni, E Grosso and C Poggiani. 'Effects of Inositol Supplementation in a Cohort of Mothers at Risk of Producing a NTD Pregnancy'. *Birth Defects Research Part A: Clinical and Molecular Teratology* 91, no. 11 (2011): 962–5.

Cedergren, MI. 'Maternal Morbid Obesity and the Risk of Adverse Pregnancy Outcomes'. *Obstetrics and Gynaecology* 103, no. 2 (2004): 219–24.

Center for Reproductive Rights. *US Center for Reproductive Rights Declarations* (New York, 1992–2013).

Chalmers, B. 'Psychosocial Factors and Obstetric Complications'. *Psychology and Medicine* 13 (1983): 333–9.

——'Types of Life Events and Factors Influencing Their Seriousness Ratings'. *Journal of Social Psychology* 121 (1983): 283–95.

——*African Birth: Childbirth in Cultural Transition* (Sandton, South Africa: Berev Publications, 1990).

——'Terminology Used in Early Pregnancy Loss'. *British Journal of Obstetrics and Gynaecology* 99 (1992): 357–8.

——'WHO Appropriate Technology for Birth Revisited'. *British Journal of Obstetrics and Gynaecology* 99 (1992): 709–10.

——'Western and African Conceptualizations of Birth'. *Psychology and Health* 12 (1996): 1–10.

——'Implementing the Baby Friendly Hospital Initiative'. *Journal of the Society of Obstetricians and Gynaecologists of Canada* 20 (1997): 271–9.

——'Psychosomatic Obstetrics and Gynaecology in the New Millennium: Some Thoughts and Observations'. *Journal of Psychosomatic Obstetrics and Gynaecology* 19 (1998): 62–9.

——'Multicultural, Multidisciplinary, Psycho-Social Obstetric Care'. *Journal of Obstetrics and Gynaecology of Canada* 21 (1999): 975–9.

——'Over-Reliance on a Medical Approach to Care: Some Thoughts for Consideration'. *Journal of the Society of Obstetricians and Gynaecologists of Canada* 21, no. 11 (1999): 1081–6.

——'What Do International Health Consultants Need to Know?' *Journal of the Society of Obstetricians and Gynaecologists of Canada* 21 (1999): 556–63.

——'What Should International Health Consultants Know?' *Bulletin of the World Health Organization* 77 (1999): 97.

——*Training Manual for Use by Traditional Birth Attendants in Southern Sudan, for UNICEF Operation Lifeline Sudan* (UNICEF Operation Lifeline Sudan, 2001).

——'How Often Must We Ask for Sensitive Care before We Get It?' *Birth* 29, no. 2 (2002): 79–82.

——'The Baby Friendly Hospital Initiative: Where Next?' *British Journal of Obstetrics and Gynaecology* 111, no. 3 (2004): 198–9.

——'The Case for Perinatal Psychologists'. *Perinatology* 6, no. 6 (2004): 320–5.

——'Globalization and Perinatal Health Care'. *BJOG* 111, no. 9 (2004): 889–91.

——'Maternity Care in the Former Soviet Union'. *British Journal of Obstetrics and Gynaecology* 112 (2005): 495–9.

——'How Ethical Is International Perinatal Research? Challenges and Misconceptions'. *Birth* 34, no. 3 (2007): 191–3.

——'Shame on Us!'. *Birth* 38, no. 4 (2011): 279–81.

——'Childbirth across Cultures: Research and Practice'. *Birth* 39, no. 4 (2012): 276–80.

——'Breastfeeding Unfriendly in Canada?' *Canadian Medical Association Journal* 185, no. 5 (2013): 375–6.

——'Cultural Issues in Perinatal Care'. *Birth* 40, no. 4 (2013): 217–19.

——*Birth, Sex and Abuse: Women's Voices under Nazi Rule* (London: Grosvenor House, 2015).

Chalmers, B and BM Chalmers. 'Post-Partum Depression: A Revised Perspective'. *Journal of Psychosomatic Obstetrics and Gynaecology* 5 (1986): 93–105.

Chalmers, B and S Dzakpasu. 'Interventions in Labour and Birth and Satisfaction with Care: The Canadian Maternity Experiences Survey Findings'. *Journal of Reproductive and Infant Psychology* 33, no. 4 (2015): 374–87.

Chalmers, B, S Dzakpasu, M Heaman, J Kaczorowski and the Maternity Experiences Study Group. 'The Maternity Experiences Survey: An Overview of Findings'. *Journal of Obstetrics and Gynaecology of Canada* 30 (2008): 217–28.

Chalmers, B and GJ Hofmeyr. 'The Gestation of a Childbirth Education Diploma'. *Journal of Psychosomatic Obstetrics & Gynaecology* 10 (1989): 179–87.

Chalmers, B and D Jeckaite. 'Giving Birth in Two Maternity Hospitals in Lithuania'. *Birth* 37, no. 2 (2010): 116–23.

Chalmers, B, J Kaczorowski, E Darling, M Heaman, D Fell et al. and the Maternity Experiences Study Group of the Canadian Parental Surveillance System of the Public Health Agency of Canada. 'Cesarean and Vaginal Birth in Canadian Women: A Comparison of Experiences'. *Birth* 37, no. 1 (2010): 44–9.

Chalmers, B, J Kaczorowski, B O'Brien and C Royle. 'Rates of Interventions in Labor and Birth across Canada: Findings of the Canadian Maternity Experiences Survey'. *Birth* 39, no. 3 (2012): 203–10.

Chalmers, B and A Levin. *Humane Perinatal Care* (Tallinn, Estonia: TEA Publishers, 2001).

Chalmers, B, C Levitt, M Heaman, B O'Brien, R Sauve et al. and the Maternity Experiences Study Group of the Canadian Perinatal Surveillance System. 'Breastfeeding Rates and Hospital Breastfeeding Practices in Canada: A National Survey of Women'. *Birth*. 36, no. 2 (2009): 122–32.

Chalmers, B and V Mangiaterra. 'Appropriate Perinatal Technology: A WHO Perspective'. *Journal of the Society of Obstetricians and Gynaecologists of Canada* 23 (2001): 574–5.

Chalmers, B, V Mangiaterra and R Porter. 'WHO Principles of Perinatal Care: The Essential Antenatal, Perinatal and Postpartum Care Course'. *Birth* 28 (2001): 202–7.

Chalmers, B and J McIntyre. 'Integrating Psychology and Obstetrics for Medical Students: Shared Labour Ward Teaching'. *Medical Teacher* 15, no. 1 (1993): 35–40.

——'Do Antenatal Classes Have a Place in Modern Obstetric Care?' *International Journal of Psychosomatic Obstetrics and Gynaecology* 15 (1994): 119–23.

Chalmers, B, J McIntyre and D Meyer. 'South African Obstetricians' Views on Caesarean Section'. *South African Medical Journal* 82 (1991): 161–4.

Chalmers, B and D Meyer. 'Adjustment to the Early Months of Parenthood'. *International Journal of Prenatal and Perinatal Studies* 1 (1990): 229–40.

——'Babies with Abnormalities: Reactions of Mothers'. *International Journal of Prenatal and Perinatal Studies* 1 (1990): 13–29.

——'What Men Say about Pregnancy, Birth and Parenthood'. *Journal of Psychosomatic Obstetrics and Gynaecology* 17 (1996): 47–52.

Chalmers, B, H Muggah, D Samarskaya and E Tkachenko. 'The Canada–WHO–St Petersburg Maternal Child Health Program'. *Journal of Society of Obstetricians and Gynaecologists of Canada* 20 (1998): 43–51.

Chalmers, B, H Muggah, M Samarskaya and E Tkatchenko. 'What Women Say about Antenatal Care in St Petersburg, Russian Federation'. *Journal of Psychosomatic Obstetrics and Gynaecology* 20 (1999): 1–10.

Chalmers, B and K Omer-Hashi. 'What Somali Women Say about Birth in Canada'. *Journal of Reproductive and Infant Psychology* 20 (2002): 267–82.

——*Female Genital Mutilation and Obstetric Care* (Vancouver, BC: Trafford Publishers, 2003).

Chalmers, B and R Porter. 'Assessing Management of Normal Labour: The Bologna Score'. *Birth* 28, no. 2 (2001): 79–83.

Chalmers, B, R Porter, D Sheratt and A Peat. *Essential Antenatal, Perinatal and Post-Partum Care Training Manual*, ed. B Chalmers (Copenhagen: WHO Regional Office for Europe, 1999).

Chalmers, B and D Qulieva. 'A Report of Women's Birth Experiences in Baku, Azerbaijan'. *Journal of Psychosomatic Obstetrics and Gynaecology* 25 (2004): 3–14.

Chalmers, B, M Samarskaya, E Tkatchenko and H Muggah. 'Women's Experiences of Birth in St Petersburg, Russian Federation Following a Maternal-Child Health Intervention Program'. *Birth* 25, no. (1998): 107–16.

——'What Women Say about Post-Partum Care and Breastfeeding in St Petersburg, Russian Federation'. *Journal of the Society of Obstetricians and Gynaecologists of Canada* 21 (1999): 127–37.

Chalmers, B, M Sand, H Muggah, L Oblivanova, N Almazova et al. 'Contraceptive Knowledge, Attitudes and Use among Women Attending Health Clinics in St Petersburg, Russian Federation'. *Canadian Journal of Human Sexuality* 7 (1998): 129.

Chalmers, I, M Enkin and M Keirse. *Effective Care in Pregnancy and Childbirth* (Oxford University Press, 1989).

Charpak, N, Z Figueroa and JG Ruiz. 'Kangaroo Mother Care'. *Lancet* 351 (1998): 914.

Charpak, N, JG Ruiz-Palaez and Y Rey-Martinez. 'Kangaroo Mother Program: An Alternate Way of Caring for Low Birth Weight Infants? One Year Mortality in a Two Cohort Study'. *Pediatrics* 94 (1994): 804–10.

Cheyney, M, P Burcher and S Vedam. 'A Crusade against Home Birth'. *Birth* 41, no. 1 (2014): 1–4.

Childbirth Connection. *The Rights of Childbearing Women* (New York, 2012).

Clinton, H and B Obama. 'Making Patient Safety the Centerpiece of Medical Liability Reform'. *New England Journal of Medicine* 354 (2006): 2205–8.

Cochrane Library. The Cochrane Database of Systematic Reviews, available at www.cochranelibrary .com/cochrane-database-of-systematic-reviews/index.html (accessed 17 April 2015).

Cone, SK, S Short and G Gutcher. 'From "Baby Barn" to the "Single Family Room Designed NICU": A Report of Staff Perceptions One Year Post Occupancy'. *Newborn Infant Nursing Review* 10, no. 2 (2010): 97–103.

Cooke, RW. 'Factors Affecting Survival and Outcome at 3 Years in Extremely Preterm Infants'. *Archives of Diseases in Children* 71 (1994): F28–31.

D'Amour, D and I Oandasan. 'Interprofessional Education for Patient-Centred Practice: An Evolving Framework'. In *Interdisciplinary Education for Collaborative, Patient-Centred Practice: Research and Findings Report*, ed. I. Oandasan, D. D'Amour, M. Zwarenstein et al. (Ottawa, ON: Health Canada, 2004).

Declercq, E and B Chalmers. 'Mothers' Reports of Their Maternity Experiences in the USA and Canada'. *Journal of Reproductive and Infant Psychology* 26, no. 4 (2008): 295–308.

Declercq, E, C Sakala, MP Corry et al. *Listening to Mothers: Report of the First National U.S. Survey of Women's Childbearing Experiences* (New York: Maternity Center Association, 2002).

——*Listening to Mothers II: Report of the Second National US Survey of Women's Childbearing Experiences* (New York: Childbirth Connections, 2006).

Declercq, E, R Young, H Cabral and J Ecker. 'Is a Rising Cesarean Delivery Rate Inevitable? Trends in Industrialized Countries, 1987 to 2007'. *Birth* 38, no. 2 (2011): 99–104.

Dennis, L. *Characteristics of Pregnant Women as Predictors of Utilization of Prenatal Care Services and Satisfaction with Those Services in St Petersburg Russia* (Bloomington: Indiana University Press, 1995).

Dennis, CL and E Hodnett. 'Psychosocial and Psychological Interventions for Treating Postpartum Depression'. *Cochrane Database of Systematic Reviews* 4 (2009).

DeRegil, ML, G Fernandez, AC Dowswell, T Rosas and P Juan. 'Effects and Safety of Periconceptional Folate Supplementation for Preventing Birth Defects'. *Cochrane Database of Systematic Reviews* 10 (2010).

Dodd, JM, RM Grivell, CA Crowther and JS Robinson. 'Antenatal Interventions for Overweight or Obese Pregnant Women: A Systematic Review of Randomised Trials'. *BJOG* 117, no. 11 (2010): 1316–26.

Domanico, R, DK Davis, F Coleman and BO Davis. 'Documenting the NICU Design Dilemma: Comparative Patient Progress in Open-Ward and Single Family Room Units'. *Journal of Perinatology* 31, no. 4 (2011): 281–8.

Douglas, VK. 'Childbirth among the Canadian Inuit: A Review of the Clinical and Cultural Literature'. *International Journal of Circumpolar Health* 65, no. 2 (2006): 117–32.

Downe, S, K Finlayson, O Tuncalp and A Metin Gülmezoglu. 'What Matters to Women: A Systematic Scoping Review to Identify the Processes and Outcomes of Antenatal Care Provision That Are Important to Healthy Pregnant Women'. *BJOG* 123, no. 4 (2015): 529–39.

Editorial. 'Achieving Respectful Care for Women and Babies'. *Lancet* 385, no. 9976 (2015): 1366.

Enkin, M, M Keirse and I Chalmers. *A Guide to Effective Care in Pregnancy and Childbirth* (Oxford University Press, 1989).

Enkin, M, M Keirse, M Renfrew and J Neilson. *A Guide to Effective Care in Pregnancy and Childbirth*, 3rd edn. (Oxford University Press, 2000).

Escobar, GJ, B Littenberg and DB Petitti. 'Outcome among Surviving Very Low Birthweight Infants: A Meta-Analysis'. *Archives of Diseases in Children* 66 (1991): 204–11.

Fabic, MS and Y Choi. 'Assessing the Quality of Data Regarding Use of the Lactational Amenorrhea Method'. *Studies in Family Planning* 44, no. 2 (2013): 205–21.

Family Care International. *Action for the 21st Century: Reproductive Health and Rights for All* (New York, 1994).

Fleischer, BE, K VandenBerg et al. 'Individualized Care for Very Low Birthweight Premature Infants Improves Medical and Developmental Outcome in the Neonatal Intensive Care Unit'. *Clinical Pediatrics* 10 (1995): 523–9.

Flenady, V and T Wilson. 'Support for Mothers, Fathers and Families after Perinatal Death'. *Cochrane Database of Systematic Reviews* 1 (2008).

Fox, R, S McMullen and M Newburn. 'UK Women's Experiences of Breastfeeding and Additional Breastfeeding Support: A Qualitative Study of Baby Cafe Services'. *BMC Pregnancy & Childbirth* 15 (2015): 147.

Freedman, L and M Kruk. 'Disrespect and Abuse of Women in Childbirth: Challenging the Global Quality and Accountability Agendas', *Lancet*, early online publication 23 June 2014.

Gagnon, AJ and J Sandall. 'Individual or Group Antenatal Education for Childbirth or Parenthood, or Both'. *Cochrane Database of Systematic Reviews* 3 (2007): CD002869.

Garcia, J, M Redshaw, B Fitzsimons et al. *First Class Delivery: A National Survey of Women's Views of Maternity Care* (London: Audit Commission, 1998).

Gibbons, L, JM Belizán, JA Lauer, AP Betrán, M Merialdi et al. *The Global Numbers and Costs of Additionally Needed and Unnecessary Caesarean Sections Performed per Year: Overuse as a Barrier to Universal Coverage* (Geneva: WHO, 2010).

Gilbert, E. *Female Genital Mutilation: Information for Australian Health Professionals, Victoria* (Victoria: Royal Australian College of Obstetricians and Gynaecologists, 1997).

Goer, H and A Romano. *Optimal Care in Childbirth: The Case for a Physiologic Approach* (Seattle, WA: Classic Day Publishing, 2012).

Goksan, S, C Hartley, F Emery, N Cockrill, R Poorun et al. 'FMRI Reveals Neural Activity Overlap between Adult and Infant Pain'. *eLife* 4 (2015); e06356.

Gold, KJ, VK Dalton and TL Schwenk. 'Hospital Care for Parents after Perinatal Death'. *Obstetrics & Gynecology Clinics of North America* 109, no. 5 (2007): 1156–66.

Government of Canada. *Report of Royal Commission on Aboriginal Peoples* (Ottawa, ON, 2006).

Gramling, L, K Hickman and S Bennett. 'What Makes a Good Family-Centered Partnership between Women and Their Practitioners? A Qualitative Study'. *Birth* 31, no. 1 (2004): 43–8.

Green, J, HA Baston, SC Easton and F McCormick. *Greater Expectations: The Inter-Relationship between Women's Expectations and Experiences of Decision Making, Continuity, Choice and Control in Labour, and Psychological Outcomes. Summary Report* (Leeds, UK: Mother & Infant Research Unit, University of Leeds, 2003).

Green, J, VA Coupland and JV Kitzinger. *Great Expectations: A Prospective Study of Women's Expectations and Experiences of Childbirth*, 2nd edn. (London: Books for Midwives Press, 1998).

——'Expectations, Experiences and Psychological Outcomes of Childbirth: A Prospective Study of 825 Women'. *Birth* 17 (1990): 15–24.

Grey, JE and DA Goldmann. 'Medication Errors in the Neonatal Intensive Care Unit: Special Patients, Unique Issues'. *Archive of Disease in Childhood: Fetal and Neonatal Education* 89 (2004): F472–3.

Griffin, T and M Abraham. 'Transition to Home from the Newborn Intensive Care Unit: Applying the Principles of Family-Centered Care to the Discharge Process'. *Journal of Perinatal & Neonatal Nursing* 20, no. 3 (2006): 243–51.

Hack, M, HG Taylor, N Klein, R Eiben, C Schatschneider et al. 'School-Age Outcomes in Children with Birthweights under 750 g'. *New England Journal of Medicine* 331 (1994): 753–9.

Hall, A, A MacCloed, C Counsell, L Thomson and L Mutch. 'School Attainment, Cognitive Ability and Motor Function in a Total Scottish Very-Low-Birthweight Population at Eight Years: A Controlled Study'. *Developmental Medicine and Child Neurology* 37, no. 12 (1995): 1037–50.

Hall, D and G Kirsten. 'Kangaroo Mother Care: A Review'. *Transfusion Medicine* 18 (2008): 77–82.

Hannah, ME, WJ Hannah, SA Hewson et al. 'Planned Caesarean Section versus Planned Vaginal Birth for Breech Presentation at Term: A Randomised Multicentre Trial'. *Lancet* 356 (2000); 1375–83.

Harvey, S, J Jarell, R Brant, C Stainton and D Rach. 'A Randomized, Controlled Trial of Nurse-Midwifery Care'. *Birth* 23 (1996): 128–35.

Harvey, S, C Snowdon and D Elbourne. 'Effectiveness of Bereavement Interventions in Neonatal Intensive Care: A Review of the Evidence'. *Seminars in Fetal and Neonatal Medicine* 13, no. 5 (2008): 341–56.

Hatem, M, J Sandall, D Devane, H Soltani and S Gates. 'Midwife-Led versus Other Models of Care for Childbearing Women'. *Cochrane Database of Systematic Reviews* 4 (2008): CD004667.

Haynes, R de Regt, HL Minkoff, J Feldman and RH Schwartz. 'Relation of Private or Clinic Care to the Caesarean Section Birth Rate'. *New England Journal of Medicine* 315 (1986): 619–24.

Healthcare Improvement Scotland. 'The Scottish Woman-Held Maternity Record', 2013, available at www.healthcareimprovementscotland.org/our_work/reproductive,_maternal_child/woman_held_maternity_record/swhmr_maternity_record.aspx

Heiberg, E, S Skurtveit, E Helsing and B Chalmers. 'Women's Experiences of Giving Birth in Northwest Russia in 2000 and 2002 and in Northern Norway 2000'. *Acta Obstetrica et Gynecologica Scandinavica* 86, no. 3 (2007): 373–5.

Hellerstein, S, S Feldman and T Duan. 'China's 50% Caesarean Delivery Rate: Is It Too High?' *BJOG* 122, no. 2 (2015): 160–4.

Henley, A and J Schott. 'The Death of a Baby before, during or shortly after Birth: Good Practice from the Parents' Perspective'. *Seminars in Fetal & Neonatal Medicine* 13, no. 5 (2008): 325–8.

Heredia-Pi, I, EE Servan-Mori, V Wirtz, L Avila-Burgos and R Lorenzo. 'Obstetric Care and Method of Delivery in Mexico: Results from the 2012 National Health and Nutrition Survey'. *PLoS ONE* 9, no. 8 (2014): e104166.

Hodnett, ED, S Gates, GJ Hofmeyr and C Sakala. 'Continuous Support for Women during Childbirth'. *Cochrane Database of Systematic Reviews* 10 (2012): CD003766.

Hofmeyr, J, C Nikodem, W-L Wolman, B Chalmers and T Kramer. 'Companionship to Modify the Clinical Birth Environment: Effects on Progress and Perceptions of Labour and Breastfeeding'. *British Journal of Obstetrics and Gynaecology* 98 (1991): 756–64.

Homer, CS, M Griffiths, PM Brodie, S Kildea, AM Curtin et al. 'Developing a Core Competency Model and Educational Framework for Primary Maternity Services: A National Consensus Approach'. *Women & Birth: Journal of the Australian College of Midwives* 25, no. 3 (2012): 122–7.

Hong, YR and JS Park. 'Impact of Attachment, Temperament and Parenting on Human Development'. *Korean Journal of Pediatrics* 55, no. 12 (2012): 449–54.

Horta, BL, R Bahl, JC Martinés and CG Victora. 'Evidence on the Long-Term Effects of Breastfeeding'. World Health Organization, Geneva, 2007.

Hueston, W and M Rudy. 'A Comparison of Labour and Delivery Management between Nurse-Midwives and Family Physicians'. *Journal of Family Practice* 37 (1993): 449–54.

Immigration and Refugee Board of Canada. 'Venezuela: Implementation and Effectiveness of the 2007 Organic Law on the Right of Women to a Life Free of Violence'. In *Refworld* (Ottawa, ON: Immigration and Refugee Board of Canada, 2008).

Joy, SB De and K Bittner. 'Obesity Stigma as a Determinant of Poor Birth Outcomes in Women with High BMI: A Conceptual Framework'. *Maternal Child Health Journal* 19 (2015): 693–9.

Kahn, KE, S Wayburne and M Fouch. 'Baragwanath Premature Unit: An Analysis of the Case Records of 1,000 Consecutive Admissions'. *South African Medical Journal* 28, no. 22 (1954): 453–6.

Keedle, H, V Schmied, E Burns and H Dahlen. 'Women's Reasons for, and Experiences of, Choosing a Homebirth Following a Caesarean Section'. *BMC Pregnancy and Childbirth* 15, no. 206 (2015).

Keirse, M. 'Commentary: The Freezing Aftermath of a Hot Randomized Controlled Trial'. *Birth* 38, no. 2 (2011): 165–7.

——'Just ROAR: Rely on Acronym Rhetoric. Roundtable Discussion on the Language of Birth'. *Birth* 39, no. 2 (2012): 163–4.

Kennell, J. 'The Humane Neonatal Care Initiative'. *Acta Paediatrica* 88 (1999): 367–70.

Kennell, J and M Klaus. 'The Perinatal Paradigm: Is It Time for a Change?' *Clinical Perinatology* 15 (1988): 801–3.

Klaus, M and J Kennell. *Parent-Infant Bonding*, 2nd edn. (St Louis: Mosby, 1982).

——'The Doula: An Essential Ingredient of Childbirth Rediscovered'. *Acta Paediatrica* 86, no. 10 (1997): 1034–6.

Klaus, M, J Kennell, S Robertson and R Sosa. 'Effects of Social Support during Parturition on Maternal and Infant Morbidity'. *British Medical Journal* 293 (1986): 585–7.

Klein, M, R Liston, W Fraser et al. and the Maternity Research Group. 'Attitudes of the New Generation of Canadian Obstetricians: How Do They Differ from Their Predecessors?' *Birth* 38, no. 2 (2011): 129–39.

Ko, N, J Darnell, E Calhoun, K Freund, K Wells et al. 'Can Patient Navigation Improve Receipt of Recommended Breast Cancer Care? Evidence from the National Patient Navigation Research Program'. *Journal of Clinical Oncology* 32, no. 22 (2014).

Kobler, K and R Limbo. 'The Tie That Binds: Relationships in Perinatal Bereavement'. *American Journal of Maternal/Child Nursing* 35, no. 6 (2010): 16–21.

Kong, GWS, TKH Chung and IH Lok. 'The Impact of Supportive Counselling on Women's Psychological Wellbeing after Miscarriage: A Randomised, Controlled Trial'. *BJOG* 121, no. 10 (2014): 1253–62.

Kotaska, A. 'Commentary: Routine Cesarean Section for Breech: The Unmeasured Cost'. *Birth* 38, no. 2 (2011): 162–4.

——'Guideline-Centered Care: A Two-Edged Sword'. *Birth* 38, no. 2 (2011): 97–8.

Kraman, S and G Hamm. 'Risk Management: Extreme Honesty May Be the Best Policy'. *Annals of Internal Medicine* 131 (1999): 963–7.

Kramer, MS, F Aboud, E Mironova, I Vanilovich, PW Platt et al. and the Promotion of Breastfeeding Intervention Trial (PROBIT) Study Group. 'Breastfeeding and Child Cognitive Development: New Evidence from a Large Randomized Trial'. *Archives of General Psychiatry* 65, no. 5 (2008): 578–84.

Kramer, MS, B Chalmers, E Hodnett, Z Sevkovskaya, I Dzikovitch et al. and the PROBIT Study Group. 'Promotion of Breastfeeding Intervention Trial (Probit): A Cluster-Randomized Trial in the Republic of Belarus'. *Journal of the American Medical Association* 285 (2001): 413–20.

Kramer, MS and R Kakuma. 'Optimal Duration of Exclusive Breastfeeding'. *Cochrane Database of Systematic Reviews* 8 (2012).

Lagerkrantz, H, E Nilsson, I Redham and P Hjelmdahl. 'Plasma Catecholamines Following Nursing Procedures in a Neonatal Ward'. *Early Human Development* 14 (1986): 61–5.

Lancet. 'It Happened to Me: Responses to the Stillbirth Series'. *Lancet* 377, no. 9779 (2011): 1720.

Lawrence, RA and RM Lawrence. *Breastfeeding: A Guide for the Medical Profession*, 7th edn. (St Louis: Elsevier Mosby, 2011).

Lawson, GW. 'Report of a Breech Cesarean Section Maternal Death'. *Birth* 38, no. 2 (2011): 159–61.

Levin, A. 'The Mother-Infant Unit at Tallinn Children's Hospital, Estonia: A Truly Baby Friendly Unit'. *Birth* 21, no. 1 (1994): 39–44.

——'Where Are You Going, Neonatal Medicine? Letter to Editor'. *Intensive and Critial Care Nursing* 11 (1995): 49–52.

——'Viewpoint: Humane Neonatal Care Initiative'. *Acta Paediatrica* 88 (1999): 353–5.

Levin, A and B Chalmers, 'Strengthening Neonatal Intensive Care'. Available at www.perinat.ee/ materjal/UN_letter_4_20130829.doc (accessed 20 February 2014).

Lewin, S, S Munabi-Babigumira, C Glenton, K Daniels, X Bosch-Capblanch et al. 'Lay Health Workers in Primary and Community Health Care for Maternal and Child Health and the Management of Infectious Diseases'. *Cochrane Database of Systematic Reviews* 3 (2010): CD004015.

Library and Archives of Canada. Muscowequan Residential School Box 56, File 28, 30 June 1997.

Lindegger, G and LM Richter. 'HIV Vaccine Trials: Critical Issues in Informed Consent'. *South African Journal of Science* 96 (2000): 313–7.

Long, JG, JF Lucey and AG Philip. 'Noise and Hypoxia in the Intensive Care Nursery'. *Pediatrics* 65 (1980): 143–5.

Lu, MC. 'Recommendations for Preconception Care'. *American Family Physician* 76, no. 3 (2007): 397–400.

Ludington, SM. 'Energy Conservation during Skin-to-Skin Contact between Premature Infants and Their Mothers'. *Heart and Lung* 19 (1990): 445–51.

Ma, K. 'Attachment Theory in Adult Psychiatry, Part 1: Conceptualisations, Measurement and Clinical Research Findings'. *Advances in Psychiatric Treatment* 12 (2006): 440–9.

MacDorman, M, F Menacker and E Declercq. 'Trends and Characteristics of Home and Other Out-of-Hospital Births in the United States 1990–2006'. *National Vital Statistics Report* 58, no. 11 (2010): 1–7.

Macfarlane, AJ, B Blondel, AD Mohangoo, M Cuttini, J Nijhuis et al. and the Euro-Peristat Scientific Committee. 'Wide Differences in Mode of Delivery within Europe: Risk-Stratified Analyses of Aggregated Routine Data from the Euro-Peristat Study'. *BJOG* 123, no. 4 (2016): 559–68.

Magee, SR, C Battle, J Morton and M Nothnagle. 'Promotion of Family-Centered Birth with Gentle Cesarean Delivery'. *Journal of the American Board of Family Medicine* 27, no. 5 (2014): 690–3.

Maslow, A. *Motivation and Personality* (New York: Harper, 1943).

McClellan, MS and WA Cabianca. 'Effects of Early Mother-Infant Contact Following Cesarean Birth'. *Obstetrics and Gynecology* 56 (1980): 52–5.

Meffe, F, C Claire Moravac and S Espin. 'An Interprofessional Education Pilot Program in Maternity Care: Findings from an Exploratory Case Study of Undergraduate Students'. *Journal of Interprofessional Care* 26, no. 3 (2012): 183–8.

Melzer, K, Y Schutz, N Soehnchen et al. 'Effects of Recommended Levels of Physical Activity on Pregnancy Outcomes'. *American Journal of Obstetrics and Gynecology* 202, no. 266 (2010): e1–6.

Mercer, JS, DA Erickson-Owens, B Graves and MM Haley. 'Evidence-Based Practices for the Fetal to Newborn Transition'. *Journal of Midwifery & Women's Health* 52, no. 3 (2007): 262–72.

Merewood, A, LB Chamberlain, JT Cook, BL Philipp, K Malone et al. 'The Effect of Peer Counselors on Breastfeeding Rates in the Neonatal Intensive Care Unit: Results of a Randomized Controlled Trial'. *Archives of Pediatrics and Adolescent Medicine* 160, no. 7 (2006): 681–5.

Midmer, D, A Biringer, JC Carroll, A Reid, L Wilson et al. *A Reference Guide for Providers: The Alpha Form – Antenatal Psychosocial Health Assessment Form* (University of Toronto 1996).

Midwives Alliance North America. 'What Is a Midwife?', available at http://mana.org/about-midwives/what-is-a-midwife (accessed 24 June 2015).

Millar, HC, EA Randle, HM Scott, D Shaw, MN Kent et al. 'Global Women's Health Education in Canadian Obstetrics and Gynaecology Programs: A Survey of Program Directors and Senior Residents'. *Journal of Obstetrics and Gynaecology of Canada* 37, no. 10 (2015): 927–35.

Miller, KJ, C Couchie, W Ehman, L Graves, S Grzybowski et al. 'Rural Maternity Care'. *Journal of Obstetrics and Gynaecology of Canada* 34, no. 10 (2012): 984–91.

Milloy, JS. *A National Crime: The Canadian Government and the Residential School System, 1979–1986* (Winnipeg, MB: University of Manitoba Press, 1999).

Montero, S, J Sanchez, C Montoro, M Crespo, A Jaén et al. 'Experiences with Perinatal Loss from the Health Professionals' Perspective'. *Revista Latino-Americana de Enfermagem* 19, no. 6 (2011): 1405–12.

Moore, ER, GC Anderson, N Bergman and T Dowswell. 'Early Skin-to-Skin Contact for Mothers and Their Healthy Newborn Infants'. *Cochrane Database of Systematic Reviews* 5 (2012).

Muraskas, J and K Parsi. 'The Cost of Saving the Tiniest Lives: NICUs versus Prevention'. *Virtual Mentor* 10, no. 10 (2008): 655–8.

Murdock, D. 'Handling during Neonatal Intensive Care'. *Archives of Disease in Children* 59 (1984): 957–61.

Nagpal, J, A Sachdeva, R Sengupta Dhar, VL Bhargava and A Bhartia. 'Widespread Non-Adherence to Evidence-Based Maternity Care Guidelines: A Population-Based Cluster Randomised Household Survey'. *BJOG* 122 (2015): 238–48.

National Aboriginal Health Organization. *Cultural Competency and Safety: A Guide for Health Care Administrators, Providers and Educators* (Ottawa, ON, 2008).

National Collaborating Centre for Women's and Children's Health. 'Antenatal Care: Routine Care for the Healthy Pregnant Woman', 2008, available at www.Nice.Org.Uk/Nicemedia/Live/11947/40145/40145.Pdf.

National Health Service. 'Pelvic Pain in Pregnancy', UK government, available at www.nhs.uk/conditions/pregnancy-and-baby/pages/pelvic-pain-pregnant-spd.aspx (accessed 24 April 2015).

National Institute for Health and Care Excellence (NICE). 'Intrapartum Care: Care of Healthy Women and Their Babies during Childbirth', 2007 BC, available at www.nice.org.uk/guidance/cg190 (accessed 20/2/2017).

——'NICE Guideline: Routine Care for the Healthy Pregnant Woman' (March 2008).

——'Weight Management before, during and after Pregnancy: Quick Reference Guide', 2010, available at www.Nice.Org.Uk/Nicemedia/Live/13056/49929/49929.Pdf and www.Nice.Org.Uk/Guidance/Published?Type=Guidelines (accessed 21 July 2014).

New Brunswick Department of Health. 'New Brunswick Trauma Program', available at http://horizonnb.ca/home/facilities-and-services/provincial-programs/new-brunswick-trauma-program/injury-prevention/intentional-injury/child-abuse-neglect.aspx (accessed 24 June 2015).

New York State Department of Health. *Breastfeeding Mothers' Bill of Rights* (Albany, 2010).

Nikodem, VC, D Danziger, N Gebka, AM Gülmezoglu and GJ Hofmeyr. 'Do Cabbage Leaves Prevent Breast Engorgement? A Randomized, Controlled Study'. *Birth* 20, no. 2 (1993): 61–4.

Nordic and Quebec Working Group. 'BFHI Initiative in Neonatal Units'. In *Conference and Workshop on the Expansion of the Baby Friendly Hospital Initiative* (Uppsala, Sweden, 2011).

Northway, WH. 'Bronchopulmonary Dysplasia: Twenty-Five Years Later'. *Pediatrics* 89 (1992): 969–73.

Novick, G. 'Women's Experience of Prenatal Care: An Integrative Review'. *Journal of Midwifery and Women's Health* 54, no. 3 (2009): 226–7.

Nuzum, D, S Meaney and K O'Donoghue. 'The Impact of Stillbirth on Consultant Obstetrician Gynaecologists: A Qualitative Study'. *BJOG* 121, no. 8 (2014): 1020–8.

Nyqvist, KH. 'Breastfeeding Support in Neonatal Care: An Example of the Integration of International Evidence and Experience'. *Newborn Infant Nursing Review* 5, no. 1 (2005): 34–48.

O'Brien, K, M Bracht, K Robson, XY Ye, L Mirea et al. 'Evaluation of the Family Integrated Care Model of Neonatal Intensive Care: A Cluster Randomized Controlled Trial in Canada and Australia'. *BMC Pediatrics* 15 (2015): 210.

——'Evaluation of Family Integrated Care (FiCare): A Cluster Randomized, Controlled Trial in Canada and Australia.' In *Pediatric Academic Societies Meeting* (Baltimore: 2016).

O'Driscoll, T, L Kelly, L Payne, N St. Pierre-Hansen, H Cromarty et al. 'Delivering Away from Home: The Perinatal Experiences of First Nations Women in Northwestern Ontario'. *Canadian Journal of Rural Medicine* 16, no. 4 (2011): 126–30.

O'Leary, CM, L Heuzenroeder, EJ Elliott and C Bower. 'A Review of Policies on Alcohol Use during Pregnancy in Australia and Other English-Speaking Countries, 2007'. *Medical Journal of Australia* 186, no. 9 (2007): 466–71.

O'Leary, J and C Thorwick. 'Father's Perspectives during Pregnancy, Postperinatal Loss'. *Journal of Obstetrics, Gynecology, and Neonatal Nursing* 35, no. 1 (2006): 78–86.

Oakley, D, T Murland, F Mayes, R Hayashi, B Petersen et al. 'Comparisons of Certified Nurse-Midwives and Obstetricians'. *Journal of Nurse-Midwifery* 40 (1995): 399–409.

Oandasan, I and S Reeves. 'Key Elements of Interprofessional Education, Part 2: Factors, Processes and Outcomes'. *Journal of Interprofessional Care Supplement* 1 (2005): 39–48.

Ogloff, J and R Schuller. *Introduction to Psychology and Law: Canadian Perspectives* (University of Toronto Press, 2001).

Ornstein, M, A Ohlsson, J Edmonds and E Asztalos. 'Neonatal Follow-Up of Very Low Birthweight/Extremely Low Birthweight Infants to School Age: A Critical Review'. *Acta Paediatrica* 80 (1991): 741–8.

Osterman, MJK and JA Martin. 'Primary Cesarean Delivery Rates, by State: Results from the Revised Birth Certificate, 2006–2012'. *National Vital Statistics Report* 63, no. 1 (2014).

Paulson, FJ, D Sharnail and MS Bazemore. 'Prenatal and Postpartum Depression in Fathers and Its Association with Maternal Depression: a Meta-Analysis'. *Journal of the American Medical Association* 303, no. 19 (2010): 1961–9.

Pelvic Obstetric and Gynaecological Physiotherapy. 'Pregnancy-Related Pelvic Girdle Pain (PGP): For Health Professionals Formerly Known as Symphysis Pubis Dysfunction (SBD)', available at http://pogp.csp.org.uk/publications/pregnancy-related-pelvic-girdle-pain-pgp-health-professionals (accessed 24 April 2015).

Pesado, C, RL Beckstrand, L Clark Callister and C Corbett. 'Postpartum Depression and Culture: MCN'. *American Journal of Maternal/Child Nursing* 35, no. 5 (2010): 254–61.

Petryshen, P, B Stevens, J Hawkins and M Stewart. 'Comparing Nursing Costs for Preterm Infants Receiving Conventional vs. Developmental Care'. *Nursing Economics* 15 (1997): 138–45.

Phelan, SM, DJ Burgess, MW Yeazel, WL Hellerstedt, JM Griffen et al. 'Impact of Weight Bias and Stigma on Quality of Care and Outcomes for Patients with Obesity'. *Obesity Reviews* 16 (2015): 319–26.

Posner, SF, DL Broussard, WM Sappenfield, N Streeter, LB Zapata et al. 'Where Are the Data to Drive Policy Changes for Preconception Health and Health Care?' *Womens Health Issues* 18, no. 6 (2008): S81–6.

Price, M and J Broomberg. 'The Impact of Fee-for-Service Reimbursement System on the Utilization of Health Services, Part III: A Comparison of Caesarean Section Rates in White Nulliparous Women in Private and Public Sectors'. *South African Medical Journal* 78 (1990): 136–8.

Public Health Agency of Canada (PHAC). *What Women Say: The Maternity Experiences Survey* (Ottawa, ON: PHAC, 2009).

——*Canadian Hospitals' Maternity Policies and Practices Survey* (Ottawa, ON: PHAC, 2012).

——*Perinatal Health Indicators for Canada 2011* (Ottawa, ON: PHAC, 2012).

——*Family-Centred Maternity and Newborn Care Guidelines* (in preparation) 2017.

Puhl, R and KD Brownell. 'Bias, Discrimination, and Obesity'. *Obesity Research* 9, no. 12 (2001): 788–805.

Pyone, T, S Adaji, B Madaj, T Woldetsadik and N van den Broek. 'Changing the Role of the Traditional Birth Attendant in Somaliland'. *International Journal of Gynaecology and Obstetrics* 127, no. 1 (2014): 41–46.

Ratti, J, S Ross, K Stephanson and T Williamson. 'Playing Nice: Improving the Professional Climate between Physicians and Midwives in the Calgary Area'. *JOGC* 36, no. 7 (2014): 590–7.

Reading, C and F Wein. *Health Inequalities and Social Determinants of Aboriginal Peoples' Health* (2009).

Redshaw, M, R Rowe, C Hockley and P Brocklehurst. *Recorded Delivery: A National Survey of Women's Experience of Maternity Care* (National Perinatal Epidemiology Unit, University of Oxford, 2007).

Renfrew, MJ, D Craig, L Dyson, F McCormick, S Rice et al. 'Breastfeeding Promotion for Infants in Neonatal Units: A Systematic Review and Economic Analysis'. *Health Technology Assessment* 13, no. 40 (2009): 1–146.

Renfrew, MJ, A McFadden, MH Bastos, J Campbell, AA Channon et al. 'Midwifery and Quality Care: Findings from a New Evidence-Informed Framework for Maternal and Newborn Care'. *Lancet* 384, no. 9948 (2014): 1129–45.

Robson, MS. 'Classification of Caesarean Sections'. *Fetal Maternal Medicine Review* 12 (2001): 23–39.

Rollins, N, N Bhandari, N Hajeebhoy, S Horton, C Lutter et al. and the Lancet Breastfeeding Series Group. 'Why Invest, and What Will It Take to Improve Breastfeeding Practices?', *Lancet* 387, no. 10017 (2016): 491–504.

Romano, AM. 'Creating a Culture of Consumer Engagement in Maternity Care', *Journal of Perinatal Education* 19, no. 2 (2010): 50–4.

Romano, AM and JA Lothian. 'Promoting, Protecting and Supporting Normal Birth: A Look at the Evidence'. *Journal of Obstetric, Gynecology and Neonatal Nursing* 37 (2008): 94–105.

Roudebush, JR, J Kaufman, BH Johnson, MR Abraham and SP Clayton. 'Patient- and Family-Centered Perinatal Care: Partnerships with Childbearing Women and Families' *Journal of Perinatal & Neonatal Nursing* 20, no. 3 (2006): 201–9.

Royal College of Obstetricians and Gynaecologists, Royal College of Midwives and National Childbirth Trust. *Making Normal Birth a Reality: Consensus Statement from the Maternity Care Working Party* (London: Maternity Care Working Party, 2007).

Rush, J. 'A Randomized, Controlled Trial of the Effects of the Bath in Labour', PhD dissertation, University of Toronto, 1999.

Saxell, L, S Harris and L Elarar. 'The Collaboration for Maternal and Newborn Health: Interprofessional Maternity Care Education for Medical, Midwifery, and Nursing Students'. *Journal of Midwifery and Women's Health* 54, no. 4 (2009): 314–20.

Schachter, CLO, CA Stalker, E Teram, GC Lasiuk and AA Danilkewich. *Handbook on Sensitive Practice for Health Care Practitioners: Lessons from Adult Survivors of Childhood Sexual Abuse* (Ottawa, ON: PHAC, 2008).

Scheidt, C, N Waller, J Wangler, A Hasenburg and A Kersting. 'Mourning after Perinatal Death: Prevalence Symptoms and Treatment – A Review of Literature'. *Psychotherapie Psychosomatik Medizinische Psychologie* 57, no. 1 (2007): 4–11.

Scott, J. 'Folic Acid Consumption throughout Pregnancy: Differentiation between Trimesters'. *Annals of Nutrition & Metabolism* 59, no. 1 (2011): 46–9.

Scottish Programme for Clinical Effectiveness in Reproductive Health. *Maternity Care Matters: An Audit of Maternity Services in Scotland 1998* (Aberdeen: Douglas Baird Centre for Research on Women's Health, 1999).

Sell, EJ, JA Gaines, C Gluckman and E Williams. 'Early Identification of Learning Problems in Neonatal Intensive Care Graduates'. *American Journal of Diseases of Childhood* 139 (1985): 460–3.

Shearer, B. 'Failure to Progress or Failure to Wait? In Roundtable Discussion on the Language of Birth'. *Birth* 39, no. 2 (2011): 158–9.

Siassakos, D, TJ Draycott, JF Crofts, LP Hunt, C Winter et al. 'More to Teamwork Than Knowledge, Skill and Attitude: EBM Reviews – Cochrane Central Register of Controlled Trials'. *BJOG* 117, no. 10 (2010): 1262–9.

Simkin, P. 'Non-Pharmacological Methods of Pain Relief During Labour'. In *Effectiveness and Satisfaction in Pregnancy and Childbirth*, ed. M Enkin, I Chalmers and M Keirse (Oxford Medical Publications, 1989).

Simkin, P, M Stewart, B Shearer, JC Glantz, J Rooks et al. ' Roundtable Discussion on the Language of Birth'. *Birth* 39, no. 2 (2012): 156–64.

Singh, S and G Posner. 'Doctors Behaving Badly and the Tyranny of Peer Pressure'. *Journal of Obsterics and Gynaecology of Canada* 37, no. 12 (2015): 1113–15.

Skibniewski-Woods, D. 'A Review of Postnatal Debriefing of Mothers Following Traumatic Delivery'. *Community Practice*. 84, no. 12 (2011): 29–32.

Smith, C, JB Brown, M Stewart, K Trim, T Freeman et al. 'Ontario Care Providers' Considerations Regarding Models of Maternity Care'. *Journal of Obstetrics & Gynaecology Canada* 31, no. 5 (2009): 401–8.

Smith, J, F Plaat and N Fisk. 'The Natural Caesarean: A Woman-Centred Technique'. *BJOG* 115 (2008): 1037–42.

Smithgall, LM. *Perceptions of Maternal Stress and Neonatal Patient Outcomes in a Single Private Room versus Open Room Neonatal Intensive Care Unit Environment* (East Tennessee State University Press, 2010).

Society of Obstetricians and Gynaecologists of Canada. 'Joint Policy Statement on Normal Birth'. *Journal of Obstetrics and Gynaecology of Canada* 30, no. 12 (2008): 1163–5.

——'Improving Sexual and Reproductive Health: Integrating Women's Empowerment and Reproductive Rights', available at http://iwhp.sogc.org/uploads/File/ISRH_booklet_web.pdf (accessed 16 July 2011).

——'International Women's Health Programme: Sexual and Reproductive Rights and Health', available at http://iwhp.sogc.org/index.php?page=sexual-reproductive-rights&hl=en_US (accessed 12 March 2013).

——'Female Genital Cutting: Clinical Practice Guidelines'. *Journal of Obstetrics and Gynaecology of Canada* 35, no. 11 (2013): e1–18.

Sonfield, A. 'Popularity Disparity: Attitudes about the IUD in Europe and the United States'. *Guttmacher Policy Review* 7, no. 4 (Fall 2007): 349–67.

Sroufe, LA. 'Attachment and Development: A Prospective, Longitudinal Study from Birth to Adulthood'. *Attachment and Human Development* 7 (2005): 349–67.

St-André, M, PN Reebye and J-V Wittenberg. 'Infant Mental Health in Canada: Initiatives from British Columbia, Quebec and Ontario'. *Journal of the Canadian Academy of Child and Adolescent Psychiatry* 19, no. 2 (2010): 116–19.

Starrs, A. 'A Lancet Commission on Sexual and Reproductive Health and Rights: Going beyond the Sustainable Development Goals'. *Lancet* 386, no. 9999 (2015): 1111–2.

Stevens, B, P Petryshen, J Hawkins, B Smith and P Taylor. 'Developmental vs. Conventional Care: A Comparison of Clinical Outcomes for Very Low Birthweight Infants'. *Canadian Journal of Nursing Research* 28 (1996): 97–113.

Stewart, M. 'Talking to, and about, Women in Labour: In Roundtable Discussion on the Language of Birth'. *Birth* 39, no. 2 (2011): 157–8.

Stjernqvist, K and W Svenningsen. 'Ten Year Follow-Up of Children Born before 29 Gestational Weeks: Health, Cognitive Development, Behaviour and School Achievement'. *Acta Paediatrica* 88 (1999): 557–62.

Stratulat, P, O Bivol, M Stratila et al. 'Evaluarea Rezultatelor Implementarii Technologiilor Programului National De Ameliorare a Asistentei Medicale Perinatale in Republica Moldova'. *Buletin de Perinatologie* 3 (2002): 3–41.

Sutton, K and B Chalmers. 'Contraception and Pregnancy Options'. In *Human Sexuality*, ed. C Pukall (Toronto: Oxford University Press, 2014).

Symington, AJ and J Pinelli. 'Developmental Care for Promoting Development and Preventing Morbidity in Preterm Infants'. *Cochrane Library* (2009).

Tafari, N and SM Ross. 'On the Need for Organized Perinatal Care'. *Ethiopian Medical Journal* 11 (1973): 93–100.

Transforming Maternity Care Vision Team. '2020 Vision for a High-Quality, High-Value Maternity Care System'. *Women's Health Issues* 20, no. 1 (2010).

UK/UNICEF. '*UNICEF UK Baby Friendly Initiative: Guidance for Neonatal Units*', available at www.unicef.org.uk/Documents/Baby_Friendly/Going%20Baby%20Friendly/neonatal%20guidance%202015.pdf (accessed 16 January 2016).

UNICEF. '*UNICEF Southern Sudan Monthly Report*', July 2005, available at http://Reliefweb.Int/Report/Sudan/Unicef-Southern-Sudan-Monthly-Report-Jul-2005.

——'*The State of the World's Children*', available at www.unicef.org/sowc/ (accessed 11 April 2014).

United Nations. *The United Nations Convention on the Rights of the Child* (New York, 1989), available at www.Unicef.Ca/En/Policy-Advocacy-for-Children/About-the-Convention-on-the-Rights-of-the-Child.

——'*Reproductive Rights*', available at www.un.org/en/development/desa/population/theme/rights/index.shtml (accessed 1 June 2014).

United Nations General Assembly. *Draft Outcome Document of the United Nations Summit for the Adoption of the Post-2015 Development Agenda*, A/69/L.85, 2015.

University of Toronto. Centre for Interprofessional Education, at http://ipe.utoronto.ca/overview (accessed 20 April 2015).

Victora, C, R Bahl, A Barros, G Franca, S Horton et al. and the Lancet Breastfeeding Series Group. 'Breastfeeding in the 21st Century: Epidemiology, Mechanisms and Lifelong Effect'. *Lancet* 387, no. 10017 (2016): 475–90.

Villar, J, E Valladares, D Wojdyla, N Zavaleta, A Shah et al. 'Caesarean Delivery Rates and Pregnancy Outcomes: The 2005 WHO Global Survey on Maternal and Perinatal Health in Latin America'. *Lancet* 367, no. 9525 (2006): 1819–29.

Vogel, L. ''Do It Yourself' Births Prompt Alarm'. *Canadian Medical Association Journal* 183, no. 6 (2011): 648–50.

Vogel, JP, MA Bohren, Ö Tuncalp, OT Oladapo and AM Gülmezoglu. 'Promoting Respect and Preventing Mistreatment During Childbirth'. *BJOG* 123, no. 5 (2016): 671–4.

Wagner, M. *Pursuing the Birth Machine: The Search for Appropriate Birth Technology* (Australia: ACE Graphica, 1994).

Waldenstrom, U, I Hildingsson, C Rubertsson and I Radestad. 'A Negative Birth Experience: Relevance and Risk Factors in a National Sample'. *Birth* 31 (2004): 17–27.

Wallin, L and M Eriksson. 'Newborn Individual Development Care and Assessment Program (NIDCAP): A Systematic Review of the Literature'. *Worldviews on Evidence-Based Nursing* 6 (2009): 54–69.

Walsh, WF, KL McCullough and RD White. 'Room for Improvement: Nurses' Perceptions of Providing Care in a Single Room Newborn Intensive Care Setting'. *Advances in Neonatal Care* 6, no. 5 (2006): 261–70.

Warren, SL, L Huston, B Egeland and LA Sroufe. 'Child and Adolescent Anxiety Disorders and Early Attachment'. *Journal of the American Academy of Child and Adolescent Psychiatry* 36 (1997): 637–44.

Westrup, B, A Kleberg, K von Eichwald, K Stjernqvist and H Lagerkrantz. 'A Randomized Control Trial to Evaluate the Effects of the Newborn Individualized Developmental Care and Assessment Program in a Swedish Setting'. *Pediatrics* 105 (2000): 66–72.

White, RD. 'Single-Family Room Design in the Neonatal Intensive Care Unit: Challenges and Opportunities'. *Newborn Infant Nursing Review* 10, no. 2 (2010): 83–6.

——'Recommended Standards for Newborn ICU Design', 2013, available at www.nature.com/jp/journal/v26/n3s/full/7211587a.html.

White Ribbon Alliance. *The Respectful Maternity Care Charter: The Universal Rights of Childbearing Women* (Washington, DC, 2011).

Whitworth, M and T Dowswell. 'Routine Pre-Pregnancy Health Promotion for Improving Pregnancy Outcomes'. *Cochrane Database of Systematic Reviews* 4 (2009).

World Health Organization. WHO Health for All Database, available at www.euro.who.int/en/data-and-evidence/databases/european-health-for-all-database-hfa-db.

——*Preamble to the Constitution of the World Health Organization* (Geneva: WHO, 1946).

——*Code of Marketing of Breastmllk Substitutes* (Geneva: WHO, 1981).

——'Appropriate Technology for Birth'. *Lancet* 8452 (1985): 436–7.

——*Having a Baby in Europe* (Copenhagen: WHO, 1985).

——*Essential Newborn Care and Breastfeeding* (Copenhagen: WHO Regional Office for Europe, 1997).

——*Female Genital Mutilation: A Joint WHO/UNICEF/UNFPA Statement* (Geneva: WHO, 1997).

——*Second Meeting of Focal Points of Reproductive Health/Health of Women and Children in the European Region* (Geneva: WHO, 1998).

——*Workshop on Perinatal Care Proceedings* (Venice: WHO, 1998).

——*Essential Antenatal, Perinatal and Postpartum Care Course* (Copenhagen: WHO Regional Office for Europe 2002).

——*Global and Regional Estimates of Violence against Women: Prevalence and Health Effects of Intimate Partner Violence and Non-Partner Sexual Violence* (Geneva: WHO, 2013).

——'World Health Organization (WHO) Framework for Action on Interprofessional Education and Collaborative Practice', 2013, available at www.who.int/hrh/resources/framework_action/en/ (accessed 20 April 2015).

——'Safe Motherhood: Mother-Baby Package – Implementing Safe Motherhood in Countries'. WHO Maternal Health and Safe Motherhood Programme, 2013, available at http://whqlibdoc.who.int/hq/1994/WHO_FHE_MSM_94.11_Rev.1.pdf (accessed 19 February 2017).

WHO/UNICEF. *Protecting, Promoting and Supporting Breastfeeding: The Special Role of Maternity Services, a Joint WHO/UNICEF Statement* (Geneva: WHO and UNICEF, 1989).

——*Global Strategy for Infant and Young Child Feeding* (Geneva: WHO and UNICEF, 2003).

Wilson, LM, AAJ Reid, DK Midmer et al. 'Antenatal Psychosocial Risk Factors Associated with Adverse Postpartum Outcomes'. *Canadian Medical Association Journal* 154 (1996): 785–99.

Winberg, J. 'Mother and Newborn Baby: Mutual Regulation of Physiology and Behavior: A Selective Review'. *Developmental Psychobiology* 47 (2005): 217–29.

Witt, WP, K Litzelman, ER Cheng, F Wakeel and ES Barker. 'Measuring Stress before and during Pregnancy: A Review of Population-Based Studies of Obstetric Outcomes'. *Maternal Child Health Journal* 18, no. 1 (2014): 52–63.

Yeo, CL, S Choo and LY Ho. 'Chronic Lung Disease in Very Low Birthweight Infants: A 5 Year Review'. *Journal of Pediatrics and Child Health* 33 (1997): 102–6.

Yoo, HI, BN Kim, MS Shin, SC Cho and KE Hong. 'Parental Attachment and Its Impact on the Development of Psychiatric Manifestations in School-Aged Children'. *Psychopathology* 39 (2006): 165–74.

Zanardo, V, G Svegliado, F Cavallin, A Giustardi, E Cosmi et al. 'Elective Cesarean Delivery: Does It Have a Negative Effect on Breastfeeding?' *Birth* 37, no. 4 (2010): 275–9.

Zwelling, E and CR Phillips. 'Family-Centered Maternity Care in the New Millennium: Is It Real or Is It Imagined?' *Journal of Perinatal and Neonatal Nursing* 15, no. 3 (2001): 1–12.

Index